RUSSIA'S SISTERS OF MERCY AND THE GREAT WAR

RUSSIA'S SISTERS OF MERCY AND THE GREAT WAR

More Than Binding Men's Wounds

LAURIE S. STOFF

UNIVERSITY PRESS OF KANSAS

To RSS, MS, and MDS

Published by the University Press of Kansas (Lawrence, Kansas 66045),
which was organized by the Kansas Board of Regents and is operated and funded by
Emporia State University, Fort Hays State University, Kansas State University,
Pittsburg State University, the University of Kansas, and Wichita State University

Library of Congress Cataloging-in-Publication Data
Stoff, Laurie, author.
Russia's Sisters of Mercy and the Great War : more than binding men's wounds / Laurie S. Stoff.
pages cm. — (Modern war studies)
Includes bibliographical references and index.
ISBN 978-0-7006-2125-5 (cloth : alk. paper) — ISBN 978-0-7006-2165-1 (ebook)
1. World War, 1914–1918—Medical care—Russia. 2. Nurses—Russia—
History—20th century. 3. Nurses—Russia—Biography. 4. Military nursing—Russia—
History. 5. Women and war—Russia—History. 6. World War, 1914–1918—Russia.
7. World War, 1914–1918—Participation, Female. I. Title.
D807.R9S76 2015
940.4'75092520947— dc23
2015023667

British Library Cataloguing-in-Publication Data is available.

Printed in the United States of America

10 9 8 7 6 5 4 3 2 1

The paper used in this publication is recycled and contains 30 percent
postconsumer waste. It is acid free and meets the minimum requirements
of the American National Standard for Permanence of Paper for Printed
Library Materials Z39.48-1992.

CONTENTS

ACKNOWLEDGMENTS

I would like to express my deepest gratitude to the individuals and institutions that provided me with support during the process of research and writing this book. Funding for travel to collections and research was provided by the American Councils for International Education Title VIII Research Scholar Program Grant, the Louisiana Tech University International Summer Faculty Development Grant, the Louisiana Tech University Summer Research Grant, and the University of Illinois Summer Research Lab program, as well as the Department of History at Louisiana Tech University. I am grateful to the fantastically helpful librarians on staff at the University of Illinois Library in its Slavic and East European Collections and Services, who were invaluable in providing me with assistance in locating materials. In particular, I thank Jan Adamczyk, who not only went out of his way on a number of occasions to help me track down the obscure sources that I required, but always did so with a smile and usually a good joke. The archivists at Stanford University's Hoover Institution Archives were similarly extremely accommodating and helpful, assisting me in locating sources and images held in the superb Political Poster Collection housed there. The staff of the Russian State Military-Historical Archive in Moscow also provided me with access to vitally important documents for this project.

The writing process was made possible by a Louisiana Board of Regents Support Fund Award to Louisiana Artists and Scholars (ATLAS) Grant, providing me with a year of release from teaching and service to focus on preparation of the manuscript. I am indebted to William Willoughby, who helped me prepare numerous grant proposals and continually encouraged me to push forward with my research plans despite many obstacles. Many individuals provided me with valuable feedback on various aspects of the emerging manuscript. Specifically, I would like to thank Christine Hallett, Marianna Muravyeva, Karen Petrone, Rochelle Ruthchild, Joshua Sanborn, and David Stone, as well as the reviewers for *Aspasia, The International Yearbook of Central, Eastern, and Southeastern European Women's and Gender History* for their suggestions. I am eternally grateful to Denise Youngblood, who read the entire manuscript and provided me with extremely useful commentary and advice, as well as mentoring, friendship, and support for the last ten years. I would also like to thank the members of the editorial board of *Russia's Great War and Revolution*, who saw various iterations of shorter pieces that were incorporated in the manuscript and gave me constructive criticism as well. Among them, Boris Kolonitskii was extremely helpful to me in this project, sharing his tremendous insight into the war and revolutionary period generally and Russian nursing specifically, as well as his extensive collection of images, many of which appear in this book. Additionally, to Melissa Stockdale I express my great thanks for her valuable commentary, for directing me to a number of critical sources, and for her wonderful camaraderie in the Moscow archives and library. Additionally, I would like to express my gratitude to my former colleagues at Louisiana Tech University and my current colleagues at Arizona State University for feedback and general collegial support. Thanks in particular to Stephen Webre, who was an excellent mentor and provided me with extensive support during my tenure at Lousiana Tech to allow me to pursue my research goals.

On a more personal level, there are many people in my life to whom I owe enormous debts of gratitude for their material and emotional support. My husband, John Benschoter, has been the most supportive and understanding spouse an academic could ever hope for, allowing me to pursue my career goals while providing the most amazing care for our family. My immediate and extended family and friends have been similarly supportive and encouraging. I dedicate this book to the important women in my life: my mother, Roslyn Stoff, and my grandmother, Mildred Stoff, both of whom provided me with indefatigable role models, and my daughter, Meghan Stoff, who will carry their memories with her into the future.

INTRODUCTION

NURSING IN THE GREAT WAR: THE RUSSIAN EXPERIENCE

The Great War is salient in the history of warfare in a number of ways, including how women experienced the war. The pervasive nature of the hostilities generated an extraordinary degree of female involvement. Most notably, women were affected by and became involved in war on a level never before encountered in history. Russia's women, like those of many of the other belligerents, participated in the war effort on a mass scale, working in various capacities both at the front and in the rear. They joined numerous voluntary organizations created to meet wartime needs. Most of these women were not attached to the army but worked through civilian governmental and nongovernmental organizations such as the Union of Zemstvos and Union of Towns (organizations of local government bodies that provided a variety of services) and the Russian Society of the Red Cross. Women's groups around the country organized committees dedicated to "women's war work." The major women's organizations engaged in a variety of war-related endeavors, from military supply to caring for war victims, refugees, orphans, and prisoners of war. Thousands more women volunteered their time, energy, and resources in activities such as sewing soldiers' clothing and linens, cutting bandages, making care packages for troops, staffing travelers' aid stations for soldiers in transit, and working in shelters, soup kitchens, orphanages, and other facilities for the homeless and disabled. Women also performed a number of vital auxiliary services for the Russian armed forces. Peasant women were recruited to dig trenches for the troops. Women worked as cooks, supply clerks, drivers, and scouts both behind the lines and in the advanced positions. Some women even managed to participate in combat.[1]

Although women engaged in a variety of wartime activities, the most popular form of female service was nursing. The female nurse has been a fixture in modern warfare since Florence Nightingale made her famous entry into medical service during the Crimean War in the mid-nineteenth century, appearing frequently as a secondary player in war narratives dominated by male combat activities. While she was never the star, the nurse's supporting role was nonetheless essential to the military machines conducting the wars. Indeed, the participation of women in wartime nursing had become a standard feature of Western conflicts by the end of the nineteenth century. And while Nightingale became an international celebrity, the Russians quietly contributed hundreds of women to its military hospitals during the Crimean conflict, who engaged in service provision in more dangerous areas very close to the fighting, establishing an important precedent for the use of women in future conflicts.

During World War I the number of female nurses expanded exponentially, to match the scope and scale of the hostilities. All of the nations that engaged in the conflict mobilized large numbers of women to undertake medical care during the Great War, and Russia was no exception. There the wartime nurse became a figure of national prominence, the female equivalent of the patriotic male soldier, dedicated to the causes of tsar and fatherland. Engagement in wartime medical service was seen as an appropriate activity for women from every walk of life, from the empress herself and her daughters to the simplest peasant. In Russia women's participation in medical service came primarily through the auspices of civilian organizations mobilized to augment military medical services, which were woefully inadequate and needed extensive assistance to treat the millions of wounded and ill soldiers that resulted from the conflict. Without women's participation in medical services, the nation would have been unable to execute the war. Nurses also served Russia's civilian population, as the war precipitated a series of public health crises: epidemic diseases spread quickly through the war zone and the home front, millions became homeless refugees facing starvation and illness, and thousands of children lost their parents. By 1917 the number of women serving as "sisters of mercy," as Russian nurses were called, exceeded thirty thousand.[2] In fact, nurses carried out much of the medical care during the war, outnumbering doctors more three to one. These numbers are only exceeded by those of combat medics and orderlies, which approached sixty thousand, but whose medical training significantly lagged behind that of nurses. Therefore, much of the medical aid provided to both the Russian military and its civilian population was carried out by women.[3]

Despite the vital contributions of these women to the war effort, they have largely been overlooked by the historical record. Partially to blame is the traditional perception of war and military activity as male preserves. Indeed, it has been argued that "the defining characteristic of war is its masculinity."[4] More specifically, after the conclusion of World War I, the construction of a "myth of the war experience"[5] celebrated male achievements in what was seen as a specifically masculine endeavor to the great neglect of female participation. Over the past several decades, however, scholars of women and gender have worked to demonstrate the importance of women to war and of war to women. In particular, the wartime activities of Western women have received serious scholarly attention.[6] The same cannot be said with regard to Russian participation, which has often been overlooked in favor of that on the western front. The problematic nature of the war in relation to the Russian Revolution, which brought to power a communist regime that could not celebrate the heroes of a "bourgeois imperialist" war, adds to the limited number of studies of Russia during World War I.[7] In the words of Jane Marcus, this "historical repression of the Eastern Front in favor of the story of Western Europe in histories of the war" has meant that "the Eastern Front is the female 'other' of World War I."[8] The combination of female subject matter and the geographic location of that subject matter in Eastern Europe have increased the scholarly isolation of Russian women's participation in World War I.[9] Once again, Russian wartime nurses were upstaged by their Western counterparts; the writings of British World War I nurse Vera Brittain are widely known, but few know the stories of Russian sisters of mercy. Even works that specifically investigate medical service in Russia during this period overlook nurses.[10] Although a number of publications have recently emerged in Russia that focus on sisters of mercy in general,[11] to date, there are no in-depth studies devoted exclusively to the phenomenon of Russian wartime nursing during the Great War.

To redress this neglect, this work presents an analysis of women's wartime nursing experiences during the First World War in Russia. Focusing on the stories of Russia's sisters of mercy of the Great War, it establishes their relevance not only to the war narrative but also to a number of issues of historical development, including gender, nationalism, liberalism, feminism, and war. Specifically, this study investigates the motivations that spurred women to join the war effort as nurses; the nature and specific aspects of their service; the multiple structural and cultural factors that acted as determinants of experience; the relationship of women's medical services to the tsarist government, the military, and the civilian organizations responsible for wartime medical care; the interaction between nurses and the men for whom they cared and with whom they served; the ways that wartime nurses were perceived in popular imagination; and the international context of Russian women's wartime nursing service of the Great War. What is revealed through an investigation of these experiences is often striking, composed of heretofore untold and compelling stories, filled with danger and deprivation, excitement and opportunity, sorrow and trauma, scandal and controversy.

This book deliberately focuses on experience, treating the war period as a major transformative moment in Russia's development with intrinsic historical relevance, instead of as a prelude to or explanation for successive events, specifically the revolutions of 1917. This is especially significant considering the impact of the war in Russia during the war period itself, which was often more devastating and destructive than in other belligerents. Considering that the majority of the fighting was done on the eastern front, the majority of casualties, the most material damage, greatest dislocation of population, and largest and most deadly spread of epidemic diseases occurred there as well. Thus, while it does grapple with important questions such as why and how Russia was hindered in the provision of efficacious medical service and how this affected the war effort, the book does not approach these questions as an attempt to provide answers to larger inquiries that have dominated many historical studies of the war, specifically, that seek to use the war and Russia's failures therein to explain the 1917 revolutions. This is not to say that these are not worthy investigations, but they are different kinds of inquiries, and they often take as their departure point the assumption that the outcomes of tsarist collapse, and even the Bolshevik Revolution, were inevitable. As a result, aspects of the war that do not appear directly as causation factors are overlooked, creating a somewhat myopic view and failing to account for the ways that people actually experienced the war, people who did not have any knowledge of what the final outcome would be. My attempt, therefore, is to present a study of war experiences as products of the war and of the particular historical context in which they were produced.

This work also presents an opportunity to add Russian voices to the literature on nursing and World War I, while highlighting the distinctiveness of Russian war experiences. Although it shared many features of women's medical service in other nations, and Russian sisters of mercy often reacted to wartime experiences in ways that were similar to their Western counterparts, Russian nursing during this conflict was profoundly different. Indeed, the entire Russian war experience diverges considerably from the conventional wisdom about the war shaped by the western front. Specifically, in contrast to the oft-stagnant warfare of the western front, with large stretches of immovable trenches and a fairly stable connected system of auxiliary support services, the war on the eastern front was very different. There, combat, and indeed nearly all related war activity, was highly mobile and it was often impossible to draw clear distinctions between "front" and "rear." The inadequacy of the static model of the First World War based on the western experience has been challenged by scholars of the eastern front in an attempt to demonstrate the vastly differently kind of war fought in Russia.[12] This corrective needs to be applied to the picture of wartime nursing as well. Officially, female medical personnel of the Russian Red Cross and its subordinate organizations were supposed to remain three to four miles from the actual fighting, as in Western nations. Such procedural regulations were completely impractical on the Russian front and thus rarely followed. It was necessary for many nurses to serve directly in the battle zones, in mobile dressing stations, ambulatory transport units, and flying columns (*letuchky*), described by nursing scholar Christine Hallett as "mobile hospitals housed in makeshift accommodation or tents, carried on cumbersome wooden horsedrawn wagons, but often moving almost as rapidly as an army."[13] Thus, while most Western nurses were assigned to stationary hospitals located at a considerable distance from the battlefields, many Russian nurses served very close to the fighting and were subject to conditions similar to those of combatants. Although Russian sisters who served in rear facilities are not ignored, the focus of this study is on the experiences of frontline nurses. Moreover, Russian nursing should be differentiated from Western nursing in places such as Great Britain and the United States, in that it was not professionalized.

Rather, it remained a charitable and quasi-religious activity, characteristics that worked to shape Russian nursing experience throughout the war period.

The study of women's wartime nursing in Russia during the Great War is salient to a number of significant aspects of historical development and contributes to our understanding of the nature of war, gender, and Russian history in general. Perhaps most importantly, because both armed conflict and nursing are perceived as distinctly gendered activities, this study indicates much about the relationship between women and war and the dynamism of ideas about gender. Scholars have long considered the gendered implications of the Great War to be of primary importance. The debate over the impact of the war on gender roles covers a range of arguments, from an emancipatory experience for women to one that solidified the sexual division of labor and restored patriarchy.[14] This work seeks to demonstrate the extent to which it is necessary to, in the words of Billie Melman, "take stock of the mutations in the borderlines of femininities and masculinities."[15] Wartime nursing moved women beyond conventional gender conceptions into nebulous and even distinctly male realms, revealing porosity in the sexual divisions of labor. As sisters of mercy, women took on roles considerably more active than the passive binding of men's wounds. The red crosses they wore on their uniforms did not shield them from depravation, danger, and even death. They experienced extreme cold, constant fatigue, infectious diseases, deadly artillery fire, and aerial bombardment. They took on public leadership roles, often in command of men. They came into contact with aspects of life considered inappropriate for women. In many ways, the experiences of female medical personnel share much with those of male combat personnel. Simultaneously, although wartime nursing was promoted as an appropriate service for women, predicated on notions of women's natural capacity for caring and nurturing, nurses' experiences reveal that such conventions were not always applicable, welcome, useful, or even possible within the context of frontline medical service. Thus, the experiences of sisters of mercy challenge the perception of nursing as a uniquely feminine endeavor shaped by essentialist notions. This, combined with their experiences at the front that mirror those of male soldiers, points to the shared humanity of the effects of war and indicate the fallacy of understanding the war as a primarily masculine experience and one defined by combat.

Such commonalities, however, should not lead to the assumption of a uniform "myth of the female war experience" that ascribes a single model to women's wartime experiences. Rather, as this study seeks to demonstrate, factors such as class and social status, nationality, political ideology, and religion worked as determinants of wartime nursing experience, revealing significant differences in the ways women and war intersected and interacted. The stratified nature of Russian society, with clear divisions between the dominant and subordinate, the privileged and nonprivileged, was reflected among nursing staff. Yet wartime nursing also demonstrates the extent to which imperial social structures were in flux, allowing greater interaction between those of different social strata and identities, and how nursing worked to influence such flexibility.

While the exigencies of war may have allowed, even obligated, women to act in ways outside of normative femininity and appropriate roles for their sex, class, and social status, such behavior was not always welcomed, even temporarily, much less as a permanent feature of Russian society. Particularly, the operation of women in the very public, very male sphere of war was problematic for many, raising anxieties and tensions that were borne out in negative associations that would plague Russia's sisters of mercy throughout the war. Ultimately, gendered dichotomies and associations were not completely subverted, nor were imperial social structures and cultural values overturned during the war. Indeed, the constraints of those factors seriously hindered efficacious service provision and contributed to Russia's colossal problems in successful waging of the war. At the same time, the war offered new opportunities for action for women. Russia's wartime nurses are thus exemplars of that nation's larger struggle with modernity and indicate a central paradox of female wartime service, one in which the full participation of citizenry, including women, was required but not necessarily desired, and which caused considerable concern by demonstrating the extent to which conventional gender assumptions, social structures, and cultural norms had become unhinged.

SOURCES OF EXPERIENCE

In order to highlight experience, the sources consulted in this work consist largely of the writings of the women who served as sisters of mercy themselves, as well as those who observed and commented on their activities, recorded in memoirs, diaries, reminiscences, and contemporary periodicals. The focus on experience dictates that the voices of the women who served as nurses themselves feature prominently. They are essential for describing their motivations for enlisting, the context and conditions of their service, the activities in which they engaged, their reactions to the war, their relationships with one another, and their interactions with the men for whom they cared and with whom they served. These records vary considerably, as indicated previously, and are dependent on a number of factors. They also, like all historical sources, suffer from some serious limitations and problems. Perhaps most importantly, they are not sufficiently representative of the diverse population that served as nurses. Despite the presence of women from a variety of social backgrounds in wartime nursing, because enlistment in the Red Cross was limited predominantly to literate women, most wartime nurses came from the educated classes. Therefore, the vast majority of their own recorded evidence about them comes from writing either by or about the women of Russia's upper and middle strata, and primarily from ethnic Russians. Not only does this apply to memoirs and other personal recollections, but also to periodicals. During the war, a number of published accounts of women's nursing experiences appeared in Russia and were generally integrated into official efforts to promote the war effort. The prowar journals of the period often featured stories about women serving as nurses. Yet these publications had a tendency to focus on the experiences of more prominent individuals and members of the elite. This does not mean, however, that their reflections or experiences were uniform. In fact, one discerns significant differences between those from well-connected aristocratic backgrounds as compared to those of the nonprivileged sectors and even the lower gentry. We are also fortunate to have a few examples from citizens of other nations who served in Russia, providing different perspectives.

Time and place of publication are also significant factors. Many of the records were produced during the war itself and published in Russia, which means they had been passed successfully through government censorship. Therefore, these sources tend to be very prowar, even propagandistic, and often formulaic. Names of individuals, places, and other information were often removed, ostensibly for reasons of military security. Moreover, nurses' writings published as wartime propaganda tended to focus on the men they cared for, rather than on their own experiences.

This makes them useful in providing information about nurses' interactions with and impressions of the men with whom they came into contact during the war. But they also omit many things, particularly negative portrayals of nurses or soldiers, or criticism of the war effort. Russian troops are uniformly strong, patriotic, stoic, and kindhearted, if at times simple and childlike. Officers are brave and chivalrous. Nurses are compassionate, dedicated, and competent, but the stories, in many cases, do not feature their experiences as much as they concentrated on the real "heroes," the men in combat.

The written sources on Russian wartime nurses are further delimited by the revolutions of 1917. After the war, unlike in Western nations, the publication of war reminiscences fell off sharply, as a result of the new Soviet government's stance against the "imperialist" war, which was not something to be celebrated in public memory. During the Soviet period, few postwar accounts of World War I nurses were published in Russia; rather, the majority appeared among the Russian community in emigration, which created its own "myth of war experience."[16] Politically, this made a difference, as the émigré population was generally anti-Bolshevik, some even decidedly pro-tsarist. Some memories were recorded long after the fact, often by women who left Russia following the revolution and reminisced from abroad. Undoubtedly, the distance (both chronologic and geographic) from the event led to inaccuracies, omissions, and embellishments in the accounts. Moreover, some were kept as private records, never intended for public consumption, and were only published after the participant had passed away or was advanced in age. Some, in fact, were never published, retained in archival collections.

In addition to these firsthand accounts, this study also makes use of contemporary writings and images, particularly those found in periodicals published during the war, in an attempt to analyze the ways that sisters of mercy were conceived in the public imagination. Of primary importance are the numerous "illustrated" journals that carried photographs, artistic representations, stories, poetry, and other images of nurses. Other sources also contained representations of nurses, which reflected the opinions of members of Russian society about these women and thus entered the public discourse. Additionally, many other printed visual images of nurses, including those presented in posters, postcards, and *lubki* (illustrated broadsides), were produced as part of Russia's patriotic culture of the war, both those that reflected officially sanctioned views of nurses as well as those that were more controversial. These, too, must be used with some care, as they reflect cultural attitudes and particular notions about gender and sexuality that did not necessarily reflect reality or have significant impact on nursing experience.

Despite such shortcomings, which require the use of scholarly caution, these sources are valuable as reflections of the experiences of women in medical service. In combination with critical analysis, to set these subjective experiences firmly within the historical context, this study also includes an examination of archival records concerning medical service during the war. These include the unpublished and published documents of the agencies that engaged in medical service provision during the war, primarily the Russian Society of the Red Cross and other organizations such as the Union of Zemstvos and the Union of Towns. These documents serve to corroborate some of the things written by the nurses themselves, disprove others, and reveal aspects that the individuals were unaware of, while providing a larger backdrop for their activities and allowing us to view their experiences as part of the general effort to conduct the war.

***

This book is arranged thematically, divided into eight chapters, plus an introduction and conclusion. Each chapter begins with a short vignette from the story of a nurse who served in Russia during the Great War, then moves to analyze specific aspects of wartime nursing. Chapter 1 establishes the context of Russian wartime nursing before the Great War, elaborating on the structural development of the activity from the mid-nineteenth century through the period immediately preceding the outbreak of World War I in 1914. Ideas about gender had decisive influence on the early development of wartime nursing, both in its promotion and opposition.

Chapter 2 describes the structural history of wartime nursing during World War I, examining the specific ways that women's medical service was mobilized, organized, and administered. The chapter is based primarily on the published and unpublished documents and records of the various Russian agencies, organizations, and individuals that engaged in or supervised medical services during World War I. This chapter also examines the way that structural features affected the actual provision of service and details the myriad problems faced by the Russian authorities in attempting to treat millions of soldiers and civilians during the war. Again, gender was a primary factor in shaping the mobilization and organization of nursing service during the war, and it comes to the fore in the ways that women's medical service was conceived and implemented, in the ways authorities attempted to administer and control it, and ultimately, as an obstacle in effective service provision.

The next three chapters focus on the wartime nursing experiences of the women who engaged in this kind of service. Chapter 3 establishes who these women were, their social and economic backgrounds, their levels of education, their motivations for enlisting as nurses, and their expectations about wartime nursing. It then examines the experiences of these women as influenced by specific structural factors that were significant determinants, including class and social status, nationality, and religion. In so doing, it indicates the subjectivity of nursing experience while establishing the importance of shared structural factors, and it clearly demonstrates the inadequacy of a single model of female wartime experience. Ultimately, such an examination reveals that while wartime nurses continued to be shaped and constrained by the persistence of traditional structures of identity that could not be transcended even in the chaotic upheaval of the war, their actions worked to affect change on those very structures, as the war increased mobility, flexibility, and opportunity, giving women the chance to engage in activities and behaviors that were not usually possible under peacetime conditions in Russian imperial space.

Chapter 4 demonstrates the ways that the experiences of women's wartime nursing belies the masculine "myth of war" by examining the similarities between women's medical service in the war and male combat (and medical) service. It also reveals the blurring of boundaries between conceptions of masculinity and femininity and the contravention of conventional notions of womanhood associated with nursing by examining the ways in which women, as wartime nurses, engaged in nontraditional behaviors and activities. Moving this argument beyond corporeal experience into the realm of the psychological impact of the war, chapter 5 offers additional insights about the porosity of gendered divisions in discussing the limitations of women's emotional and psychological value as wartime nurses in the brutal context of modern warfare, and further demonstrates the close connections between female nursing and male combat experiences. These chapters rely primarily on the records left by the nurses themselves (which are less numerous and more difficult to locate than those of nurses who served with Western nations), using their own voices but analyzing them within the context of the war and early twentieth-century Russian society. While recognizing the limitations and problems associated with such sources (lack of complete information, generalization, bias, intent, exaggeration, and time elapsed since the events, among others), these chapters attempt to examine the experiences, as the subjects' histories, in the context of both the historical circumstances of the war and the subjects' own understandings of what they experienced.

The intersections and interactions between female nursing personnel and the men with whom they came into contact during their wartime medical service are the focus of chapter 6. An examination of the writings of both men and women reveals the multiple ways that nurses constructed perceptions of the soldiers, officers, doctors, male nurses, and orderlies they encountered daily. The chapter similarly explores relationships between nurses and their patients, and between nurses and the male medical personnel who served with them. Additionally, the multiple ways in which men viewed and imagined nurses are analyzed, as well as the expressions of the explicit and implicit understandings of the nature and function of wartime nursing and women's roles within war.

Focusing on cultural representations of wartime nurses, chapters 7 and 8 examine the impact of their activities on those that observed and places them within the cultural context in which they were operating. In investigating how nurses were imagined in Russian society, these chapters look primarily at the cultural meanings of wartime nurses as expressed through the images and discourse that appeared in various media during the war. These include the prolific textual and visual representations of wartime nurses, which appeared in contemporary periodicals, brochures, posters, postcards, cartoons and caricatures, paintings, films, and *lubki*. Such an investigation reveals the complexities of such representations, which do not fit neatly into traditional ideas about the ways nurses were imagined, that is, as passive sources of comfort to wounded men. Chapter 7 focuses on the positive representations, largely expressed through official publications and other sources meant for public consumption, often with a clearly prowar intent. Chapter 8 explores the negative ways that sisters of mercy were imagined during the war, examining the "bad" nurses, those that were perceived as self-aggrandizing or dissolute women using wartime nursing for personal gain. These were not the images that appeared in sources of patriotic culture; rather, they were presented through rumor, speculation, and sources meant for private rather than public consumption. In so doing, the chapter attempts to explain the creation and dissemination of such portrayals within the context of the war, class and social structure, and gendered assumptions.

The conclusion summarizes the development of Russian wartime nursing after the fall of tsarism in 1917. It offers some ideas about the meaning of Russian wartime nursing during World War I and the extent to which it established precedents for the future use of women in military medical capacities. Indeed, no serious attempt to wage war in the years following the Great War would be considered *without* the extensive participation of women.

All translations from Russian that appear in this text are my own, unless otherwise noted. In transliterating names from the original Russian, I have used the standard Library of Congress system, with the exception of conventionally Anglicized names of prominent figures such as Tsar Nicholas (instead of Tsar Nikolai). Names of personages are provided in as complete a form as I was able to locate, but contemporary reports often failed to include names of persons (particularly first names) and places or to give precise (or any) dates, and they frequently neglected to identify military units, often for reasons of wartime security. Thus, where only first initials or last names are provided in the text, it is because the full names were unavailable. Since nearly all the action described in this work took place prior to 1918, dates are given according to the Julian (Old Style) calendar that was in use in Russia during this period, which lagged thirteen days behind the Gregorian calendar used in the West. The various fronts referred to in the text are on what the Western powers labeled the eastern front, but in Russia they were designated the northern, western, southwestern, and Romanian fronts, stretching from Riga to the Black Sea. Geographical locations are given according to their contemporary Russian names, with more prominent places in formerly Russian-held areas followed in parentheses by their current, linguistically appropriate names, when these are known.

1

CONTEXT AND CONTROVERSY

TAT'IANA VARNEK: SOCIALITE TURNED SISTER

After completing her secondary education in the spring of 1912, with no particular plans for the future, Tat'iana Varnek, a young Saint Petersburg noblewoman, spent a leisurely summer at her family's country estate on the north shore of the Black Sea. There she swam, played tennis, went on outings and picnics with family and friends, and engaged in other leisure activities. During that time, she learned that several of her schoolmates had decided to "do something useful" and had enrolled in nursing training courses. Under the strong influence of her close friend Anya Dumitrashko, Varnek decided to join them. In the fall of 1912 she returned to Saint Petersburg and entered courses at the Kaufman *obshchina,* one of the most prestigious nursing communities in Russia, with four hundred other elite women. A prominent member of the State Duma (Russian parliament) spoke at the commencement ceremony for the courses. He emphasized that the experience of the Russo-Japanese War (1904–1905) had demonstrated the need for "real nurses, not volunteers," thus establishing the importance of creating a cadre of trained reserve sisters of mercy to draw on should Russia be embroiled in another conflict.[1]

In keeping with this goal, students were subjected to rigorous training. They were required to attend both lectures and practical lessons every day and to practice their skills continuously. Varnek remembered,

> The program was very large. And very strict. . . . We were constantly followed around by the staff sisters. Before Christmas we took our examinations, oral and practical. Studying proved to be very strenuous, especially practical lessons, which were very difficult,

> and had to be done in a very short time. . . . At home, Anya Dumitrashko and I harassed poor Zhenia (my younger brother), who good-naturedly put up with it. Every time he would see us, he would say, "Again it is bandager and bandager." We would wrap him up in bandages endlessly, unwrap him, and wrap him up again.

The most challenging subject was anatomy, which required a tremendous amount of time for study. Varnek and her friends were lucky, however, in that their gymnasium had required anatomy courses. Because they had already taken exit examinations in this subject, all they had to do was review. This was not true of many of the other women in the courses, despite the fact that all possessed secondary education. As a result, more than half of the students failed their exams, and the number of prospective nurses entering the hospital practicum was less than two hundred.[2]

On successfully passing her exams, Varnek was assigned to the Obukhovskii City Hospital, which treated patients from the lower ranks of Saint Petersburg society, in particular the poor, vagrants, and drunks. She described the conditions in this facility as "terrible":

> overrun with the ill, the hospital was huge and very old, so that it seemed that the walls absorbed all of the smells into them. The air was horrible, the linens poor and the blankets were old, all were grey, there were no comforts, there was never enough of anything, we even lacked enough thermometers, and the furious duty nurse never took her eye off of us and scolded us all the time.

Tat'iana was assigned to the surgical ward, which contained the more serious cases, most of whom had little chance of survival. The smell of the hospital was so pervasive that even when she was not in the facility it seemed to linger on her body and clothing, despite numerous attempts to wash it away and to cover it with perfume. A number of the other nurses in training could not withstand the conditions and left the *obshchina.*

Varnek herself found it very difficult, but she continued to work for more than a month. Then she too decided to quit, not as a result of her inability to endure the hardships associated with the work, she insisted, but rather because she claimed to have lost interest. Instead, she wanted to concentrate on her studies at the Drafting School of the Imperial Society for the Promotion of the Arts, where she had been simultaneously enrolled. She also resented the fact that nursing had cut into her social life, lamenting that her work in the hospital had left her so exhausted that she missed her "first season of the best balls and outings." After her friend Anya withdrew as well, the two young women spent their free time visiting museums, skating, playing tennis, "having lots of fun and forgetting about nursing." Varnek maintained this carefree lifestyle through the summer of 1914, which she once again spent amusing herself at her family's Black Sea estate, unconcerned about the looming prospect of war. "We went on excursions, swam, went boating, played tennis, and worked in the garden a little bit, most importantly, gathering fruit. My responsibility was to look after the roses, to prune them and collect some for the bouquets that decorated the house. We lived without care."[3]

THE RUSSIAN WARTIME NURSING TRADITION: ORIGINS

Tat'iana Varnek was like many young women of Russia's privileged elite, who, in seeking to be useful to their country, enlisted in nursing courses in the years prior to the outbreak of World War I. Yet, as Varnek's story clearly indicates, for many such women nursing was not seen as a long-term endeavor or a professional occupation but rather a pastime to pursue only when it did not interfere with social engagements or other interests. The activity was far from professionalized or regularized, despite the fact that the desire to create a cadre of "real nurses" was long-standing among many members of the Russian medical community. Although many did not see nursing as a serious endeavor, a number of women had devoted themselves to the profession, entering the *obshchiny* as permanent members (they became designated as "staff sisters") and working in hospitals on a consistent basis. Many of these women, unlike Varnek and her cohorts, were completely dedicated to nursing. Moreover, these women were not merely members of the upper class engaging in charitable work on a voluntary basis. Rather, they were often individuals who had no other source of income—they were supported by the *obshchiny* and by their labors. From the mid-nineteenth century a number of medical professionals and ardent supporters of female nursing had pressed for efforts to be undertaken in this vein. These views were further catalyzed by the negative experiences of the Russo-Turkish (1877–1878) and Russo-Japanese (1904–1905) wars, which revealed serious inadequacies in provision of medical services. However, despite such attempts, nursing in Russia had not been transformed into a professional occupation but remained a semiprivate, quasi-religious, charitable, and voluntary activity. Moreover, the numbers of trained nursing personnel remained low in the years just prior to the outbreak of hostilities in 1914, hovering around four thousand. These factors are crucial to understanding the way that nursing functioned during the Great War.

The origins of Russian nursing lie in women's participation in charitable and religious traditions, which date back to the seventeenth and eighteenth centuries and became increasingly significant in the nineteenth century. The impetus to participate in charitable work came largely from Russia's Orthodox religious traditions, which stressed self-sacrifice and giving, especially for women, as the primary means for them to express their devotion. Charity work, as Adele Lindenmeyr indicates, "was the most accessible form of public activity for women in the nineteenth and early twentieth centuries." The Russian Orthodox Church promoted charity, including caring for the ill, as a primary component of piety. For women, in particular, participation in this kind of work was a unique path to salvation that also afforded them prestige. Women of means could establish their own religious or quasi-religious communities (*obshchiny*), which catered to the needs of the less fortunate. Those without wealth at their disposal could dedicate their lives to the care of the ill and poor by joining such communities. These activities were explicitly sanctioned by the autocracy, the Russian Orthodox Church, and Russian society in general, and received considerable support and patronage from the highest levels, including the dowager empresses and other female members of the imperial family. Charity work was not, however, limited to women of the elite. Over the course of the nineteenth century, it increasingly came to include women from a variety of social backgrounds.[4]

The charitable quasi-religious status of nursing in Russia is extremely significant. The Russian name for nurses, "sisters of mercy" (*sestry miloserdiia*), clearly reflects this notion. The word *miloserdiia* can be variously translated as "mercy" or "charity," and one scholar has even suggested that the term is best rendered as "loving-kindness," as a reflection of its Latin origin (*misericordia*) as well as the essentialist connotations of women as naturally life-giving and motherly.[5] The terminology was borrowed from the French, who used first the title *soeurs de charité, de la misericorde* in the seventeenth century. Societies of these sisters were founded by Louise de Marillac and St. Vincent de Paul to administer to the ill and poor in Europe. They were not considered to be full monastic orders, nor were they lay organizations, but rather they received a unique religious legal status. The "external" charitable efforts of these women meant that they would not be confined within the walls of a convent. Nonetheless, those who became members of these communities were considered to be "women who dedicated themselves to God."[6]

The foundations for the Russian nursing tradition were laid through the establishment of homes for impoverished widows by the dowager empress, Maria Fedorovna (mother of Tsar Alexander I), in the early nineteenth century. In return for their upkeep in the homes, the widows were encouraged to devote their energies to looking after patients in poor hospitals. Eventually, several dozen women were working in groups that came to be called the Compassionate Widows of the Empress, performing a variety of important tasks, including caring for and feeding patients and assisting doctors with surgeries. These organizations operated in Moscow and Saint Petersburg, admitting into their ranks women living in the widows' homes as well as their unwed daughters, as long as those individuals displayed sufficient devotion, self-discipline, and seriousness toward their work, as well as gendered behavioral strictures that emphasized modesty and sexual purity.[7]

In additional to the charitable and religious origins of Russian nursing, it is also important to note the tradition of women participating in medical care. Although prior to the nineteenth century women did not figure among medical professionals in Russia, they did often perform the roles of folk healers (*znakharki*) and village midwives (*povitukhi*). In fact, the vast majority of peasant healers in Russia were women, and childbirth was attended exclusively by village midwives, not male physicians. Unlike in the West, as medicine became increasingly professionalized and denigrated the activities of these women, slowly forcing them out of medical practice beginning in the seventeenth century, in Russia female folk healers still played prominent roles in providing health care for rural inhabitants. This was true even when professional medical practitioners began offering their services in the countryside through the expansion of the Zemstvo (local government) system, which brought scientifically trained male physicians and feldshers (*feld'shery*, roughly equivalent to physicians' assistants or nurse practitioners, and who included both men and women) to the villages. Folk healing was also closely connected with religion, and healers were tacitly accepted even by the Russian Orthodox Church at the village level, despite their frequent invocation of magic and other means clearly at odds with institutionalized religion.[8] The state also invested in an attempt to replace the untrained village midwives (*povitukhi*), who used folk methods that were often unsanitary and unsafe, with scientifically trained midwives (*akusherki*). Their work had been officially sanctioned and professionalized since the mid-eighteenth century, when the first training courses for midwifery were established. Focusing on basic anatomy and childbirth practices, these courses aimed at providing peasant women who attended most rural births with rudimentary medical knowledge, which, it was hoped, they would put to use in the villages.[9] By the turn of the twentieth century, there were more than fifty schools and more than ten thousand *akusherki* practicing throughout the empire.[10]

Also significant to the development of female nursing was the notion that women had a "natural" inclination toward caring and healing, which had become fairly widespread in contemporary Russian opinion by the nineteenth century. These ideas had begun to be seen as essential biological characteristics following the influence of writers such as Jean-Jacques Rousseau, wherein authors promoted nurturing and caring support as women's special attributes, closely associated with their capacities as mothers. Many Russians accepted the idea that women had a special role in family and the upbringing of children, based on a natural propensity for such activities and the moral authority ascribed to women. This idea was accompanied by the view that a woman's greatest attributes were self-sacrifice, sensitivity and love, as embodied by her role as mother.[11] Nursing thus came to be seen as an extension of the activities ascribed to women based on the assumption of their natural proclivity for caring and nurturing.

It was this combination of charitable, religious activity and what had become conventional wisdom concerning women's caring and nurturing abilities that established the ideological basis for the development of women's nursing in Russia. The first community (*obshchina*) of sisters of mercy in Russia, founded in 1844 by the Grand Duchess Alexandra Nikolaeva (daughter of Tsar Nicholas I) and Princess Teresa Old'enburgskaia, came to be called the Order of the Holy Trinity. All of its members were required to be unmarried.[12] Training lasted from one to three years and, according to religious scholar A. V. Posternak, "was purely practical, and confined to the knowledge of some medical procedures and hygiene care rules."[13] Interestingly, as nursing scholar L. A. Karpycheava has found, the community was interconfessional, a mix of Russian Orthodox, Lutheran, and Catholic members. Soon after, in 1846, another interfaith Russian community of sisters of mercy, the Community in the Name of Christ the Savior, was founded.[14]

Sisters of these communities were charged with caring for the ill in private apartments as well as in hospitals. The daily lives of these women were highly structured and disciplined, closely resembling, "in form and spirit," that in a convent. Posternak argues that in "conservative-minded Russia, where such undertakings had always been treated with great suspicion," the communities "could not be anything other than semi-monastic."[15] Indeed, not all members of Russian society agreed with the dowager empress and other supporters of women's charitable activities that these were appropriate for women. The main concern was that they were carried out in the public sphere, which some conservative members of Russian society believed was an inappropriate arena for female action, regardless of how well intentioned the endeavor. The semimonastic aspects, including strict behavioral control and complete asexuality, assuaged some of these concerns and made it possible for nursing to develop in Russia, albeit within the strict confines of religious charitable activities. Yet, as Karpycheava insists, the sister of mercy communities were not *fully* monastic, for they did not adhere to the rules of asceticism prescribed by Russian Orthodoxy and their work took place outside the walls of the *obshchiny*.[16]

RUSSIA'S FIRST WARTIME SISTERS: THE CRIMEAN WAR

Official Russian wartime nursing began during the Crimean War of 1854–1856, following closely on the heels of the deployment of women in nursing capacities first by the French "sisters of charity" and then the British, led by Florence Nightingale. Efforts to create a trained cadre of Russian women to carry out medical duties during this conflict were spearheaded by famous surgeon Dr. Nikolai Pirogov. Pirogov was highly concerned about the horrific medical conditions of the hospitals in the Crimea; enlisting the support of the Grand Duchess Elena Pavlovna (sister-in-law of Tsar Nicholas I), he convinced the military authorities to allow women to perform nursing service among the wounded. Together, they established the Order of the Exaltation of the Cross (*Krestovozdvizhenskii Obshchina*) on October 25, 1854, and sent twenty-eight sisters of mercy to the Crimea in November. While these were the first Russian women to be sent officially by the Russian government to attend to the wounded in this war, a number of the members of a Saint Petersburg community of sisters (which would come to be known as the Holy Trinity Community) and the Nikol'skii Obshchina of Moscow had gone to the Crimea early in the spring of 1854, a full eight months ahead of the dispatch of the first units of the Krestovozdvizhenskii community.[17] At that time Russian troops were fighting with Turkey, before the entrance into the war with Britain and France in the fall of 1854. And even before these sisters were sent, women were performing nursing services for Russian soldiers. These were women who traditionally traveled with armies and performed a variety of services for soldiers, from cooking to laundry, and even provided rudimentary medical care. Often they were soldiers' wives or family members, usually referred to as "camp followers" or *vivandières*. The services these women provided were essential for premodern armies, both before the creation of well-developed auxiliaries and even after, when ancillary services were often insufficient. As historian Barton Hacker has demonstrated, "from the fourteenth to the nineteenth century, if not earlier, women in armies were not only normal, they were vital. Armies could not have functioned as well, perhaps could not have functioned at all, without the service of women."[18]

Although other women cared for ill and injured men during the war, the Krestovozdvizhenskii *obshchina* was given primary responsibility for providing sisters of mercy to the military hospitals in the Crimea, and it was this group that began the formal, official tradition of wartime nursing. The community would ultimately dispatch hundreds of Russian women to care for the wounded in the conflict. One scholar has estimated that based on the more than 1,450 military honors the Russian government awarded to women for their medical service, it is safe to assume that the numbers of women who performed nursing duties during that war approximated 1,000.[19] This number exceeds the more famous example of British nurses working under Florence Nightingale by more than ten times. Moreover, their experiences were significantly different from their British and French counterparts, as the latter were confined to base hospitals, while Russian sisters served on the front lines, very close to the actual fighting.

The social backgrounds of the women who served as sisters of mercy during the Crimean varied considerably. According to historian John Curtiss, they ranged "from illiterates of humble background to members of the upper nobility."[20] They faced daunting circumstances; medical treatment was not well developed, and conditions were dangerous and unsanitary. The chief trustee of the Gogol'evskii Charity described the way he and other doctors approached the treatment of patients to Pirogov when the latter arrived in Sevastopol' in November 1854: "The closer to nature, the better. We do not use expensive medicines here. Man is simple: if he is going to die, he will die; if he is going to recover, so he will be healed." Pirogov was shocked to find that since October, more than ten thousand men had lain wounded in the military hospitals, more than half of which, "like dogs, had been thrown on the ground and on the bunks, tied up for weeks and not even fed."[21] In Simferopol the situation was no better. Pirogov described how patients lay on the floor of a stable being used as a hospital, on straw soaked with urine, blood, and pus, their wounds wrapped in dirty bandages. However, the vast majority of patients in the hospital were not there as a result of wounds received in battle, but to be treated for contagious diseases such as typhus and cholera, which claimed far more casualties than bullets or bayonets. The rate of infection was also very high for nurses. Moreover, working in field hospitals within close range of enemy fire also exposed Russian sisters of mercy to considerable danger; a number were wounded and some even killed in the fray.[22]

Despite Pirogov's enthusiasm for the use of women in wartime medical service, many men thought it unsuitable for women to be at the front. Disapproval stemmed from a number of difference sources. Those who were made uncomfortable by female participation in any public sphere activity obviously objected, but even those who had accepted them in civilian charitable capacities had great difficulty stomaching women's involvement in what was perceived as the exclusively male arena of war. There was considerable concern that women would be unable to withstand the harsh conditions of life in a military hospital. More often, objections centered on the possibility of sexual misconduct, either committed against the women or undertaken by the women themselves. One high-ranking general complained to the tsar that he could not possibly seriously consider sending women into the theater of war, as they would immediately be raped. The commander of Russian forces, General Alexander Menshikov, snidely commented to Pirogov, "I am afraid that this institution will increase the numbers of our syphilitics." The surgeon dismissed Menshikov's remarks as those typical of "old sinners," who "have studied women only *usque ad portionem vaginalem.*"[23]

These attitudes are not at all surprising considering the history of women associated with warfare, who were lumped into the category of "camp followers." While, as indicated above, these women provided a number of vitally important services for armies, camp followers had a reputation for sexual promiscuity, likely because some of them found it necessary to exchange sexual services for food or money to ensure survival. Thus, although most of the women called camp followers did not engage in prostitution and performed a number of other vital services, the label "camp follower" was fraught with pejorative connotation. Indeed, this negative reputation led to the requirement that nurses in official wartime service wear uniforms at all times. Florence Nightingale insisted that "the necessity of distinguishing them at once from camp followers is particularly obvious when they are not engaged in Hospital work."[24] Despite official sanction and uniforms, the "tainted" reputation of the camp follower continued to haunt wartime nurses.

Pirogov, however, was convinced that opposition to the presence of women in military hospitals had more to do with rampant corruption therein and fear that women would interfere with and expose such malfeasance. Moreover, it was not just that military officials were afraid that honest individuals would disrupt their schemes, but it was specifically that women could not be trusted to be discreet and would "wag their tongues," gossiping and exaggerating the problems in civilian quarters.[25] There was also a challenge to patriarchal hierarchy when female nurses intervened on behalf of patients, at times against doctors' orders. Physicians who ascribed to the "closer to nature" philosophy of medical care, often leaving men to die without much medical attention, were sometimes questioned by female nurses, who argued for the provision of care and comfort even for seemingly hopeless cases. These actions were often deeply resented by doctors, who did not welcome any intrusion in their work, particularly from women, and perceived such interventions as threatening to their authority.

Despite these critics, as well as the difficulties and dangers associated with their service, the Russian sisters of mercy of the Crimean War were noted by many as having performed their duties in an exemplary fashion. In particular, they were lauded for their ability to endure the privations of war and cope with the traumatic and often gruesome effects of combat. Nurses were put to work immediately in not only caring for sick and injured soldiers but also improving the hygiene and sanitation in medical facilities, assisting doctors in nearly every aspect of treatment, and attending to all of the additional needs of patients such as bathing, feeding, and general care. As one report from doctors M. Sokolov and F. Kiiakovskii, who served in the Crimean War, indicated, they were "motivated by the highest spirit of selflessness, compassion and humanity. They proved to be the most precious assets to the hospitals." They continued to praise the sisters, writing, "any doctor who had such a helper was sure that all the prescriptions would be performed perfectly. . . . In short, the compassionate nurses were the best helpers for the doctors and they were truly the best friends and patronesses for the patients."[26] In fact, there were many who believed that women were better suited to the work of caring for and comforting wounded and ill patients than men. Kh. Ia. Giubbenet, a doctor with the Sevastopol' garrison where many Russian nurses were also sent, remarked that "they . . . are more capable than men in these tasks . . . who are closer to the gentle feminine handiwork."[27] Furthermore, there were no reported cases of "sexual misconduct" on the part of sisters of mercy who served in the Crimea. As a result, many of the doubts and fears were disproven, and a number of members of Russian society came to accept their usefulness. The female wartime nurse thus became seen as a valuable asset and even a heroic figure.

THE LEGACY OF RUSSIAN CRIMEAN NURSING

The examples of the nurses in the Crimean conflict worked to conventionalize the tradition of employing women in military medical capacities.[28] According to Elizabeth Murray, "by providing a crucial service to her country, the Sister of Mercy had propelled Russian women, in nursing roles, for the first time, from the domestic to the public sphere, to the 'field of state service.'"[29] Yet there was no regularized utilization of women in military nursing. Instead, female nurses continued to be employed on an ad hoc basis, being allowed to participate in military medical services only in times of crisis. By the end of the Crimean War, it is estimated that Russia had approximately 327 fully trained nurses. However, most of these wartime nurses retired, with only a few remaining in service in the military hospitals located in Kiev and Saint Petersburg.[30] A few supporters, such as Pirogov, argued that the war had demonstrated the necessity of expanding women's military nursing, and urged the advancement of women's education in medical fields. He also wanted to see Russian nursing move away from its religious and charitable origins toward secularization and professionalization. "Our nurse should not be an Orthodox nun," he argued. Rather, "she must be a woman with a practical mind and a good technical background, though certainly she should retain a sensitive heart."[31]

Ultimately, Russian nursing made little headway in this direction. Military and medical authorities alike opposed professionalization. Very few were convinced by the Crimean experience that women should play a permanent role in military nursing. In particular, there was serious opposition to integrating female nurses into the military. Resistance to women's military nursing in Russia stemmed largely from the fact that with such professionalization, women would gain authority—authority that was not at all welcomed by male personnel. What vexed officials most was when nurses attempted to perform administrative functions and improve the management of hospitals, such as when nurses raised concerns about the lack of proper hygiene and sanitary conditions in military medical establishments. This was perceived as completely undesirable meddling in the running of medical facilities and unwelcome diversions from their "appropriate" duties. Female nurses had also ruffled feathers among male authorities, as Pirogov correctly predicted, when they attempted to combat the rampant corruption plaguing Russian military and medical institutions. Sisters of mercy were particularly aghast that badly needed supplies, equipment, medications, and even food were often diverted away from their intended beneficiaries by thieving hospital personnel. Nurses' attempts to stem corruption were blocked at the highest levels of Russian military medicine. As Yuri Bessonov explains, "although the authorities admitted much of the criticism, they could not give up prejudice against female capabilities in administrating and refused to accept the idea that nurses would be delegated certain responsibilities and legal rights to take part in hospital management." Even those who had praised women's work in nursing expressed this idea. The same doctors who had lauded nurses for their dedicated service to patients in the Crimean War, Sokolov and Kiiakovskii, closed their remarks with the following comments: "Nurses demonstrated all these qualities only in the beginning of their activity. However, since they had started interfering in all the parts of hospital administration, considering themselves utterly independent, they dodged performing their direct responsibilities."[32]

These kinds of sentiments established the most significant resistance to advancing women's wartime nursing. The only male medical authority who consistently promoted women in these capacities, and even insisted that they be appointed to administration positions within military medical facilities to oversee their management and ensure proper conditions, was Dr. Pirogov. His retirement immediately following the Crimean conflict, however, denied the nurses a powerful champion and left them with few defenders against the majority of the male military medical establishment who opposed professionalization. As a result, nursing was set apart from military contexts, especially after the military reforms of the 1870s, which created Russia's first regularized standing army.

The failure of professionalization of Russian nursing occurred even in spite of efforts of other promoters in high places. In 1856 Grand Duchess Elena Pavlovna attempted to use her connections as a member of the royal family to seek a greater role for women in military nursing. She submitted a proposal requesting that female nurses be utilized in military hospitals on a permanent basis. The tsar then appointed a special commission consisting of members of the medical council and top military officials to review the matter. The head of the nursing community of the Exaltation of the Cross, sister Ekaterina Bakunina, was its only female representative. While all of the members of the commission agreed on the value of women's nursing during wartime, none believed women should be granted any administrative authority. The commission began to work out rules and regulations for the implementation of female nursing personnel in military medical facilities, which were integrated into the development of a new hospital statute. This intended law incorporated some important innovations for the use of women in military nursing capacities, including appointment of a senior nurse to every hospital, including military facilities. But as a result of political contentions, largely in the form of opposition from male medical military personnel, the measures concerning female nursing personnel were never implemented. Moreover, although many in the Russian medical profession had recognized the positive impact of female nursing in military facilities, not all were convinced that such practices should continue. As Bessonov indicates, "a number of officials and chief doctors were convinced that nurses would be useless; some others even claimed that nurses would do considerable harm to hospitals once they were allowed to take care of the patients."[33] Thus Russian nursing would remain a private, charitable activity available to women in the Russian empire only through the auspices of the quasi-religious communities of sisters of mercy.

It is not altogether surprising that Russian nursing was not professionalized prior to World War I, considering its religious and charitable origins, which essentially provided it with its raison d'être. According to these roots, women who engaged in nursing did so based on a selfless desire to care for others, a quality bestowed on them by God, in emulation of the Virgin Mary. Professionalization was anathema to these principles in a number of ways. First, it recognized expertise based on learned scientific knowledge and acquired skill, rather than love, tenderness, and kindness divinely ordained and naturally attributed to women. That expertise would further endow the nurse with authority, instead of emphasizing subordination and submission to both God and man, and thus was incompatible with proscribed femininity within Orthodox patriarchal society. Moreover, in a professionalized occupation, expertise was to be compensated materially, as financial reward for applied knowledge in performance of service. This was likely seen as problematic for two reasons: (1) it is again inconsistent with the self-sacrificing mission of philanthropic nursing, and (2) payment to women for public services could be closely associated with prostitution, and thus with lack of respectability, designating it an improper activity for women. Retaining the charitable and quasi-religious elements of nursing and thereby denying nurses professional status and authority was thus seen as the "proper" way to allow women to engage in medical service. When the exigencies of war demanded the use of women from outside the "semimonastic" nursing communities, anxieties rose sharply.

THE RUSSIAN SOCIETY OF THE RED CROSS

Nonetheless, the unremitting recognition of need for medical personnel in times of national crisis meant that Russian women continued to serve as wartime nurses throughout the remainder of the nineteenth century. The Order of the Exaltation of the Cross served as the model for the creation of the nursing communities that would eventually make up the Russian Society of the Red Cross. This organization grew out of international efforts to establish a neutral body to provide medical assistance to armed forces, spearheaded by Swiss humanitarian Henri Dunant. After observing the horrific carnage of the Battle of Solferino in July 1859, Dunant pressed for improved care of wounded soldiers and was instrumental in drafting the Geneva Convention in 1863, which led to the creation of the International Committee of the Red Cross (ICRC) in 1864. On May 3, 1867, the Russian State Duma ratified the Geneva Convention and established its own agency, to be called the Russian Society for the Care of Ill and Wounded Soldiers (which was renamed the Russian Society of the Red Cross in 1876), and began establishing additional sister of mercy communities.[34] In November 1871 the Ministry of War established regulations for the assignment of sisters of mercy to the care of the ill and wounded in military hospitals.[35] By this time, there were more than twenty nursing communities in various cities throughout the empire. Caring for injured and ill soldiers was defined as part of the function of three *obshchiny*, the Exaltation of the Cross and Saint George's communities in Saint Petersburg and the "Soothing of My Sorrows" community (renamed Aleksandrov in 1881) in Moscow.[36]

Russian women's participation in medical care also expanded beginning in the second half of the nineteenth century, when they were given opportunities to become doctors. By the 1870s women's medical education had found increasing support from a number of quarters, including such unlikely places as the Chief War-Medical Inspector N. I. Kozlov and Minister of War Dmitri Miliutin. According to historian Christine Johanson, Miliutin's patronage would "prove to be a particularly significant factor in promoting women's medical education." The War Ministry would provide professional staff and clinical facilities for the training of female medical personnel, and later moved to establish women's higher medical courses within the Medical-Surgical Academy. However, fear of radicalization caused a shift in imperial policy and led to the closing of the courses.[37] This was not the only source of opposition to women physicians. Count Dmitri Tolstoi, minister of education, and A. E. Timashaev, minister of internal affairs, both worked to block the advancement of women's higher medical education, based on their belief that it would have detrimental effects on Russian society by taking women away from their primary responsibilities in the home. A. I. Georgevskii of the Ministry of Education argued that "advanced medical training would rob women of 'a sense of modesty and decency.'"[38] Somewhat ironically, considering his strong support of female wartime nursing, even Dr. Pirogov himself remained wary of expanding women's roles as physicians. Arguing against this, he insisted, "let many things remain unknown to her. She must be proud that she does not know a lot of things. Not everyone is a doctor. Not everyone must needlessly gaze on the sores of society."[39]

WOMEN'S WARTIME NURSING SERVICE: A PERMANENT FEATURE OF RUSSIAN MILITARY CONFLICT

While debate over the roles of women in the medical care profession persisted, women continued to serve as sisters of mercy through the auspices of charitable, quasi-religious communities. Women were instrumental in providing medical care during the remaining wars of the tsarist era. Thousands of women from all over the empire and from a wide variety of social backgrounds served as sisters of mercy during the Russo-Turkish War of 1877–1878. More than one hundred women with medical training had already been serving with doctors in military hospitals in Serbia, where hostilities between that country and the Ottoman empire had erupted in 1876. These included sisters of the Krestovozdvizhenskii, Georgievskii, and Pokrovskii communities, among others, including some organized by private initiatives. When Russia entered war with the Ottoman empire the next year, the numbers of Russian nurses increased significantly. This was also the first war in which graduates, as well as some students, of the Women's Higher Medical Courses served, both as doctors and as feldshers. These women operated at the same level as male doctors but were not allowed to be given the same titles or pay. Again, Russian sisters of mercy served on the front lines, even risking their lives to attend to the wounded on the battlefields on multiple occasions. Women also served in the military hospitals located in Russia, to which injured and ill soldiers were evacuated.[40] They received high praise from observers who witnessed them in action, performing difficult surgeries, administering treatments, and operating under the dangerous conditions of warfare and exposure to infectious diseases such as typhus.[41]

From a medical standpoint, this conflict was one of the most unsuccessful in history. As in the Crimean War, more lives were claimed by epidemic illness than combat fatalities. Military medical services were significantly underprepared to treat so many ill soldiers and unable to stem the spread of disease. When the hostilities between Russia and the Ottoman empire began, there were only a few hundred trained sisters of mercy qualified to work in the theater of war. It soon became readily apparent that this number was insufficient to meet the medical needs of the armed forces. To accommodate the great demand for training nursing personnel, shortened two-month courses were opened in Saint Petersburg.[42] The brief courses attracted numerous women from a variety of different social backgrounds. Even with these efforts, Russian participants in the war were overwhelmed by infection with typhus, which reached epidemic proportions from the very outbreak of hostilities.[43] The contagion soon spread to medical workers as well, infecting many sisters of mercy. In the hospital in Adrianople, for example, the epidemic decimated the nursing staff, leaving only eight sisters to treat more than four thousand patients. The situation was similar in many other medical facilities.[44]

According to Posternak, it was during this conflict that the idea of becoming a wartime sister of mercy first became "fashionable." He asserts that many were women who, although they wore "the cross on their chests, did not have the cross in their hearts"—society women who "had become jaded by entertainment and were bored with life," who went to war seeking adventure and excitement, and "interesting acquaintances." As a result, a number of the women who volunteered for medical service in this war had little idea of what wartime nursing actually entailed. They did not anticipate the serious hardships and danger they would face. The idea that women were motivated by personal reasons rather than patriotism and self-sacrifice would be repeated in the Great War. So, too, would the notion that women with more base sexual desires joined the ranks of Russia's wartime nurses during the Russo-Turkish conflict. Posternak claims that in particular, the majority of women who worked as sisters of mercy in the rear did not fit the model of the angelic, pure, devoted nurse, and those that did were "saints" in "the cities of sin." The divide between the rear, and its negative connotations, and the front, with more positive associations, will be an important theme in World War I as well. The notion that some of the women, especially "high society ladies," entered nursing service during this war with less than noble motivations was also present, as indicated by scholars such as Iurii Khechikov. He remarks on the reproach for those members of the Red Cross who, "in contrast with those selfless, shining individuals who sincerely understood the great idea of mercy in war and gave themselves for good works, there were those who used their positions for selfish goals."[45] Women who seemed to engage in wartime nursing for any reasons other than those defined by self-sacrifice and compassion, and those whose behavior failed to conform to strictures of controlled female sexuality, were open to criticism. Moreover, not all nurses regarded the experience as prestigious. One young woman working in a rear hospital in Kharkov commented, "If my family had not gone broke, I would never have come to this indignity."[46] The fact that she calls wartime nursing an "indignity" clearly reveals continued ambiguities about the reputation of nurses. These comments indicate the extent of anxieties and ambivalence caused by the increasing presence of women in public activities, and particularly in the sphere of war, and the extent to which nursing continued to be tied to its quasi-religious roots. These would be repeated and, indeed, increased during World War I.

Khechikov, however, insists that the majority of nurses were devoted to service.[47] Posternak's criticisms may stem from his position as an Orthodox priest and the comparison of civilian volunteer nurses to permanent members of the nursing *obshchiny,* with their quasi-religious character. This was not, however, the standard applied by all contemporary observers, something even Posternak himself admits. He indicates that although young women sometimes possessed less than lofty motivations, not everyone believed this to be detrimental. One regimental priest commented the young women "did not perform work poorly," despite the fact that they seemed to "approach the difficult work as if it were a holiday." Instead, he appreciated their lightheartedness and cheerful attitudes. "Their joyful laughter," he remarked, "often drowns the depressing groans of the wounded."[48] There is no indication, however, of how patients reacted to such levity.

Moreover, the idea that nursing was a respectable and important national service had become well developed in Russian society. A number of women from Russia's intelligentsia enlisted as sisters of mercy, expressing the desire to display their skills and abilities as medical professionals. Many wanted to demonstrate their ability to operate successfully in the public sphere as a means to eventually achieve equal rights with men. Iu. N. Ivanova, a scholar of Russian women's activities in military endeavors, asserts that the extreme dedication, sincerity, and hard work of these women in the difficult conditions of war "broke society's traditional view of the subordinate position and secondary importance of the roles of women."[49] This claim seems tenuous, as there is little evidence to indicate that actual change occurred with regard to women's rights or opportunities as a direct result of the activities of sisters of mercy during this war. Nonetheless, it is important to note the desire on the part of women to use wartime medical service as a means to achieve greater opportunity and rights. Again, this would be an important motivating factor in the service of Russian nurses during the Great War.

Additionally, the Russo-Turkish War established the precedent of distinguishing between the permanent members of the sister of mercy communities, who had completed the longer professional training (at least one year) and who remained part of the *obshchiny* before and after war, from those who volunteered and served exclusively during wartime. Wartime volunteers completed shortened training courses, resulting in less well developed knowledge of medical treatment compared to staff sisters. Moreover, the conditions of the Russo-Turkish War differed in significant ways from those of the Crimean War while foreshadowing events to come in World War I. Most significantly, this was the first war in which the movements of the troops were extremely rapid and frequent, requiring the medical units that served them to become mobile, in contrast to the stationary hospitals of the Crimean conflict. Officially, female nurses were still prohibited by law from serving in frontline positions. Conditions of the war, however, necessitated that they carry out medical care in those areas, very near to and sometimes even on the battlefields.[50] The impossibility of drawing clear lines between the front lines and the rear had already become apparent in this conflict. Now women would serve in mobile dressing stations, field hospitals, and other temporary facilities that would move quickly along the front. Work in temporary medical facilities was much more difficult, demanding, and dangerous, especially because they were closer to combat activity.

Further foreshadowing difficulties that would also surface in World War I, relations between the Red Cross and the military medical authorities were troubled during this conflict. During the Russo-Turkish War, a number of agents of the Russian Red Cross did not believe that the organization was obliged to provide assistance to the military establishment, citing instances where individual representatives of the Red Cross refused to comply with requests for supplies and equipment for military medical facilities.[51] Problems of interaction between the two organizations were exacerbated by the fact that the Red Cross was supposed to act as subordinate to military medical authorities but was often unable to provide the necessary assistance in the theater of war. Although the Red Cross was well financed (with a budget of more than 9 million rubles), it was ill equipped to handle the pressures of a mobile war. Specifically, the organization had little idea how to set up ambulatory medical units that operated very close to the fighting, provide accommodations for convalescing patients at the front, or establish safe evacuation routes for patients unable to return to the battlefields. Lack of previous planning and misunderstanding of the nature of the conflict meant that these issues had to be resolved spontaneously, which led to many mistakes and loss of precious time determining the best courses of action. Nurses were caught in the middle of these "learning experiences."[52]

Despite the terrible conditions and great danger, once again Russian women were lauded for their valuable contributions to the war effort. The example of women's actions in medical capacities during the Russo-Turkish War was also important in shoring up arguments in defense of the ability of women to work as physicians in the Russian empire. Ultimately, these would be successful, and in 1880 the tsar signed a decree that granted graduates of women's higher medical courses the right to be designated as women doctors and to practice medicine independently. This victory proved to be short-lived, however, as the assassination of the reformist Alexander II, and the accession to the throne of his conservative son Alexander III, led to the revocation of this decree. All women's higher education courses were officially halted, and not until after Alexander III's death would women once again be given the opportunity to train as doctors, beginning in 1895.[53] Despite these setbacks, women were given some additional opportunities to become medical professionals as feldshers. Training schools for feldshers enrolled increasing numbers of women into their courses in the last decade of the nineteenth century. By 1910 more than 70 percent of Russian students in these courses were women.[54]

Women's nursing activities were not curtailed during the conservative backlash under Alexander III. Following the Russo-Turkish War, the permanent or "staff" sisters returned to their nursing communities in Russia and continued to provide care for ill and wounded Russians during peacetime. Some even became involved in foreign wars, serving as impartial medical personnel in the conflicts of the late nineteenth century, including the Italian campaign in Abyssinia in 1896 and the British Boer War in South Africa in 1899.[55] The Russian Society of the Red Cross took control over all wartime nursing activities in 1897. Although the Russian Red Cross was officially affiliated with the ICRC, it operated as a completely independent entity. By 1900 there were 81 separate sister of mercy communities with more than 1,600 nurses serving in them, with another 600 in training and approximately 600 in reserves (they had completed formal training and left their *obshchiny* but were prepared to be called up for duty should the need arise). However, such a quantity was still insufficient to provide medical service for such a large country, as recognized by the deficiencies experienced in the previous war.[56]

Despite exhortations from the Red Cross that the numbers of sisters of mercy be increased in order to handle the next crisis, little was actually done before the outbreak of the Russo-Japanese War in 1904. However, two mobile field hospitals established in Port Author were staffed by small contingents of nurses as early as 1898. The first full unit of sisters of mercy was sent to the Far East on January 28, 1904. The prosecution of the war, however, was plagued with difficulties. Aside from military defeats resulting from a serious underestimation of the enemy, the provision of medical service was significantly hampered by problems in getting sufficient materials, equipment, and personnel to field hospitals in the Far East. Located extremely far from the distribution centers of European Russia, the journey there usually took approximately thirty-five days.

There is some debate among scholars regarding the effect of the war on the status of wartime medical service and, particularly, the Red Cross. Khechikov asserts that despite these difficulties, in comparison with the previous conflict, during the Russo-Japanese War the Red Cross was restored to a position of strength and functioned not only as an important assistant to the military medical establishment but also as a formidable independent organization.[57] Posternak, however, points out that while the organization did its best to provide care for the ill and injured, including generously allocating funds to medical service, there was a strong impression among some observers that despite the ample financial resources at the organization's disposal (it raised 20 million rubles from private donations alone), the administration often chose to spend money on luxury for itself.[58] Observing Russian medical practices during the war, U.S. Navy surgeon Raymond Spear confirms this view. While asserting that the Russian Red Cross was "the largest and most powerful of its kind in the world," he noted that "there has been much scandal caused by the misappropriation of the society's funds and large sums of money have gone astray."[59] Moreover, it is clear that the Red Cross was not able to perform the tasks of medical service provision alone, and its efforts were augmented, as they would be again and to a much greater degree in World War I, by civilian organizations, including the Zemstvos, private companies, social groups, and civil committees, which sent funds and materials to help with the establishment of infirmaries and hospitals, and even organized and sent units of personnel to assist with providing medical aid.[60]

Estimates on the total number of sisters of mercy employed during this conflict vary from two thousand (Posternak) to five thousand (Spear). For these women, however, the experience was an uneven one. The nurses, as in previous wars, came from a variety of social and educational backgrounds; because the Russian Red Cross had not yet established a literacy requirement, the women varied from those with university educations to those who were practically illiterate. So, too, was the diversity of training and experience of nurses in these hostilities. Many were staff sisters who had been part of nursing communities for years, including some veterans of previous conflicts. Some had undergone training for as long as four years before being sent into wartime service. Others, because of the great demand for female medical personnel necessitated by the unexpectedly high numbers of casualties, had to be sent into service after significantly truncated training, lasting as little as six weeks. Even the pay of sisters of mercy during this conflict varied greatly, ranging from five to thirty rubles a month, contingent on the funding of the *obshchiny*. Those assigned directly by the military authorities could receive as much as ninety rubles a month, plus expenditures.[61] And while the Russian women who served as sisters of mercy in this conflict were praised by many observers, foreign and Russian alike, for their sacrifice, devotion, courage, and fortitude, they came out somewhat lacking when compared to Japanese nurses, who greatly impressed observers with their excellent organizational and technical skills, appearing as models of efficiency and professionalism.[62]

Furthermore, the Russo-Japanese War augured serious difficulties that would arise again in the Great War. These included clashes over authority between the Red Cross, the nursing communities, and military medical establishment, as well as between nurses and military and medical personnel. Officially, the Red Cross was supposed to maintain authority over the assignment and work of sisters of mercy. In reality, the individual nursing communities had tremendous influence over where nurses were sent. But once in service, military medical authorities exercised near complete control over nurses. Military doctors had the ability to dismiss nurses they deemed unfit for service, a decision they often made based on personal dislikes rather than true measures of ability. Many military medical authorities remained unconvinced that women had a place in army sanitary services, particularly in mobile field units that operated on the front lines, and expressed suspicion of the nurses that came under their command. They were also insistent that sisters of mercy, despite their civilian status, follow the dictates of military discipline and authority.[63] There were those who questioned the motives of some women in joining the war effort, another problem that would persist into the First World War. Indeed, one Russian doctor of the Great War reflected that it was during the Russo-Japanese conflict that "the good name of the sister of mercy was severely undermined," as a result of some, he lamented, who had become sisters out of a "thirst for adventure and frivolity" rather than out of "necessity of serving a historic cause."[64]

Another important precedent was established during this conflict: the "obsession," as Posternak labels it, of the volunteer nurse to serve at the front rather than in rear medical establishments. The chief commissioner of the Russian Society of the Red Cross in the Far East, Senator Kaufman, complained of nurses that "the idea that the real work is not in the rear, but rather the need for them is where the fighting is going on—constantly haunts them and prevents them from working peacefully in the places where they have been assigned."[65] The urge was so strong among some nurses that they often feigned illness or personal tragedy in order to be granted leave from rear hospitals. But instead of returning home they illicitly made their way to units operating in areas such as Harbin, close to the battlefields. This would continue to be a problem during the Great War.

Moreover, debate continued regarding the wisdom of placing women in such close proximity to the dangerous conditions of combat. Most agreed that Russian women could perform the tasks required in these settings, and indeed, they played valuable roles in medical service as well as provision of comfort and support for soldiers. Spear noted that Russian women were clearly physically capable of handling the rigors of life at the front (something he attributed to a commonly held Western conception of Russian women as sturdier and hardier than their Western counterparts). Yet he expressed reservations about placing them in harm's way, stating, "they should not be exposed on the firing line," risking the loss of valuable resources for the army.[66] A number of women who served as sisters of mercy during the Russo-Japanese War would experience significant psychological distress and difficulty adjusting to the harsh conditions of frontline medical service. The moral propriety of nurses was also a significant aspect of wartime nursing during this conflict. Nurses were still held to rigid standards of sexual behavior, but it was recognized that despite their efforts to remain aloof and proper, female nurses faced unwanted advances from male personnel. In particular, officers gained a bad reputation for overt harassment of sisters of mercy, resulting in an aversion on the part of nurses to assignment in officer wards. All of these issues would resurface when the empire went to war again in 1914.

The experiences of the wars of the late nineteenth century clearly indicated the need for a well-developed organization of medical service to augment military provisions, ready to be implemented from the moment hostilities began. In the period immediately preceding the Great War, planning efforts for what many considered to be an inevitable conflict included further development of medical services, now deemed to be essential for the successful waging of war. Despite this ideological commitment, few actual resources were devoted to this task. A category of "reserve" sisters of mercy was created following the Russo-Japanese War, and young educated women (particular those such as Tat'iana Varnek, who had just completed secondary education) were encouraged to enter the communities of the Red Cross to receive appropriate medical training in case war broke out and their skills would be needed. Through these efforts, the Red Cross had successfully increased the number of sisters of mercy in the *obshchiny* to around four thousand in the years immediately before the war. But this fell far short of the prewar goal of ten thousand nurses, which the organization had determined were required for the successful provision of medical services to the Russian population even in peacetime conditions.[67] This left much work to be done once the guns of August sounded in 1914.

CONCLUSIONS

The outbreak of war in the summer of 1914 caught Tat'iana Varnek completely by surprise, as it did much of the Russian nation. She remarked that she "did not sense the approaching storm" and in fact only learned of the mobilization order three days after it had been promulgated. At that point, she decided to reenter nursing service out of a sense of national duty. But because she had not finished her practicum and had not received a diploma, she was worried that she would not be accepted as a sister of mercy. The great demand for female medical personnel, however, meant that few women with any kind of training would be turned away. She was told to report to the Kaufman *obshchina* in Saint Petersburg immediately, which she did, arriving on September 2, 1914. She was assigned to the Aleksandrovskii Hospital in order to finish her practicum, where she worked until September 19, after which she received her designation as a sister of mercy and then was dispatched to the front on September 23.[68]

Of course, Russia was not the only country to realize the need for trained female medical personnel during military conflict, and wartime nursing had developed significantly by the time of the outbreak of the First World War in a number of other nations. As in Russia and France, the nursing traditions in a number of other European countries had their roots in the religious traditions of the early nineteenth century but developed significantly away from that influence by the end of the century. In Germany women of the elite entered nursing as a charitable activity from the middle of the nineteenth century, when the German Red Cross established sisterhoods similar to the *obshchiny* of Russia. While the Crimean War established the tradition of female wartime nursing in France, Britain, and Russia, in Germany it came a bit later, as a result of that country's experiences in the wars of 1866 and 1870, and continued to develop thereafter.[69]

In the United States a similar trajectory had been followed after the devastating experiences of the Civil War, which led to the foundation of the American Red Cross and the pioneering efforts of Clara Barton. The development of women's nursing came as a result of common ideological underpinnings regarding gender: the general assumption that had come to predominate in the nineteenth century that nursing was a proper activity for women based on essentialist characteristics of femininity. Writing in 1911 for the *American Nursing Journal,* Colonel John Hoff of the U.S. Army summed up this sentiment well:

> God made the nurse, woman; and from the beginning the practice of this art has never reached perfection in any other hands. I speak advisedly, as for the last quarter of a century, it has been part of my duty to train men of the hospital corps to take care for the ill and injured of our army. Training in anything, of course, adds greatly to efficiency; but the calling must be congenial if the best results are to follow. Man has no real vocation as a nurse. Some there are who adopt nursing as an occupation . . . but they never have the divine touch which marks woman as especially chosen for this work.[70]

Nursing was also perceived as the proper counterpoint to male patriotic activity. Providing care for wounded soldiers was understood as the best way that women could serve their countries in times of war. These ideas, however, had not been permanent features of European societies but rather were developed, in many ways deliberately, by national efforts to engage women in national duty. For example, in France the occupation had not been seen as particularly feminine or patriotic but instead a dirty, sordid affair with little value—until a successful propaganda campaign by the Red Cross transformed nursing into a proper female vocation and a means by which women could demonstrate their devotion to *la patrie*.[71]

Somewhat remarkably, within a span of merely a half a century, what was once a male endeavor considered strictly off-limits to women (at least to respectable women), performed in a space designated exclusively masculine where it had been unthinkable to introduce (again, respectable) women, had been transformed into a service that not only was deemed appropriate for women but also, for the most part, now was seen as honorable, dutiful, and best undertaken by women as a result of their specific "nature." Despite reservations concerning the ability of women to endure the rigors of war, most early twentieth-century societies had come to view nursing as something specifically feminine, and necessary, even in the male zone of war. Thus, while war itself continued to be considered "men's work," nursing, even in wartime, had come to be understood as "women's work," and respectable women's work at that.

2

MOBILIZING MEDICAL SERVICE

KHRISTINA SEMINA: DOCTOR'S WIFE TURNED SISTER

As soon as news of the outbreak of war reached her, Khristina Semina proposed the idea of enrolling in a nurses' training course to her husband, Ivan. The latter refused unequivocally. As a regimental doctor in Baku, Ivan was intimately familiar with military medical service. He did not believe his wife possessed the strong constitution needed to handle the "blood and pieces of human flesh," and he worried she would become infected with typhus. He insisted that she stay at home, primarily so that he would not have to worry about her well-being. As soon as he left for the front, however, Semina deliberately disobeyed her husband and entered the local nursing courses. The military doctor at the enlistment point expressed similar concerns that the demands of wartime nursing would be too great for a noblewoman who had never "worked." Khristina insisted, convincing the doctor to allow her to sign up for training, and began attending lectures at the local hospital immediately after.

The first set of lectures Semina attended was on care for the ill and wounded. The second covered anatomy. She and her fellow sisters-in-training would gather after the lessons and drill each other on the knowledge they had acquired during the day. She recalled that after only a week of classes, many of the women "already considered themselves to be experienced nurses." Before Semina had to chance to complete the courses, she received a letter from her husband, asking her to come join him where he was stationed, in Tiflis (present-day Tbilisi, Georgia). Khristina was torn—she badly wanted to finish her training, but having gone against her husband's will, she could not explain why she wanted to stay in Baku. She went to one of the doctors teaching the courses to ask his advice. The doctor told her the most important thing was her husband; she should go to him immediately, as this was her duty as a wife. She readily agreed and left that evening to join Ivan.

In Tiflis she secretly continued attending nursing courses while her husband was away at work. Meanwhile, Doctor Semin struggled to complete the organization of his unit, hindered at every turn by corruption and shortages and plagued by incessant internal theft and robbery of vitally important equipment and supplies, which he was powerless to stop. He was also highly vexed that the administrative nature of his job prevented him from practicing medicine, instead demanding that he act as a bureaucrat. He complained that he did nothing but endlessly sign papers, none of which he understood because they were so tangled and confusing, and all of which seemed to have been falsified. He was so distraught that he contemplated leaving his position as head of the transport unit to become a junior doctor in a field hospital. Ivan's desperation soon led him to depression, alcohol abuse, and eventually suicide later in the war.

When Semin's unit finally received orders to leave for the front, despite the fact that it still lacked a complete complement of supplies and equipment (although it was a transport unit, it had no carts to carry the wounded), the doctor urged his wife to return to Baku for her safety. Khristina complied, but once home, she reenrolled in the nursing courses she had originally attended. She completed the coursework and began a practicum in the local hospital. After successfully finishing all of the training, she was awarded a certificate and named a sister of mercy. Although Semina was very proud of this accomplishment and eager to put her new skills to work for the wounded, her family was much less impressed. Her sister-in-law accused her of wanting to go to the front to seek personal glory, merely to obtain medals, while her brother-in-law implied that her motives were more sexual in nature, spurred by a desire to flirt with officers. Semina was deeply offended by their insinuations and specifically lashed back at her brother-in-law Yasha, chiding him for his own "low morality," which had earned him a reputation as a notorious womanizer. She further rebuked him for failing to perform his patriotic duty by evading enlistment using personal connections to receive an exemption despite his good health and appropriate age for military service. Yasha laughed off the suggestion that he go to the front, replying, "If all the men go off to war, who will remain to entertain the women?! Poor things, the dears will die of boredom!"

After receiving her diploma, Semina was presented with a list of locations that badly needed nursing personnel and was asked to choose one for assignment. The doctor who ran the training courses even offered her a position in his surgical hospital. She refused all of these options, instead insisting on being dispatched to Sarykamysh (present-day Sarıkamış, Turkey), in Russian-controlled territory where her husband was now stationed. Despite the doctor's exhortations to go where the need was greatest, Khristina insisted on joining Ivan. When she arrived in Sarykamysh (to the great surprise and dismay of her husband), she applied to the local hospital asking to be put to work there. But the head doctor had no place for her, as the facility already had a full complement of nurses. Burning with the desire to be useful, she decided to accompany her husband's medical transport unit on its missions to collect the wounded from frontline dressing stations and bring them back to the hospital for further treatment. After one experience in the bitter cold, however, with temperatures dipping to forty below zero, she found this activity too difficult. She spent much of her remaining time in Sarykamysh, sitting idly in her husband's quarters. After several weeks, the city was evacuated of all nonmilitary personnel in anticipation of a Turkish siege. The order had come while Ivan was out with his transport unit. Desiring to await his return, Semina resisted evacuation orders and remained in the city. When he failed to come back after several days, she was forced to leave alone. She went to the city of Kars, where she found a position as a nurse in a mobile field hospital. There, she filled a badly needed position in a staff that was desperately far from complete. She insisted, however, that the chief doctor leave her name off the staff list, telling him, much to his chagrin, that she would leave at the first word of her husband who had been missing since the evacuation of Sarykamysh. Indeed, after serving only a few weeks, she left on her own volition, despite the pleas and admonitions of the chief doctor, to try to find her husband.[1]

THE PROBLEMS OF MOBILIZATION

With the outbreak of hostilities in August 1914, the Russian government began the laborious process of mobilizing the population for the war effort. Initially, neither military nor medical authorities fully understood what was required for the successful prosecution of such a war. Problems with production and distribution of goods, equipment, and arms; difficulties in carrying out conscription and transportation of soldiers; and obstacles in the organization and provision of medical services immediately caught Russian officials off guard. Although the Russian Military-Sanitary Administration had undertaken a process of major reform after experiencing significant problems during the Russo-Japanese War of 1904–1905, many of the lessons they took from that conflict either were not applied to or would not be useful for this new war.[2] Shortages of everything, including medical personnel, became readily apparent when the war began, even though many officials had recognized that more trained nursing personnel was essential after the experience of the war with Japan. But the Russian government had not correctly anticipated the vast numbers of medical personnel, facilities, equipment, and supplies that would be required to successfully prosecute a world war. The extensive scale of the war coupled with the lack of experience and reluctance to utilize civilian sources of support often hindered efficient provision of medical services. This would prove to be very troublesome for the Russian armed forces, which suffered very high casualties during this conflict. By September 1917 the number of Russian troops wounded in the war was approximately 2.5 million. Another 2.3 million soldiers had fallen ill as a result of the spread of highly contagious epidemic diseases, including typhoid fever, typhus, cholera, and dysentery, as well as other illnesses such as pneumonia or scurvy. For many men, these illnesses proved fatal. Typhoid fever and typhus (two different diseases) averaged a 22 percent mortality rate, while cholera was fatal for 33 percent of those it infected. Typhus also had a tendency to recur among patients who were previously infected and had recovered from its effects.[3] Moreover, these illnesses also affected the civilian population, who fell victim to the spread of epidemic disease facilitated by the dislocations caused by the conflict. The result was a breakdown in public health and major discontent, which contributed to a growing lack of confidence that the tsarist system could meet the needs of its people.

RUSSIAN WARTIME NURSING IN AN INTERNATIONAL CONTEXT

Russia was not alone in underestimating the medical needs of its military and civilian populations. None of the belligerents were prepared for the magnitude of total war. Despite the presence of trained professional nurses in many of these places, the medical needs of the First World War were so great that all of these nations were forced to employ large numbers of volunteer nurses through their respective societies of the Red Cross, as well as professional nurses attached to their armies. Great Britain perhaps had the greatest success in this endeavor. British volunteer nurses, called VADs (voluntary aid detachment nurses), supplemented wartime medical service performed by professional nurses, who served as part of the British military, and together, they numbered more than 90,000. The total number of men who served in the British armed forces during the war was roughly 8.7 million. In other belligerents, however, the ratio of medical personnel to combatants was significantly lower. In Germany, by the fall of 1918, 28,000 volunteer nurses had augmented the service of several thousand professional nurses working behind the lines, providing medical aid to an army of 11 million.[4] Although France had begun to train military nurses in 1909, at the time of the outbreak of the Great War the country had fewer than one hundred such women. Eventually, the French army was able to increase this number to 30,000 to serve 8 million men mobilized for battle, but this number was insufficient to satisfy the demand for medical personnel. As a result, that country relied heavily on Red Cross volunteers, recruiting more than 63,000 women to work in wartime nursing.[5] Although not all of the women were actually put to work in nursing capacities, and the British and French participated in the war longer than the Russians, it is striking that the numbers of their nurses far exceeded the numbers of women employed by the Russian Red Cross and its subordinate organizations. This is despite the fact that Russia fielded many more men during the war, with roughly 15 million men in its armed forces. The United States, although it did not enter the war until April 1917, was also initially ill equipped to handle the massive numbers of wounded caused by modern warfare. With only around four hundred trained nurses in the Army Nurse Corps, the United States was forced to rely heavily on the assistance of the American Red Cross. Eventually, it was able to increase that number to more than 21,000, who carried out medical assistance for roughly 4 million soldiers.[6]

The largest contrasts come when Russian wartime nursing is viewed against those nations where professionalization of nursing had already occurred prior to the outbreak of World War I: Great Britain, the United States, Germany, Australia, and Japan. By the turn of the twentieth century, a transnational organization, the International Council of Nurses, had been established to protect the interests of nurses and advocate on their behalves in these countries.[7] This kind of professional organization highlighted how in other important ways, the experiences of Russia's wartime nursing organization was quite different. By the time of the outbreak of World War I, nursing had become a respected occupation for educated women—indeed, one of the few open to women other than teaching. As Henriette Donner has argued, even the volunteer nurses who served in the British Red Cross as VADs were integrated into a system of professional nursing that was well established before the outbreak of the Great War. Donner asserts that "the V.A.D.s were poured into an already organizing environment supported by a streamlined system of organizing, training and deploying a professional voluntary sector. Indeed, the War did not cause but reflected a process of modernisation of Britain which had been underway for half a century."[8]

Even despite its significantly shorter experience in the war, the United States had a number of advantages not possessed by the tsarist empire. The Americans had time prior to their entry into the war to observe French medical services and, as a result, had devised an elaborate plan for a base hospital system. While the US government had implemented austerity measures, depriving the military of the funds to implement such a plan, the Red Cross came to the rescue by providing the necessary funding and augmenting the base hospital system with its own facilities. The Americans also had at their disposal thousands of trained professional nurses, who could be drawn on as reserves. Many of these women had worked alongside doctors in stateside hospitals before the war. As Lettie Gavin explains of the American Red Cross, "its staff was composed of men and women who had worked together in civilian life and were familiar with each other's abilities and methods."[9] While the Russian Red Cross often dispatched small groups of nurses from the same *obshchina* to common points of service, it was rare that the medical personnel had experience working as a unit prior to the crisis of the war. Nor was the Russian Red Cross able to exist without significant financial support from the state. By contrast, Russian wartime nursing remained more akin to its origins in French nursing, which similarly remained a private endeavor directed by the French Red Cross and seen as voluntary, charitable work rather than professional service.[10]

Another significant difference was the experience of Russian nurses who worked in close proximity to the fighting. Although all the belligerents, including Russia, had regulations that prohibited women from working on the frontlines near active combat activities, the realities of war made this impossible. As a result, there were a number of nurses who actually performed their medical services in locations dangerously near, and sometimes even on, the battlefields. Thus, even some French, German, and Austrian women were required to work in field units and dressing stations on the front lines. In fact, to meet these needs, late in the conflict, in 1917, the French government began to officially allow women to serve in the forward positions, despite the fact that some had actually been doing so since the start of the war.[11] In these capacities, the wartime experiences of nurses from other nations share much with those of Russian sisters of mercy. They endured extremes of temperature, long working hours and constant fatigue, depravations, and exposure to fatal diseases and sometimes even deadly danger. They saw the same effects of modern weaponry on the bodies of their patients and had to cope with the emotional and psychological distress caused by witnessing the destruction and death of so many. Unlike the situation in Russia, however, frontline nurses made up a very small percentage of women in medical service in other belligerents. Most British, French, German, Italian, and Austro-Hungarian women served in hospitals located far behind the lines. Thus, although many worked in very harrowing and demanding conditions, few operated directly in the line of fire. Medical service on the eastern front—indeed, the entire war experience—was profoundly different from that on the western front. In the East the entire notion of a division between front and rear was nearly impossible to maintain, as combat turned villages into battlefields and the war zone shifted extremely quickly. It was not at all uncommon for Russian women to serve in positions that were frequently fired on by enemy forces or bombed by enemy planes; they even administered medical care to men while still on the battlefields. Moreover, in areas where fighting between Russian and Central Powers forces occurred, epidemic diseases were rampant, spreading much more quickly and claiming many more lives than in the West, as a result of a general breakdown in public health in Russia.[12] As a result, their experiences were often quite different than those of nurses of other belligerents.

THE RED CROSS, THE GOLDEN EAGLE, AND RUSSIAN CIVIL SOCIETY IN THE CRISIS OF WORLD WAR I

In addition to lack of professionalization of nursing services and the perils of dangerous and demanding work on the front lines, Russia encountered other problems in effectively making use of human and material resources, which were specific to the tsarist empire. These stemmed at least partially from the somewhat underdeveloped nature of nongovernmental services associated with civil society. The autocratic government and its supporters had long resisted national mobilization, despite pressure from military circles, which argued for its necessity. As Joshua Sanborn has indicated, "mobilization as a regular feature of political and social life was the last thing that the besieged autocracy wanted. By definition, autocracy does not rest upon a base of popular support, much less active public participation."[13] This is not to say that Russia completely lacked any form of civil society. While scholars continue to debate the extent to which prerevolutionary efforts to create a true civil society were successful, a number of works have demonstrated that one had begun to congeal prior to the war and continued to grow during the conflict.[14] Indeed, the crisis of total war made resistance to civilian efforts impossible to maintain any longer, and as Sanborn demonstrates, "from 1914 on, the state engaged in mass politics in order to achieve mass mobilization."[15] The war made clear that much of the impetus, initiative, and action had to come from the civilian population.

Although the war would soon indicate the need to allow civil society efforts to function where governmental ones fell short, the process of growth in these areas was by no means smooth. In fact, the crisis of the war initially led the tsarist administration to attempt greater centralization and control. The autocracy remained suspicious of private initiatives, loath to relinquish responsibility to unofficial efforts, even while being forced to rely on them. As soon as the conflict began, the tsarist government recognized opportunities to expand executive power. The legislative function of the Duma (the representative body of Russia) was completely bypassed, as laws were funneled directly to the tsar through the loyal and staunchly conservative Council of Ministers. In the first year of the war, the Duma met only twice. To address the wartime medical needs of the Russian military and the civilian population affected by the conflict, the tsarist government created a number of central organs. Ensuring control over and loyalty from such entities, they were almost always directed by members of the imperial family, although the Duma created several bodies to address these needs as well.[16]

In September 1914, in an effort to centralize military medical service provision, the tsar appointed his cousin, Prince Alexander Ol'denburgskii, supreme head of an entirely new wartime military agency, the Sanitary and Evacuation Section. As such, Ol'denburgskii was charged with overseeing "all organs, organizations, societies and personnel of the sanitary and evacuation service, both the theater of military operations, and in the interior of the empire."[17] The position gave him power almost completely without oversight, for he reported directly to the commander in chief of the armed forces, Grand Duke Nikolai Nikoleavich, and the tsar himself, bypassing the minister of war and the Council of Ministers. The implication was that all medical services would come under the control of the armed forces. Curiously, however, efforts toward greater centralization of health care provision through the creation of a Main Administration for State Health Protection (as envisioned by prominent academic physician and member of the State Council, Dr. G. E. Rein), which would bring all medical organization, including the Red Cross, under the auspices of a central health administration, did not come to fruition. In particular, Prince Ol'denburgskii continually opposed the idea, which undoubtedly would have meant a loss of power for him.[18] In attempt to maintain central control over wartime medical services, the Russian Society of the Red Cross, which Ol'denburgskii also headed, was assigned sole responsibility for the medical needs at the front, with exclusive authority to operate across the line of demarcation that separated the active war zone from the rest of the country. All other organizations providing medical services were limited to evacuating soldiers away from the front and treating them in the rear. The central government's original desire was to cut off the rest of the country from the regions directly affected by the war.

As soon as the war began, the inadequacies of imperial institutions became readily apparent. To fill the void, a proliferation of civilian organizations took up wartime activities. These included the voluntary organs of the Union of Zemstvos and the Union of Towns (collectively known as Zemgor), which came to play a vital role in the provision of wartime services. Directed by liberal professionals, these were an amalgam of local efforts, charged with medical, sanitary, and food-provisioning duties for both the military and civilian populations. According to historian William Gleason, Zemgor efforts were "the most concrete manifestation of the public drive to save Russia from military collapse" and "represented the widespread public desire to contribute to the war effort as a unified nation."[19] Despite the good intentions and positive impacts of these groups, the autocracy remained decidedly wary of them and tried its best to maintain control over them. As a result, the Union of Zemstvos and the Union of Towns were placed under the "flag" of the Red Cross; the government intended for them to operate in a subordinate position and in the rear only. Moreover, these organizations and their personnel suffered from turbulent relationships with the central government, the Red Cross, and with one another. Perhaps most importantly, the Russian Imperial Army expressed resistance and was even hostile to aid from civilian quarters.

The various conflicts between these groups indicate that the interpretation of a purely dichotomous conflict, civil society versus autocracy, is insufficient in explaining the problems of wartime service provision in Russia. In many instances, the source of conflict emanated from friction between and within governmental agencies, between different civilian organizations, and between individual personnel of both. Indeed, the vocabulary used by scholars with regard to notions of "civil society" may be inadequate to accurately describe the case of late imperial Russia, wherein it is difficult to delineate clearly between "governmental" and "nongovernmental" organs. The lines of tsarist control and private initiative were not clearly drawn. Members of the imperial family were involved in numerous "semi-official" philanthropic efforts. The Russian Society of the Red Cross itself was not an autonomous "civil society" institution operating free of state control. In fact, it may be better characterized as a "quasi-state" agency with a philanthropic mission. The organization, with its roots in the Order of the Exaltation of the Cross established by the Grand Duchess Elena Pavlovna (Tsar Nicholas I's sister-in-law), continued to be very closely associated with, and indeed run by, the imperial family. When World War I began, it was nominally headed by the dowager empress, Maria Feodorovna, Tsar Nicholas II's mother, and directed by his cousin, Prince Ol'denburgskii. Many of its administrative positions were appointed by the tsar and his representatives. The society also received much of its funding from the central government and was supported by significant private donations from members of the imperial family.

Close connections with the imperial family and the state did not mean, however, that the Russian Red Cross always operated under direct government control. Nor did those ties spare the organization from rocky relations with the central government and the military establishment. Furthermore, the nursing personnel of the Red Cross and other medical organizations were composed of women who entered nursing service voluntarily and certainly were not considered state employees. The nursing communities of the Red Cross had permanent personnel, designated as "staff sisters," who entered into wartime service with significant training and background in nursing, and who were paid for their labor but were still largely considered charity workers with quasi-religious status. But during the war, women were accepted into the Red Cross as nurses without becoming permanent members of the *obshchiny*, and designated as "civil" or "wartime sisters of mercy" and "volunteer sisters" (roughly equivalent to the VADs of the British medical services). Although these women tended to come from the educated segments of Russian society, they were by no means politically or even socially homogeneous. While some were staunch supporters of the autocracy and aristocracy, many others were part of the liberal and even radical opposition. Among their numbers were members of civil society organizations, such as philanthropic organizations, professional associations, and the media, while others had no particular affiliations. They did not always conform to official efforts to control their actions and conduct during the war, which often brought them into conflict with authorities. Moreover, many of the nurses who served Russia during the First World War did so through the auspices of other organizations, such as the medical facilities and units operated by the Zemgor. Although these organizations were heavily dominated by liberals who generally stood in opposition to the tsarist regime, mistrusting its initiatives and seeking to reform it or eliminate it altogether, women who became nurses did not necessarily identify with these politics. And while many recognized the important contribution made by these groups in treating the millions of victims of the war, the tensions between the central government (as well as the military) and the civilians providing aid continued to exist throughout the war.[20] These conflicts presented some of the most significant problems in service provision, which required a vast effort derived from many diverse and competing elements of society that were nearly impossible to coordinate in a unified way.

Regardless of its intentions, the tsarist government's efforts to maintain central control would prove impossible, and ultimately it would not be able to retain dominion over the provision of medical services. In fact, it would become heavily reliant on the assistance provided by local and civilian agencies in order to administer to soldiers, their families, refugees, and others affected by the hostilities. The services provided by these groups were so essential for the war effort that when the Union of Towns, dissatisfied by being relegated to secondary status, demanded it be considered a full-fledged Red Cross organization, providing it with all of the rights given to the Red Cross, this was granted without hesitation. This included funding from the government treasury, free use of the railway system, the right to use the sign of the Red Cross, and all other privileges enjoyed by the organizations of the Red Cross.[21] As the front lines shifted constantly, it became readily apparent that this division of front and rear spheres of activity was not only impractical but also detrimental to the war effort. Indeed, it became virtually impossible to distinguish between the "front" and the "rear." To compensate, the Zemgor unions were given permission to expand their activities to the battlefields, over the loud protests of the military authorities. Additionally, though somewhat reluctantly on the part of the tsarist administration, the Unions were also handed some functions that had previously been exclusively the purview of the Red Cross.[22]

The recognition of the necessity of civilian organizations, however, did not end their turbulent relations with the central government. As indicated above, the personnel of the local unions were notoriously anti-tsarist. Reciprocally, the leadership of the Military-Sanitary Administration remained fairly antagonistic toward these groups. According to John Hutchinson, one of the most hostile was the chief military-sanitary inspector, A. Ia. Evdokimov, who "continually maintained, in the face of mounting evidence to the contrary, that the army's medical staff could cope with all the eventualities and resisted not only the services offered by the newly created civilian organizations but even in some cases the help of the Russian Red Cross."[23] The result was significant mistrust, obfuscation, and even, at times, open hostility between agencies engaged in service provision. The women who became wartime nurses often were caught in the middle of these conflicts, or even active participants in them.

All of these problems indicate the significant challenges associated with mobilization of civilian populations required in total war. They were further complicated by, specifically with regard to administration of wartime nursing, serious hindrances based on issues of gender. Indeed, as indicated previously, wartime nursing was predicated on essentialist notions about female nature, which associated women with caring and nurturing. Concomitantly, contemporary notions of femininity and female sexuality were causes of great concern, especially when placed into the male context of the theater of war. As a result, Russian authorities, and society in general, held sisters of mercy to narrowly conceived expectations of behavior and action. These strictures often served to constrain the ability of the medical authorities to make efficacious use of women in wartime nursing service. They also limited the activities of the women themselves, often in ways that prevented them from effective provision of care. Furthermore, these ideas also shaped the views of the professionals who provided the impetus for the growth of civil society and directed the civilian efforts in the provision of medical services during the war as part of the Zemgor organizations. As scholars such as Laura Engelstein have demonstrated, Russian liberalism was founded on distinctly gendered conceptions of the public sphere and public roles. Thus, while Russian liberals demanded greater autonomy of activity and participation for men in the public sphere in making decisions about the way the state and society would be governed and structured, and greater authority of male professionals in determining the rules that dictated social control, they explicitly excluded women from their demands, conforming to a gendered division of public and private that relegated women to the domestic sphere and deemed them incapable of independent action free of male custodianship.[24] Indeed, as historians Choi Chatterjee and Karen Petrone have argued, most Russian liberal men refused to see women as "self-actuating civic subjects."[25] In particular, by continuing to apply essentialist concepts of femininity and imposing rigid sexual moral standards on women, both the state and those who controlled the burgeoning civil society worked to restrict women's actions and their abilities to contribute to the war effort effectively.

WARTIME NURSING IN THE GREAT WAR: RECRUITMENT, TRAINING, ORGANIZATION, ADMINISTRATION

As soon as the war began, the Russian Red Cross appealed to all of the existing sisters of mercy in the empire to enter war service. Yet the number of trained nurses who enlisted was severely insufficient to meet the medical needs created by the war, despite the steps that had been taken to increase the numbers of sisters of mercy prior to the war. The extensive scale of the hostilities, in which millions of soldiers and civilians would require medical attention, soon made clear that those efforts had been significantly insufficient. Because the war necessitated a dramatic increase in female personnel, the Russian Red Cross began immediate efforts to train more female nurses. Beginning in September 1914 the Red Cross established shortened training courses lasting two months.[26]

By the end of that year, the Red Cross had created 150 schools with ten thousand students in attendance. There were also practical courses for nurses set up in eighty hospitals, twelve ambulatory units, and ten pharmacies run by the Red Cross.[27] As a result of these efforts, by 1917 the number of sisters of mercy serving in various medical facilities around the country had reached more than thirty thousand.[28]

Despite shortages, the Red Cross insisted that not all women could become sisters of mercy. Enlistment was limited to literate women with at least some secondary education, and assignment to medical services required formal training conducted by the local communities of the Red Cross, or at least in facilities that operated according to established Red Cross standards. Fearful of assigning to service women without sufficient training and experience, the administration of the Russian Red Cross ruled that only women who had completed training conducted by the official *obshchiny* of the Red Cross could bear the designation "sister of mercy" and wear the uniform with Red Cross insignia. Furthermore, only these individuals were given the right to receive compensation from the organization for their work.[29] Women who did not meet these criteria were accepted as voluntary aids until they could complete officially sanctioned medical training. The training of sisters of mercy was supposed to be rigorous, focusing on both the theoretical and practical aspects of medical service. Students attended a series of lectures by local doctors and specialists, studied anatomy and physiology, and were required to successfully pass examinations in these subjects prior to being allowed to continue with the practical lessons, working on patients in local medical facilities. The coursework and examinations were sufficiently difficult, particularly those in anatomy, that many of the women who enrolled in courses were unable to complete them.

In addition to their medical training, sisters of mercy of the Russian Red Cross were held to very high standards of conduct, based on conceptions of "appropriate" female behavior. As detailed in the previous chapter, since the time of the Crimean War the deportment of Russian nurses had been of primary concern to both military and civilian authorities alike. According to the rules of conduct devised by the Red Cross, all Russian sisters of mercy were supposed to be of the "highest moral caliber" and possess "internal spiritual purity."[30] From the inception of the original Order of the Exaltation of the Cross, a standard of propriety had been set in an attempt to prevent sexual interaction between male military or medical personnel and sisters of mercy. Indeed, in some cases, this seemed to be a higher priority than quality of medical care. Red Cross authorities closely scrutinized the women who enlisted in its nursing communities and training courses. Women who did not adhere to these standards of propriety risked expulsion from the *obshchiny*.

Prior to being conferred with the honorific "sister of mercy" and being sent to perform medical service, newly trained wartime nurses had to undergo close inspection by Red Cross authorities. This was usually conducted by the "trustee" of the *obshchina*, usually a noblewoman who performed the roles of both patroness and supervisor of the community, and who was ultimately responsible for the conduct of the women in its ranks. Trustees often required enlistees to undergo "tests" of their character and behavior. Sister of mercy Tat'iana Varnek detailed how the Baroness Ikskul', the trustee of the Kaufman *obshchina*, invited a number of the volunteers to tea, having instructed the new recruits to wear their civilian clothing rather than their nursing uniforms. Those she deemed "too cheeky" or insufficiently modest in their dress, or who used cosmetics or other beauty products, were asked to leave the community. For the remainder of the women in the *obshchina*, Varnek asserted, merely the news of this tea was enough to ensure that the baroness did not have to repeat the exercise.[31]

After completing training, sisters could be assigned to a variety of different kinds of medical facilities and establishments. The Red Cross and its subordinate organizations, as well as the Russian military, all operated hospitals located in the rear, field, and permanent hospitals along the front; hospital and sanitary trains used to both treat and transport wounded and ill soldiers from the forward positions to the interior; and a number of mobile units, including field infirmaries, dressing and feeding stations, and *letuchky* (flying columns). Nurses could also be assigned to military hospitals of both the Russian army and navy. Undergoing training in courses overseen by a specific agency did not necessarily mean that nurses would be assigned to medical facilities operated by the same organization. Nurses were supposed to be sent where the greatest need for their services existed. However, this did not always occur for a variety of reasons, ranging from inefficient and uncoordinated organization to sisters' own initiatives to control the place and type of service to which they were assigned.

Officially, female medical personnel of the Russian Red Cross and other organizations providing medical service were supposed to remain three to four miles from the actual fighting. This included not only sisters of mercy but also women doctors, whose presence in frontline units was considered "undesirable" and, therefore, was supposed to be restricted to relieving male doctors in rear hospitals when the latter were sent to the forward positions.[32] Instead, male orderlies and medical students were originally designated to staff medical units that operated near and on the battlefields. Such procedural regulations were completely impractical, however, considering the rapidity with which the front lines moved and the great need for medical personnel at the front. These policies were quickly abandoned in the early months of the war when it became clear that it would be impossible for frontline units, even *letuchky,* to function without the presence of female medical personnel in their ranks. As a result, most *letuchky* were staffed with between two and four nurses, as well as two medical students or feldshers, one doctor, and twenty-five to thirty medics or orderlies. At least initially, medical and military authorities preferred to send "staff" sisters of mercy, that is, those who had received the longer prewar training and were permanent members of nursing communities prior to the outbreak of the conflict, to serve in frontline medical units. This, too, would be impossible to maintain, and many wartime sisters also went to the front as part of the mobile medical facilities and transports that were vital to the Russian war machine.

Sisters of mercy and volunteer nurses were assigned not only to medical units for the treatment of wounded soldiers at the front and in the rear. They also served in feeding stations and mobile infirmaries established along the front, as well as civilian hospitals and infectious and contagious disease facilities located in the rear. Many of these catered to the civilian population, which suffered from hunger and illness as a result of the war. Sometimes civilians were even wounded by cross fire when their villages and lands were turned into battlegrounds between enemy forces. The dislocations caused by the war created millions of refugees, and the Red Cross and Zemgor agencies undertook the tremendous task of attempting to care for these civilians in the wake of a near complete breakdown of public health.

Russian medical services continued to be plagued by deficiencies of personnel despite the efforts to increase the number of trained nurses. Although the initial response to the call for volunteer medical workers was so overwhelming that many women had to be turned away,[33] official sources continue to complain about shortages throughout the war. Many volunteers were rejected because of insufficient education, failure to successfully complete nursing courses, or "political unreliability,"[34] rather than overabundance of personnel. It was only toward the end of Russia's participation in the war effort (in the summer of 1917) that the reduction of female medical personnel at the front could even be considered, and even then, the idea was to shift their service from care of wounded soldiers to treatment of the millions of civilians infected with epidemic diseases.[35] Indeed, if there is one thing that most accounts of the medical services during the war agree upon, it is that Russia suffered from chronic understaffing of treatment facilities, especially at the front. Shortages were at least partially a result of the time it took to train personnel and transport them from the interior to medical establishments in the war zone. Further complicating the difficulties was the rapidity with which troops and sites of battle moved. In many instances, nurses arrived at field hospitals and other frontline medical units only after the most critical need had passed.

In an attempt to meet the demand for medical personnel, the Red Cross eventually shortened the term of nursing courses to six weeks. Yet even this proved insufficient, and nursing training courses continued to be established around the country throughout the war in attempt to fill the need for sisters of mercy. Moreover, the central administration of the Russian Red Cross found it difficult to control the process of preparing new wartime nurses. The supervisor of medical units on the northern front, Dr. S. K. Solov'ev, commented that training courses "grew up like mushrooms" around the country, but that many were unofficial in nature and that it was often difficult to ascertain whether the women were receiving appropriate medical instruction.[36] Although the Red Cross insisted training be conducted through its *obshchiny,* this was not always possible. In order to distinguish between nurses who had completed the abridged two-month or six-week courses from those who had gone through the longer (usually no less than one year) regular prewar training, the organization applied separate designations. The latter were referred to as "staff sisters" or "reserve sisters," depending on whether they were assigned to active duty or placed in reserve medical units, while the former were termed "wartime sisters," a distinction that also included different pay scales.[37] "Staff" sisters were to be paid thirty-five to forty rubles a month, and they received room and board, including allowances for meals in the officers' mess, from their local Red Cross administration.[38] Sisters of mercy of wartime designation were to receive thirty rubles per month, as well as room and board, again with meals equal to those to which officers were entitled. This was also extended to wartime nurses who were assigned to service in naval facilities, as decreed by the tsar in October 1914, with their compensation set at thirty rubles per month.[39] Solov'ev insisted that this pay inequity was entirely unjust, as those who completed the shorter wartime training courses became just as indispensable to the provision of medical service as the permanent staff nurses and performed equally well in their duties.[40] In September 1915 the pay for sisters of mercy of the Russian Red Cross serving on the northern front was increased to fifty rubles.[41] By 1917 the inequities were addressed by granting all nurses who had been serving in the war for at least one year continuously a stipend of seventy-five rubles a month.[42]

Not only did inequities exist with regard to distinctions between types of nurses, but they also cut across the various agencies providing medical services. Nurses working for the Zemgor establishments were sometimes compensated at higher rates than their counterparts who served through the auspices of the nursing communities of the Red Cross and in military facilities. The Union of Towns, from the very outbreak of war in 1914, paid its nurses fifty rubles per month and allotted them an additional hundred rubles for expenses (a one-time payment made on their assignment to wartime service). The same year, the Union of Zemstvos designated remuneration for nursing personnel serving in its medical facilities at forty rubles a month. Sisters serving on hospital trains run by either organization received a monthly income of fifty rubles, and they were given an additional fifteen rubles for housing if they did not receive accommodations as part of their service.[43]

NURSES IN WARTIME SERVICE

After being mobilized, trained, and dispatched into service, wartime nurses were assigned to work in medical facilities either at the front or in the rear. While many of the facilities in the rear were civilian-run, those located in the war zone were military medical entities. In joining the staff of such units, Russian sisters of mercy were supposed to submit to the regulations established by the Ministry of War in 1871. These had not been updated in the forty-year period leading up to World War I and were republished unchanged in 1914. These rules indicated that nurses serving in military medical facilities operated under the authority of the command personnel of those establishments, as well as the senior staff sister of the facility, who was responsible for all lower-ranked nurses therein. All sisters were subordinate to doctors, but head nurses were given considerable authority, despite the reservations expressed by critics of female nursing. In addition to assisting doctors with medical treatment of patients, they were also expected to supervise the work of all of the junior nurses, feldshers, and orderlies; oversee the preparation of food in hospital kitchens; ensure the unit was sufficiently equipped and supplied; and maintain order in the facility, making certain all the rules and regulations were followed by all medical personnel.[44]

Junior nurses were also ascribed a variety of tasks as members of military medical facilities. They were, according to doctors' orders, to distribute medicine to patients; apply hot mustard plasters, cold compresses, and poultices; and clean and redress wounds. They had to ensure that bed linens were clean and changed on a regular basis, paying particular attention to those of patients with wound leakage. When patients had visitors, nurses were supposed to make sure they did not pass any contraband material, or anything not approved by the doctors, to the ill or wounded men. Sisters of mercy were also responsible for ensuring patients were fed, which included quality control over the food served to them and sometimes even preparation of meals. They also had to carefully supervise the distribution of alcohol among patients (wine and other spirits were often prescribed by doctors as part of medical treatments). Additionally, nurses were charged with regulating the temperature of the wards, keeping them free of noxious odors, and ensuring that the air inside was fresh. At night, they were to make sure the corridors were well lit and oversee the work of night caretakers, keeping a close watch on patients who were particularly serious cases or whose conditions were in danger of deterioration.[45] These, of course, were idealistic requirements. In reality, faced with constant scarcity of everything from supplies to personnel, as well as heavy flows of patients that often lasted for days on end, the facilities often found such demands difficult to meet, especially in locations very close to the fighting.

Treating the millions of wounded and ill soldiers and civilians affected by the war proved a severely daunting task, fraught with difficulties both at the front and in the rear. Supply, distribution, transportation, and other logistical difficulties were further complicated by troubled interactions with both military and civilian authorities. Despite the severe shortages of personnel and the inability of the army to provide medical services without the assistance of organizations such as the Red Cross and the

Zemgor Unions, the military authorities had difficulty accepting the presence of civilian organizations in the war zone. Such reluctance was not completely unfounded; these entities were not without their shortcomings and problems. The Russian Red Cross in particular had been unable to shed the poor reputation it had earned in some circles prior to this conflict, often remaining associated with corruption, ineptitude, and acting to curry political favor instead of concentrating on providing badly needed medical service to the Russian population. Dr. Solov'ev expressed this view in a lengthy report to the general commissioner of the Red Cross, echoing the ideas expressed by other officials and observers of the organization's activities. By the last year of the conflict, Solov'ev, along with other military medical officials, had come to regard the Russian Red Cross as a "weak entity" that had "lost its constructive energy" after an initial outburst of action early in the war. He accused the organization of preferring to "rest on undeserved laurels" rather than undertaking responsible action to help the army with its medical needs. The doctor further complained that the organization lacked any ability to adapt new planning strategies once its original plans had proved inadequate for the task of caring for millions of wounded and ill soldiers.[46] The overly bureaucratic nature of the Russian Red Cross beleaguered the organization and meant that the smallest actions required permission from some higher authority. Such approval was often painstakingly long in coming, preventing medical personnel from carrying out important actions when immediately necessary. Other times, the higher authorities of the Russian Red Cross passed responsibility between themselves so many times that orders were never relayed to lower entities awaiting vitally important permission.[47]

A myriad of other serious problems hindered the organization's ability to provide medical services from the outset. At the beginning of the war, the Red Cross had very few frontline units. Military commanders were often reluctant to send nonmilitary organizations and personnel into the war zone. Without sufficient numbers of Red Cross units at or near the front, and with the Red Cross, at least initially, being the only nonmilitary organization allowed to cross the line of demarcation, even other groups equipped to offer medical support for the army found themselves unable to extend that aid until they received permission to enter the war zone. This also made it difficult to transport wounded men from the front to medical facilities behind the lines. This problem was complicated by the fact that many of the mobile medical units were only able to perform cursory triage and provide temporary care for wounded and ill soldiers and civilians. According to the medical war plans, this was the sole purpose of such units. Patients who needed further care were to be transported to interior medical facilities, more permanent and extensive establishments in the rear, to get further treatment and to recover. Yet this was often impossible, as advances and retreats of troops often cut off these mobile units from roads and railways, forcing them to hold patients much longer, even though they were ill equipped to handle their treatment. Weeks would often go by before the wounded could be evacuated to necessary facilities. Other times, mobile medical units were unable to get to casualties, who often remained on the battlefields during prolonged attacks. Visiting the front, Mikhail Rodzianko, president of the Duma, was appalled by "the highly unsatisfactory state of the medical transport service." At the Warsaw-Vienna railway station, he encountered thousands of wounded men on the platform in the rain receiving little to no medical attention, some with wounds that had remained undressed for five days.[48] Kseniia Iur'eva, a nurse in a mobile hospital stationed near Dvinsk, was appalled to learn that one of her patients, a soldier named Ivan, needed both of his legs amputated after five days of lying in the snow where he had fallen wounded on the battlefield.[49] Moreover, getting the wounded from the battlefields to medical facilities even at the front was problematic. Doctors and other medical authorities were loath to send their personnel into combat zones during periods of intense activity for fear that they would lose them to enemy fire. The members of sister Lidiia Zakharova's mobile hospital unit were extremely unhappy that heavy enemy fire prevented them from going to retrieve wounded soldiers from a riverbank where a battle was taking place. "Sitting here, as if we have no hands, when there it is necessary to help!" one of the young medics exclaimed.[50]

The Red Cross encountered further difficulties in distributing services evenly and getting nursing personnel to where they were needed most. Medical personnel complained that they were idle for significant periods of time during the war. Sister of mercy Sofia Bocharskaia spoke about being without work for weeks on end at the hospital near Warsaw to which she was assigned. "We sat about, cold and idle, and felt that once more the war had escaped us," she lamented.[51] Tat'iana Varnek echoed these sentiments, finding her unit, a mobile field hospital, constantly transferred from one location to another, but only occasionally ending up assigned to a place where great need for medical care existed.[52]

Rodzianko corroborated this, reporting that on visiting one Red Cross hospital he "found six doctors and about thirty nurses doing nothing." When he asked the chief of the army medical department, General Danilov, to put them to work in providing care for the unattended wounded he had encountered, Danilov said he was unable to do so because they were to be assigned to hospital trains that had not yet completed formation.[53] In November 1914 General Danilov urgently telegraphed Prince Ol'denburgskii, the head of the Red Cross, about the incomplete staffing of hospital trains in Warsaw. Although the prince had ordered a hundred sisters of mercy to be dispatched to that city to provide medical personnel for hospital trains there, by November 19, 1914, only one small party of eighteen nurses had been sent.[54] In other instances, nurses desiring to work in certain areas applied to local medical establishments only to be turned away because there was no work for them.

At least partially to blame for this problem was the procedure by which sisters of mercy were assigned and sent to medical units. The establishment of reserves of medical personnel for each front was supposed to facilitate this process by creating a pool of available nurses ready for dispatch to the medical units that needed them, which often proved to be extremely cumbersome and inefficient. The case of the northern front illustrates this well. There, when front authorities (either military or medical) received a request for the assignment of nurses to a particular medical facility, they would send the request to the reserves, located in Petrograd, where medical personnel were supposed to be located, awaiting their orders. But if no nurses were available in the reserves, as was often the case, it was necessary to redirect the request to the main administration of the Red Cross, which would then send it on to the nearest communities of sisters of mercy. Once nursing personnel was located in the communities, they had to be sent to the reserves in Petrograd first, and only then could they be dispatched to the unit that made the initial request. The result was an inordinate length of time to complete all of the communications, the appropriate paperwork, and the actual transportation of the nurses. This proved to be a significance hindrance in getting nurses to where they were most needed, when they were most needed, during the heat of battle. Many arrived only after the greatest demand had passed. In an attempt to remedy this, another reserve of medical personnel was established in Pskov, but this did not occur until October 1916.[55]

Complicating matters further were interagency conflicts. The Red Cross and the army medical services clashed over assignment of nursing personnel to medical units. There seems to have been some considerable confusion regarding where the ultimate authority over the appointment of sisters rested. Army doctors in command of medical facilities at the front often believed that their approval was necessary to assign nurses to and release them from service in their units. The main administration of the Red Cross, however, insisted this authority lay within the purview of its officials, specifically within the *obshchiny.* Indeed, there were conflicting statutes on this specific issue. Red Cross regulations indicated that this authority was within the rights of the trustees who headed the nursing communities. But Regulation No. 181, issued by the supreme head of the Sanitary and Evacuation Section, stated that medical personnel could not be reassigned without the approval of the military commander of the medical facilities. The Red Cross insisted that its rules took precedence, while the military authorities believed their authority at the front was superior to all others.[56]

Insufficient financial and material resources also significantly hampered effective service provision. Material support for medical units was highly uneven. While some units and facilities with wealthy or well-connected benefactors were extremely well equipped and well staffed, others were deficient in necessities such as medical instruments and equipment, medicines, and other basic materials, even thermometers, as well as suffered from shortages of essential personnel. Thus, even when wounded and ill soldiers eventually made it to medical facilities for treatment, the conditions were often not much better than they had been in temporary frontline units. Philosopher Fedor Stepun, who enlisted in the army in 1914 and served as a junior officer in an artillery battery, remarked that one field hospital he visited was a terrible sight, with rain- and blood-soaked men lying unattended on stretchers or directly on the dirt floor because of the insufficiency of cots and shortage of medical personnel.[57] With insufficient funding, it was sometimes impossible to remedy these problems. Although the Russian Red Cross enjoyed patronage at the highest levels of Russian imperial society, this did not always translate into sufficient, or at least consistently reliable, financial support. The administration of the organization was bombarded with thousands of complaints of lack of funds and resources and repeatedly asked to supplement budgets of local Red Cross organs and medical facilities. The organization was not always able to fulfill such requests. General Volkov, heading the Red Cross units in Warsaw, repeatedly asked for funding through the months of October and November 1914 but was turned down on November 31, informed that the Red Cross coffers in Petrograd were empty.[58] The very next day, however, this decision was reversed, and the main administration of the Red Cross sent two hundred thousand rubles to Volkov's adjutant.[59] But by the end of December, Volkov was once again out of money and requested an additional three hundred thousand rubles from the main administration.[60]

In comparison with the wartime medical services of other belligerents, the Russian Red Cross sometimes seems significantly less advanced. For example, American facilities operated by the American Red Cross in France were equipped with medical technologies and modern equipment such as X-ray machines. Very few Russian units had these. Even more distressing in terms of meeting the needs of medical provision and saving lives was the lack of antitetanic serum, resulting in many deaths from tetanus developed from wounds.[61] Other vitally important items were also in constant short supply on the eastern front. Chloroform was only haphazardly available, forcing patients to undergo surgeries without anesthetic. Thermometers were constantly on back order as a result of a shortage of mercury. Even gauze bandages were sometimes hard to locate, especially in mobile frontline units, where medical personnel were required to substitute paper and dirty cloth to dress wounds.

The Red Cross was responsible for treating not only wounded soldiers but also those who became ill during the war, both military and civilian personnel. In particular, the campaign to stop the spread of epidemic diseases, which swept through the country on the outbreak of war, became increasingly important as the war dragged on. By early 1915 the organization had made this effort a central focus. However, many doubted its ability to effectively combat infectious disease and viewed it as a task too daunting for the poorly prepared Red Cross to undertake successfully. "The new function of the Red Cross is the battle against cholera," V. Potakhin wrote from the front to his wife in Petrograd, on January 3, 1915. "I consider this to be a big mistake, as the Red Cross appears to be completely incapable of undertaking such activities and does not possess sufficient personnel and specialized methods."[62]

Corruption was also an obstacle to sufficient funding and supply of medical units. Sofia Bocharskaia, serving in an infectious diseases hospital near Warsaw, found the institution in a state of neglect and disrepair and the patients in similarly poor condition. The hospital was suffering from an almost complete lack of equipment, deprived of even the most basic medical supplies such as thermometers and syringes. She attributed the hospital's state directly to rampant corruption. The chief doctor embezzled much of the money allocated to the hospital by the Red Cross. What supplies, food, and medicine the hospital did receive were then usually pilfered by the orderlies and much of them sold on the black market. They even stole the personal effects of the soldiers. Little had been done to stem these thefts.[63] Ivan Semin's experiences, detailed in the vignette that opens this chapter, echo these difficulties.[64]

The lack of a professionalized nursing corps with large numbers of personnel in the prewar period contributed to these problems. Wartime nurses were often sent into service with insufficient medical training. Despite the best efforts to ensure that instruction was comprehensive and rigorous, in reality many of the shortened medical courses acquainted women with only the most basic knowledge of human anatomy and cursory skills in medical treatment. Often women arrived at the front with little more than the ability to bandage wounds, which meant that they had to learn on the job, under conditions of tremendous pressure and haste. Sofia Bocharskaia recalled how she was assigned to assist with a major operation immediately after arriving at the hospital to which she was assigned, despite the fact that she had no experience with surgery whatsoever. The senior doctor insisted, however, as there were no experienced nurses on staff. He gave her the responsibility of administering anesthesia to the patient. Somehow, her lack of knowledge in this area of medical treatment did not hinder her and she claimed that she was able to carry out the task successfully. The feel of the patient's pulse steadied her through the procedure. "Far away inside me was a girl, frightened at the responsibility that had been given her," she recalled, "but she seemed small and vague, and I felt about me the movement of quick, decisive work, keeping time with the throb of the soldier's life beating his pulse."[65]

This problem of inadequate medical training was not unique to female medical personnel. In general, imperial Russia suffered from a shortage of qualified medical practitioners, even before the outbreak of the war.[66] Doctors were drafted into military service, but the insufficient numbers of trained physicians at the time the war began was a problem that persisted through the war. Young men fresh out of medical school with very limited, if any, practical experience were sent to the front as soon as the ink on their diplomas was dry. Very few, if any, had experience with military medicine. The acute shortage of surgeons meant that doctors with any surgical experience at all were assigned to operating theaters—even gynecologists, who had never performed surgery on men, let alone men wounded by modern weapons.[67]

At times, provision of medical service, particularly in the treatment of wounded soldiers, was hampered by the attitudes and actions of the troops themselves. Peasant soldiers were sometimes suspicious of modern medical techniques and treatments. They were accustomed to folk healing and natural remedies rather than scientific Western medicine. One soldier, Stepan Semenchikov, was brought into nurse Lidiia Zakharova's mobile medical unit with a terrible stomach wound that had pierced a number of his internal organs. He begged the attending physician to administer some kind of miracle powder that an old "wise" man from the nearby village had told his comrades about, which he believed would heal him. When the doctor refused, disclaiming the existence of any such substance, and ordered the soldier to remain in the field hospital for treatment, the two engaged in a heated argument. The soldier finally submitted, at least temporarily, to the doctor's demands, but when Zakharova went over to attend to him, he whispered to her that he would flee at the first opportunity presented to him. This he did, after resting for a day in the field hospital, as soon as the guard posted at the entrance had dozed off.[68] In particular, soldiers often resisted amputation of limbs, which in most cases was carried out in order to save their lives when wounded extremities became infected. But for a man who survived on physical labor, the loss of a leg or an arm was perceived to be devastating, rendering him incapable of carrying out the necessary work to support his family and essentially turning him into a useless burden on his loved ones.

Conflict between military and civilian personnel similarly created difficulties in efficacious service provision, as did clashes between the personnel of these organizations and their own authorities. Perhaps most salient to these conflicts were mistrust and misunderstanding between military and civilian entities. Military medical authorities, unsurprisingly, held certain fairly rigid expectations about the conduct of all personnel, civilian and military, placed under their command. But civilian personnel often had little conception of what life as part of military medical units at the front actually entailed. There was also conflict between the Red Cross and the military medical establishment, as well as with the other organizations carrying out medical service during the war. The turbulence at the highest levels of administration between the various organizations charged with provision of medical services has been demonstrated by scholars, as have problems with local government organizations subordinate to the Red Cross (the Zemgor facilities and units). Although some maintain that Red Cross and army medical personnel operating at the front had a "fairly good working relationship,"[69] a more careful look at the service of wartime sisters of mercy reveals that numerous misunderstandings and conflicts between the Red Cross, its personnel, and the military occurred, both at the main administrative levels and among frontline personnel. The thousands of individuals who served as medical personnel (both military and civilian) during the war were not at all in consensus about how to best minister to the health care needs of a country in crisis. More specifically, the women who became nurses did not always fall in line with official efforts and sometimes clashed with both Red Cross and military authorities, both of which were male dominated and had rigid expectations of conformity on the part of female personnel. This was particularly the case with head and senior nurses in their relations with doctors. While these women sought agency in their contributions to the war effort, officials did not welcome this kind of initiative and expressed anxiety when women stepped outside of the boundaries established for their behaviors. Indeed, both the Red Cross and the military authorities were often bound by notions of appropriate female behavior and highly concerned with the conduct of sisters of mercy, which at times seemed to take precedence over service provision. Simultaneously, many women who became nurses found it difficult or were unwilling to adhere to the demands of wartime medical service, particularly requirements of martial life and discipline.[70]

Conflicts between nurses and male medical personnel often stemmed from misunderstanding and mistrust on both sides. A number of male military medical personnel expected female civilian nursing personnel to act in accordance with military discipline and organization, while many female medical personal had unrealistic understandings of the way military medical facilities operated. As volunteers and civilians, many sisters of mercy held very different views about their service. They often insisted that they should have choice in their place and type of service. Some even believed that as civilians, despite the fact that they were assigned to military medical units, they operated outside the purview of martial authority. But male military personnel argued that all civilians, once assigned to military medical facilities, were required to accept the dictates of military life, including following orders without question. Indeed, one of the most common complaints from military medical authorities was that the sisters of mercy assigned to their medical facilities did not act in a sufficient "military" manner. Medical officials held (rather unrealistic) expectations that all personnel assigned to their command would operate according to the standards of military discipline and behavior. One should not be surprised, however, that many nurses did not adhere to such standards. These women were civilians, most of whom had never carried out any kind of state service, let alone been part of rigid institutions such as the military. Even those who came from the ranks of the staff sisters of the communities of the Red Cross were members of a civilian charitable organization. As such, they would have no familiarity with the rules of military life, nor would they enter into medical service with any idea that this would be expected of them.

The records of wartime nursing service reveal the repercussions of such failed expectations. Both the Red Cross and the military medical establishment were particularly perturbed when nurses refused to follow orders. This becomes readily apparent through the numerous messages sent from military medical units, as well as from local communities of sisters of mercy, to the main administration of the Red Cross, complaining that nurses often refused assignments, dispatched themselves to locations of service that they personally desired, or left units to which they had been ordered, of their own volition.[71] Red Cross and military officials assessed the source of this problem as "based on an incorrect understanding of their primary responsibilities" on the part of numerous female nurses. For many women, the primary motivation for entering into medical service was to serve the wounded "heroes of the battlefield." They had little interest in catering to civilian populations. Moreover, as will be discussed in greater detail in chapter 8, associations with the rear became significantly negative over the course of the war, linked to corruption, vice, opportunism, and self-aggrandizement. Some nurses would agree to serve only if they could do so in frontline units. Indeed, this seems to have been one of the most prominent features of Russian wartime nursing, as reflected in both official records and the remembrances of Russian nurses. Sister Margarita Dzekhtsevich, for example, rejected her assignment to a rear medical unit and insisted on being sent to the front instead. When her demand was refused, she left her nursing community without permission and was thereby expelled from the ranks of the Red Cross.[72] Sisters Riumina and Ornatskaia both left the Kaufman *obshchina* without permission, after their requests to be sent to the front were denied. As a result, the two were expelled from its ranks, but they were still able to enter the Georgievskii *obshchina* and somehow managed to secure official orders for frontline assignment.[73] A similar problem existed with regard to nurses' leaves, whereby sisters often left active service without formal permission to do so.

In particular, some nurses were extremely reluctant to serve in infectious and epidemic disease facilities. Organization officials were flustered when sisters of mercy failed to report for duty in such establishments, instead insisting on being sent to field hospitals or other medical units at the front that treated wounded soldiers. A number of nurses who were assigned to these kinds of treatment facilities simply refused to go. Some even took matters into their own hands when their requests for transfer were not honored, either using connections to obtain transfers to frontline medical units serving the wounded or merely dispatching themselves to desired locations. The main administration of the Red Cross urged local and regional administrators to explain clearly to nursing personnel that they were "required to provide assistance not only to wounded soldiers, but also those ill with infectious diseases" and to insist that it was unacceptable for them to refuse to serve in the contagious disease and epidemiological units.[74] Indeed, a number of nurses assigned to these facilities expressed frustration that they would be unable to carry out the romantic ideal of serving the hero wounded in battle. Sister N. Chelakova recalled that she and her companions received the news that they would be assigned to an infectious disease hospital for the treatment of glanders (a highly contagious skin disease) as if it were a "tragedy" and cried bitterly for days. They did not refuse the assignment, as a result of their "strict discipline," according to Chelakova. Yet they were despondent from the moment they arrived at the hospital, feeling as if they were "missing the war" and the opportunity to be useful to the heroic soldiers, especially since at the time of their arrival, there were no patients in the facility.[75]

Such problems, however, were not merely the result of misunderstanding of duties on the part of the nurses themselves. The risk of infection among medical personnel who were exposed to contagions through such service was very high. The records of the Russian Red Cross contain numerous reports of nurses falling ill and even dying as a result of their contact with patients in these facilities. Chelakova and her comrades expressed significant fear of infection; her friend Anya wept inconsolably, crying that she was certain she was going to die of glanders.[76] Authorities did, however, recognize the significant challenges presented by working in infectious disease facilities and attempted to address the exceptionally difficult and dangerous conditions of this work. By 1916 the Red Cross increased the pay of sisters of mercy assigned to contagious disease units by an additional fifty rubles per month.[77] The pay increase, however, was not enough to motivate many women to serve in such units. The problem of nurses assigned to infectious disease units dispatching themselves to frontline units without authorization continued throughout the war period, presenting serious problems for the commanders of those units, who often had no idea what to do with these "rogue" sisters.

Another source of conflict between sisters of mercy and military officials stemmed from the fact that the Russian Red Cross had its own rules of conduct, assignment to service, and internal discipline for nursing personnel.[78] Nurses often believed that their own obligations were to observe these dictates, as members of a civilian organization, rather than military codes of conduct. Army doctors charged with overseeing staffs of Red Cross nurses were at a loss when female nursing personnel defied orders, argued with them over treatment practices, and overall, failed to adhere to the principles of martial life. The chief doctor of the Polotskii Mobile Field Hosptial No. 3, Dr. Bezpiatov, complained bitterly that two of the nurses assigned to his hospital were impossible to work with and requested that they be replaced immediately. Bezpiatov railed against sisters Tatiana Osipova and Anna Sirenova, who had opposed him, in his view, from the very first days of their service in the hospital and had not been "imbued with the necessary strict military discipline for service in a wartime hospital." The doctor had attempted to explain to the nurses that in the military hospital, "we are all soldiers," but he claimed that he was "constantly met with a whole stream of unintelligible objections, which was intolerable from the point of view of military discipline." When confronted by the doctor, the nurses apparently responded that they were "free people, not subordinates." He insisted that the sisters either would not or could not accept the idea that they were carrying out "military service during wartime" but instead demanded special treatment.[79]

Additionally, a number of women who enlisted as sisters of mercy seemed either unable or unwilling even to abide by the standards and regulations established for wartime nursing, let alone military regulations. Red Cross authorities often bemoaned the fact that some wartime nurses failed to comprehend the nature of their service or the expectations of appropriate conduct for sisters of mercy. When nurses acted outside the boundaries of permissible behavior, or were perceived as doing so, they soon ran afoul of accusations of misconduct and risked expulsion from the ranks of the Red Cross and removal of the title of "sister of mercy." The records of the Red Cross are filled with complaints from local communities of sisters and from military officials about the "improper behavior" of nursing and requesting that these women be expelled from the ranks of the Red Cross communities and stripped of the honorific "sister of mercy."[80] Aleksandra Bogdanova, of the Krestovozdvizhenskii Obshchina, was removed from the ranks for conducting herself in a manner "inconsistent with the title of sister of mercy."[81] Sister Tamara Verba was similarly removed from her nursing community for repeated acts of insubordination and other disciplinary infractions of the regulations of the Red Cross.[82] It is safe to assume that in at least some of these cases, the behavior in question was sexual in nature, considering the strong approbations of "high moral caliber" and "purity" that were emphasized in Red Cross nursing codes of conduct. While one can understand the desire to impose strict discipline in wartime nursing, expelling such women often resulted in depriving Russian medical services of badly needed personnel. Internal order and discipline were of the highest priority. Senior and head nurses were responsible for ensuring that sisters in their units performed their duties and adhered to behavioral regulations. When this did not happen, they too were subject to expulsion. For example, problems within the Vladivostok mobile field hospital were attributed to the poor leadership of the senior nurse in that unit, Princess Kropotkina. It seems her social status did little to protect her from criticism, including accusations that she was failing to set a good personal example for the nurses in her charge.[83]

Gendered expectations shaped service experience for women in wartime nursing in such a way that duties assigned to nurses often included labor outside the provision of medical services. Indeed, because they were women, sisters of mercy were often given tasks such as cleaning and food preparation. However, this was an unrealistic assumption on the part of men, since not all women came equipped with such skills. The reality of women's lives did not always include such domestication, which was particularly true of women from the elite of Russian society, whose households usually included servants who performed physical labors in the home such as food preparation and housekeeping. Moreover, nurses did not receive training in these tasks as part of the medical courses they completed prior to entering service. Solov'ev, who clearly shared the expectation that nurses, as women, *should* be assigned these tasks, complained that while many women from privileged backgrounds had received adequate medical training, they were often unable to perform more menial duties such as cleaning and cooking.[84]

Strict regulations applied even to nurses' dress, and failure to abide by these rules was considered a serious disciplinary infraction, often with significant repercussions. Not only was the nurse's sexual behavior to be "morally upright," but her very appearance was supposed to remove any suggestions of sexuality. The Red Cross uniform, an ankle-length nondescript grey or black cotton or wool dress covered by a long white apron embroidered with a red cross and a white or black head kerchief,[85] intentionally concealed the feminine physical characteristics of her body. The long dress and apron hid any suggestion of curves made by female breasts or hips, and the head scarf covered long hair. In fact, the dress of the Russian sister of mercy differed little from that of a nun. The uniform was intended as a symbol of the organization and the high standards imposed on its wearer, a symbol of prestige that gave the wearer considerable respect, as well as mobility in the public sphere, particularly the war zone, that civilian women did not possess. Therefore, it was essential for sisters of mercy to be properly dressed. Failure to abide by these regulations had serious consequences, including removal from the ranks. For instance, sister Maria Solov'eva was expelled from the Omsk *obshchina* for her refusal to wear the complete uniform of a sister of mercy.[86] A shortage of grey wool, however, complicated matters for women enlisted in Red Cross service by making it very difficult for sisters to acquire appropriate dress, which was seen as nurses' own responsibility.[87]

More often, however, issues concerning the nursing uniform concerned those not authorized to wear it, precisely because of the freedom of action it could afford its wearer. Of particular concern was that in a number of cities along the front, women who had no connection to the organization or medical services whatsoever had been found dressed in the uniforms of Red Cross sisters. Such women were often accused of engaging in prostitution. Regulations pertaining to the wearing of Red Cross uniforms proved insufficient to stem unauthorized occurrences, and thus the organization decided to take further measures, issuing special identification "tickets" to nursing personnel and requiring them to present these documents on demand to the authorities. The Red Cross also issued an order that restricted the wearing of nurses' uniforms to assigned work periods, ordering that "walking the streets or visiting entertainment establishments in the uniform of a sister of mercy is completely prohibited."[88] Despite these regulations, nurses often did appear in public wearing their uniforms. It was nearly impossible for them to avoid doing so when assigned tasks such as transporting wounded or ill soldiers to other medical facilities or securing supplies and materials from local warehouses or depositories. These regulations thus made it difficult for nurses to carry out their work without arousing suspicion and indicated that the uniform did not always provide them with unlimited mobility in the public sphere. As such, women's abilities to provide necessary services were curtailed, proscribed by impractical social conventions that continued to foreground women's sexual purity and value it above public needs. It was also indicative of a certain level of mistrust of women, who, unguarded in the male sphere, were likely engaging in immoral activity.

CONCLUSIONS

Khristina Semina continued to serve as a nurse throughout the war, providing valuable service to many ill and wounded in the process. She worked largely on her terms, however, deciding when and where she would serve. Her story is illustrative of a number of significant issues facing Russia in its attempts to mobilize and organize medical services. It represents a microcosm of many of the problems associated with making effective use of women as wartime nurses. Her husband's efforts to organize a medical transport unit were met with constant obstacles, from shortages of basic necessities to widespread corruption. Her own desire to become a wartime nurse was thwarted by notions of female weakness, further delimited by her class, and by gendered social expectations that elevated her duty to her husband above that to her country. At the same time, her status as a noble and a civilian allowed her to operate as a free agent, to come and go as she pleased, rather than submit to authority and serve where the need for nursing personnel was greatest. The comments of her relatives reveal anxieties and suspicions about the true motives of women entering wartime nursing service centered on self-aggrandizement and sexual promiscuity held by many in Russian society. In all, her story demonstrates the opportunities, ambiguities, and difficulties associated with the mobilization, organization, administration, and provision of service of wartime nursing.

The active roles played by women in the First World War made it impossible thereafter to consider engaging in large-scale military conflict without female participation. But this experience was fraught with obstacles and difficulties, thwarted in many instances by a central government that was highly suspicious of volunteer civilian efforts while simultaneously vitally dependent on such efforts. Clearly, the demands and strains of the war on the entire country were so great that it is difficult to imagine a successful prosecution. The accumulation, organization, and distribution of enormous quantities of human and material resources needed to allow an army of 15 million men to be fed, clothed, moved, and provided with medical care took the coordination and cooperation of multiple components of Russian society, not all of which were up to the task. Despite seemingly good intentions, the great variety of individuals and groups that contributed to the war effort often disagreed on how best to carry out such assistance and, at times, came into direct conflict with one another. In retaining expectations of female behavior that were not always compatible with the demands of war, authorities sometimes actually hindered women's ability to effectively perform medical service. Inability, or unwillingness, to conform to military standards on the part of women in wartime medical service similarly caused tensions and hampered efforts to tend to the nation's ill and wounded in the war zone.

The myriad of problems that the Russian empire faced in effectively organizing and administering medical services during the Great War are revealing of larger difficulties facing the country as a result of failures of the tsarist system to cope with the challenges of a changing, modernizing world. The successful prosecution of the war required the participation of both men and women, of all classes, in public roles, roles that many Russian authorities found difficult to accept but were forced to rely on as result of the exigencies of war. Even within the disruptive context of total war, many continued to hold strict expectations of behavior, especially for women, while simultaneously, women were being asked to perform functions that clearly would have been outside their purview in peacetime conditions. Many women themselves, however, were increasingly attempting to move beyond these confines, to find places in the public sphere, to contribute to national interests, and to shape and define those interests through their own agency. Yet, at the same time, many seemed unwilling to accept the necessary discipline and hierarchy required of military life when they were dispatched to frontline medical units.

3

CLASS AND SOCIAL STATUS IN RUSSIAN WARTIME NURSING

TAT'IANA ALEKSINSKAIA: SOCIALIST TURNED SISTER

At the time of the outbreak of the Great War, doctor Tat'iana Ivanovna Aleksinskaia (née Evtikheeva) was living with her husband in Paris. The latter had been exiled as a result of his radical political activities. Aleksinskaia was also a committed socialist who expressed reluctance about participating in an "imperialist war." At least initially unaffected by the patriotic fervor that led most socialists to abandon their antiwar stance, which precipitated the dissolution of the Third International, Aleksinskaia wondered, "'Could a Socialist—ought he—to take part in war?'" It was her husband who convinced her to go to Russia to serve the troops. "Throw yourself into the activities of the war," he urged. "Spend time with the men under arms, and you will find out if the war is accepted by them, and if they have the will to fight and to conquer."[1]

Despite the fact that Aleksinskaia held a degree in medicine from the Russian Women's Higher Medical Courses, which designated her as a "woman-doctor,"[2] she was assigned as a sister of mercy to serve in a mobile hospital train operated by the All-Russian Union of Zemstvos. The train had been organized in Moscow but was constantly on the move during the war. After leaving Moscow with all necessary medical equipment and staff, it was further supplied with rolling stock in a large town near the front. The train consisted of three dozen cars: wagons for the wounded, a third-class car that functioned as both a dressing station and a dining car, a kitchen car, a first-class car that served as accommodations for the hospital staff, a wagon that contained a linen press and a dirty linen compartment, and a car for the orderlies and stretcher bearers. Eight of its wagons were set up to accommodate lightly wounded men, while fourteen were used to treat the seriously wounded. Wounded officers were put in a second-class wagon, but soldiers were placed in *tepliushki* (freight cars fitted with beds and a wood-burning stove in the middle). The train's "base" was at Brest, but it constantly moved up and down the line, going as far south as Kiev and north to Petrograd, stopping at numerous points in between. Virtually self-sufficient, Aleksinskaia described it as a "town on wheels," but like any "little provincial town," not without its problems: "its petty business, petty concerns, and petty interests." The train acted, in her words, "like a huge pump. It goes up to the firing line, is loaded with casualties, goes away to pour them out into different Russian towns, and returns to the front to take away the stream of poor mutilated bodies."[3] She was placed in charge of six cars of seriously wounded soldiers and assigned a "nurse assistant" to aid her.

The medical staff of the hospital train included thirteen individuals, eleven of whom were women, including the chief surgeon. The remaining personnel consisted of orderlies and stretcher bearers from the army medical services. The vast majority were Russian German Mennonites who were exempt from combat service based on religious objections to the taking of human life but were still required by imperial law to serve in auxiliary capacities during the war. Aleksinskaia described her fellow staff members as mostly middle-class "Russian intellectuals" who sought to be useful to their country in its time of need. The chief surgeon, a forty-year-old divorcée who had served as a Zemstvo doctor before the war, was, in Aleksinskaia's estimation, a woman whose "energy is equal to that of any man." She had little patience, however, for flirtatious behavior among the younger staff members. "She keeps a keen eye on the sentimental propensities of the girls working in her train," Aleksinskaia commented, "and intervenes, sometimes very roughly, whenever she suspects a romance in the making. Every now and then she gives them an address, in which she violently attacks what she calls somewhat contemptuously 'the sexual instinct' and revolts against the 'weakness' of women." A number of the women had served as teachers and schoolmistresses and in other provincial professional positions. One who had served as a teacher in a country school had become "hard and embittered" as a result of her experiences. "She had tilled the soil of popular education under very disadvantageous conditions, among coarse and illiterate people, and hide-bound by the oppressive authority of the bureaucracy and the police." But Aleksinskaia noted she was not without compassion, and "when she is tending the wounded, the real depths of her soul are revealed, and through her usual tone of deliberate rudeness comes the glint of a kindly word, or a tender smile, with which she puts heart into the suffering men." Another schoolmistress had "spent half her life among the peasants, teaching their children, and now that they had become soldiers, she wanted to stay with them and to work among them."[4]

THE WOMEN OF RUSSIA'S WARTIME NURSING SERVICES

Although most of the medical personnel on Aleksinskaia's train came from Russia's middle ranks, the women who entered wartime medical services in Russia came from a variety of social backgrounds, ranging from the peasantry to the imperial family. This applied to both those who were called up for service because they had already received medical training or already were part of nursing communities and those who volunteered once the war began. The most famous sisters of mercy were the Empress Alexandra and her eldest daughters, Ol'ga and Tat'iana. On the outbreak of the war, the three women entered special training courses directed by the famous surgeon Prince V. I. Gedroits. They worked as sisters of mercy caring for the wounded in the hospital established on the grounds of the palace at Tsarkoe Selo. A wing of the Winter Palace in Saint Petersburg was also converted to a military hospital. Tsar Nicholas II's younger sister Ol'ga Aleksandrovna also enlisted in the Red Cross during the war. The grand duchess Maria Pavlovna, first cousin and goddaughter of the tsar (and sister of one of Rasputin's assassins), similarly went to the front to provide medical services as part of the Russian Red Cross.[5]

The women of the imperial family and aristocracy served as examples of appropriate wartime service for Russian womanhood and were meant to inspire further enlistment in the Red Cross. With this highly effective message, for women of Russian high society, as historian Richard Stites has indicated, wearing the uniform of the sister of mercy "became a veritable status symbol." The daughter of the British ambassador to Russia, Meriel Buchanan, who also offered her services to Russia despite her foreign citizenship, commented, "Even the 'spoilt beauties of the Smart Set' . . . abandoned the round of bridge, gossip and flirtation and went to work in hospitals."[6] Vanda Stepanova, a young noblewoman from the Lithuanian territory of Russia, commented that at the beginning of the war, "when patriotism was on the rise, being a nurse was considered very good. Almost all noblewomen and young ladies entered service to care for the wounded."[7] The names and photographs of grand duchesses, princesses, baronesses, and countesses who had entered nursing service filled the pages of contemporary periodicals. Many of the wives and daughters of prominent military and government officials also became sisters of mercy. The wife of Mikhail Rodzianko, a prominent member of the Duma, enlisted as a nurse. E. M. Bubnova, the daughter of the Russian naval minister, became a nurse in the first months of the war.[8] O. M. Russkaia, the daughter of the Russian commander of the southwestern front, received medical training and volunteered as a nurse.[9] Maria (Magdalena) Skrydlova, daughter of Admiral Skrydlov, commander of the Russian Baltic fleet, had trained as a staff nurse and served in a naval hospital during the war.[10] The wife of General Gurko, chief of Russian general staff, also entered nursing service and spent much of the war in dangerous frontline units.[11]

The female relatives of Russia's cultural elite offered their services. The youngest daughter of famed Russian writer Leo Tolstoy, Aleksandra L'vovna Tolstaia, volunteered to nurse the wounded. She was initially assigned to a hospital in the rear, but she found this work did not "satisfy" her and used her influence to secure placement at the front as part of an ambulance unit organized by the Union of Zemstvos.[12] The writer Aleksandr Kuprin established an infirmary in his home, and his wife and daughter served as nurses to the wounded men sent to recover there.[13] Other noteworthy personalities such as famous actresses, singers, dancers, artists, and writers also entered medical service during the war. Ballerina A. M. Bakashova became a volunteer nurse early in the war, as did star of the imperial Russian ballet, A. P. Domenshchikova, who served much of the war at the front.[14] Singer N. V. Plevitskaia also became a nurse and cared for the wounded in the forward positions.[15]

Noblewomen without titles or high-ranking relatives also became sisters of mercy during the war. Sofia Bocharskaia enlisted in the Red Cross when the war broke out, serving in several units on the Russian western front during the war.[16] As described in chapter 1, Tat'iana Varnek left her comfortable society life and joined the Red Cross. The Kaufman *obshchina* in particular was filled with women of the Russian elite, including Ksenia Ispolatova, the niece of the chairman of the main administration of the Russian Society of the Red Cross and member of the State Council, Aleksandr Aleksandrovish Il'in. Ispolatova became close friends with Varnek when they served together on the southwestern front.[17] Not all members of the nobility were keen to see their women enter medical service, as indicated by the reservations expressed by Khristina Semina's husband and family (detailed in the opening of chapter 2). Similarly, although Vanda Stepanova desperately wanted to enroll in nurses' training courses, as many of her girlfriends were doing, as soon as the war broke out, her parents forbade it. After the region was evacuated, however, she was separated from her family and used the opportunity to enter the medical courses and served in facilities near Riga attached to the Twelfth Army.[18]

The wives and daughters of professionals and merchants, as well as women who had careers of their own, including doctors, academics, schoolteachers, members of the intelligentsia, and even revolutionaries, entered the ranks of the various civilian organizations dedicated to caring for the wounded. As poet Nadezhda Iakusheva commented, "In virtually every educated family where the daughters did not have to work for a living, the girls volunteered in the hospitals."[19] Despite the large number of women from the educated middle class and gentry who enlisted as nurses, information about them is more difficult to locate than about the elite. Theirs were not the names that were reported in the wartime press, and theirs were not the pictures featured in contemporary periodicals. However, the records of the Red Cross and the other organizations that carried out medical services clearly reflect the presence of many women who lacked titles and well-known names. Women from the nonprivileged classes were also less likely to leave behind memoirs or other written records of their service. Undoubtedly, many lacked the free time necessary to devote to composing such a work, since often they were professionals and working women. Moreover, because the war was not celebrated in Soviet memory, for those who remained in Russia following the Bolshevik Revolution, there would be little if any opportunity for the publication of such works. Indeed, this proscription applied to many of the nurses of privileged backgrounds as well, and most of those who did record their experiences had emigrated from Russia. Exceptions include Aleksinskaia's memoirs and those of Lidiia Zakharova, a middle-class mother of two from Moscow, who left her children and comfortable life in order to join a mobile field hospital at the front. During the war she was recruited by a publisher who produced a series of works specifically devoted to the war titled *Velikaia Voina* (The Great War). These books were clearly part of a prowar effort on the part of the publisher.[20]

Examples of Great War nurses hailing from Russia's laboring classes are even more difficult to locate. The Red Cross requirement of literacy for enlistment severely limited the entrance of women from the laboring classes. Furthermore, working-class and peasant women undoubtedly found it more difficult to leave home, where they were vitally important for the economic survival of their families and communities, to become wartime nurses. Since nurses were accepted on a voluntary basis, rather than conscripted like soldiers, wartime service was more feasible for those who had the means to support themselves or, at least, were not essential providers of productive labor for their families. Nonetheless, there were some who did serve, such as peasant sister M. E. Nikolaeva, who was awarded a medal for her heroic service with the Red Cross in 1915.[21] More often, it seems, women of the lower classes who served in medical capacities during the war were "staff sisters," permanent members of the communities of the Russian Red Cross. Grand Duchess Maria Pavlovna served alongside a peasant woman who had been a sister of mercy in the Russian Red Cross for more than thirty years and was a veteran of the Russo-Turkish War.[22] The senior nurse of the unit to which Tat'iana Varnek was assigned was a woman named Bol'shakova whom she described as a "*baba*" (a term for a woman from the lower classes, usually a peasant). Bol'shakova was a staff sister from the Kaufman *obshchina* who had been a member of the community for many years and had much nursing experience.[23]

Although many nurses came from the educated sectors of Russian society, they were not necessarily from well-to-do backgrounds. In fact, the records indicate that many nurses were reliant on the income they received for survival, income that was often inadequate in the face of ever-increasing costs during the war period. The main administration of the Red Cross received thousands of requests directly from nurses, or indirectly from their communities or medical units, asking to be paid after they failed to received their wages for long periods of time, or for additional material support.[24] This belies the conventional notion of the Russian wartime nurse as "society-ladies-turned-sisters" prevalent in much of the literature.[25] Undoubtedly, the deficit of personal writings by women of the nonprivileged classes has skewed the representation. Examining the archival records reveals a different picture. Often, women were unable to purchase necessary items such as warm winter uniforms and outerwear, transportation (which was their responsibility, even when being sent officially to other locations to perform medical service), and sometimes even food. Moreover, sisters of mercy of the Russian Red

Cross were required to be members of the Red Cross *obshchiny*, and many of these demanded part of the nurses' pay for "upkeep" of the communities. At times, this meant that considerable portions of the nurses' wages went into the coffers of the *obshchiny* rather than their own pockets.[26] Moreover, the Red Cross and its subordinate organizations experienced chronic funding problems, which often affected their ability to dispense payment to nurses in a timely manner. Nurses were often unpaid for long periods, particularly when transferred to new locations, when on sick leave, after returning from enemy imprisonment, and sometimes seemingly out of sheer neglect or lack of funds. Such problems were not limited to Red Cross sisters. A number of requests for money for nurses assigned to Zemgor medical units, despite the expectation that the unions would provide such support for their personnel, indicate that insufficiencies in support of nursing personnel existed in those organizations as well.

Wartime nursing service also transcended ethnic and national differences. Nationality in imperial Russia was a complex issue. The empire was composed of approximately 170 different ethnic groups. Authorities applied the term "nationalities" to all of these groups, but they used different terminology to distinguish between ethnic Russians (*russkii*), who comprised less than half of the total population, and other subjects of the Russian empire (*rossiiskii*). This is problematic, because in English both terms are translated as "Russian"; thus, when referring to non-Russian nationalities, it is important to indicate whether these were nonethnic Russian subjects of the empire or citizens of other independent states. Russian wartime nursing included both of these types of non-Russian nationalities. Complicating things further, Russian authorities regarded certain groups in both categories with suspicion and often sought to limit their participation in wartime medical services.

Many members of national groups residing under Russian imperial control served in wartime medical services. One sister, perhaps overly optimistically echoing official rhetoric about internal imperial national cohesion, commented that the female staff of her field hospital "served (in miniature) to demonstrate the solidarity of all of the nations of the Russian Empire" with "3 Poles, 2 Lithuanians, 2 little Russians [Ukrainians], 2 Estonians, a Georgian, an Armenian, a Tatar, and a Jewess." She claimed that they were tolerant of one another, despite some mutual, gentle ribbing, particularly about religious difference. Her sense of the superiority of Russian ethnicity, particularly as defined by Russian

Orthodox, was revealed by her efforts to convince the Jewish nurse to accompany them to church on Sunday and her pride in the fact that one of the Estonians had asked to visit the Russian Orthodox Church and had "followed the entire service with great interest."[27]

There were even non-Russian citizens who were motivated to serve their adopted country in its time of crisis. Florence Farmborough, a young English woman working as a governess for a Russian family, immediately volunteered as a nurse in the Russian Red Cross rather than return to Great Britain to serve her own country.[28] Mary Britnieva, an Anglo-Russian with dual citizenship, served in a hospital unit with others from Bulgaria, Italy, England, and one of the Baltic states.[29] Violetta Thurstan, a professional English nurse, left home to serve with a Russian Red Cross flying column in Poland.[30] And as indicated above, Meriel Buchanan, daughter of the British ambassador, volunteered at the Saint George's Hospital in Petrograd, despite the fact that she had absolutely no medical training and barely spoke a word of Russian.[31] In addition, a number of women whose origins were not Russian sought to serve as sisters of mercy in the Russian medical services.

Despite the multifaith and multinational character of the Russian empire, not all inhabitants were considered reliable subjects. As a result, some of the women who enlisted or attempted to enlist in wartime medical services were regarded with considerable mistrust and even rejected. Concerns over women's loyalty were reflected in a number of ways in Russian society, particularly over women whose national heritages were those of Russia's enemies in the war. While women from the nations allied with Russia during the war, such as Great Britain and France, were usually accepted into the ranks of the Russian medical services without hesitation, those from non-Entente nations, especially those whose national backgrounds were those of Russia's opponents, presented more of a problem for the authorities. This was most obviously seen in the suspicion that arose with regard to the Empress Alexandra's German origins.[32] Her status as the wife of the tsar, however, provided her with the right to serve as a nurse in the Russian Red Cross. But women without such privileged connections were not generally trusted. Cases of women of Austrian, German, and Turkish origin were not generally trusted. Even those from Italy warranted careful consideration, despite that country's initial proclaimed neutrality. Until its entrance in the war on the Entente side in May 1915, Russians were wary of Italians as a result of Italy's previous alliance with Germany and Austria-Hungary. A similar situation existed with regard to Bulgaria, which did not enter the war on the side of the Central Powers until October 1915. Before that time, several Bulgarian women were allowed to enter the Russian Red Cross and receive the designation of "sister of mercy." There was no uniform procedure regarding such cases, however.[33] The organization's policy was to review each case of non-Russian citizens applying for acceptance as wartime nurses individually in order to determine whether the woman in question could be trusted. More often than not, those with origins from enemy nations were rejected. The case of Medarda Turbiazh, a woman of Austrian heritage from Galicia, is illustrative of such wariness. Turbiazh was a doctor who appealed to the Russian Red Cross to be allowed to enter wartime medical service. Her request was denied.[34] Women with national backgrounds outside the Russian empire, even if Russian born, sometimes came under scrutiny or were even rejected, indicating that being native to Russia was not sufficient for automatic acceptance into wartime service.

These kinds of policies indicate that the nature of women's position vis-à-vis the state in late imperial Russia was somewhat precarious and dependent on a number of factors that went into determining their citizenship.[35] For women, citizenship was, as historian Nancy Cott has demonstrated through her study of marriage and American women, "not a definitive either/or proposition—you are or you are not—but a compromisable one."[36] Scholar Maureen Healy suggests that this kind of interpretation is useful for understanding citizenship in the Habsburg empire of Austria-Hungary in the period of World War I[37]—a view that can be similarly applied to the Russian empire. Determination of acceptance into Russian medical service was often based on women's demonstration of significant loyalty to the Russian state, despite their foreign heritage. The criteria used to determine such loyalty included how long the individual had lived in Russia, the religion of the individual (especially if conversion to Orthodoxy had occurred), the Russian language skills of the individual, and close associations with Russians, particularly those of the elite. For example, the Saint George's community of sisters of mercy appealed to the main administration of the Red Cross asking permission to accept a Russian-born woman of Italian heritage named Glikeria Kochi into its ranks and to allow her to be given the designation of sister of mercy after she had successfully completed the training courses and passed the examinations in the community for nursing service. In its request, the community emphasized that Kochi was of Orthodox faith, having been born in Russia and lived her entire life in the country, never venturing abroad. Apparently, these conditions were sufficient to prove Kochi's loyalty, and the Red Cross granted the request.[38]

Thus, it was not just nationality that served as a litmus test of loyalty to the tsarist regime. Religion was also considered a central component of Russian citizenship and faithfulness (as articulated in the idea of official Russian nationality: Orthodoxy, Autocracy, and Nationality) and of service in the Russian Red Cross. While there was more religious diversity in the other organizations carrying out medical service during the war, such as the Union of Zemstvos and the Union of Towns, the Red Cross was more religiously homogenous as a result of its original Christian mission. From the inception of the original community of the Sisters of the Exaltation of the Cross, nurses were instructed to "constantly keep in mind the promise to dedicate all their strength to the spiritual service of the wounded and sick" and that "they must try to ease the suffering of the sick by Christian words and prayers,"[39] something that technically could only be carried out by Christians. Russia, however, was a multifaith state, and women of other religious backgrounds desired to serve as nurses during World War I. But Russian authorities were not always trusting of those who practiced other religions, even different forms of Christianity. The Russian Orthodox Church held rather negative views of other Christian beliefs: Catholicism was regarded as apostasy, and Protestant sects were seen as little better than cults. It did not help that these other forms of Christianity were closely associated with Russia's enemies during the war (Germany with Protestantism and Austria with Catholicism). These attitudes led to considerable mistrust of women who professed these faiths. They can be seen behind the expulsion of nurses from the ranks of the Red Cross, such as Paulina Paul'son, who was removed from duty as a sister of mercy for distributing Protestant biblical literature.[40] Such views, however, ultimately impeded the organization's ability to maximize the potential of female service.

Non-Christian women desiring to become nurses presented an even greater dilemma for Red Cross authorities. In particular, many Jewish women living within the empire desired to engage in medical service during the war. The issue of Jewish identity in Russia was further complicated by the fact that it was considered not only a religion but also a nationality. Although Jews living in the Russian empire were subjects of the tsar just as all other groups were, there was tremendous suspicious regarding their loyalty. Jews were also denied a number of rights and privileges in the empire and were subjected to discrimination and persecution by a tacitly anti-Semitic government and often an openly and violently anti-Semitic population. Although Jewish men were conscripted into the armed forces, they were not trusted. And according to regulations of the Red Cross, Jews could not serve in the overtly Christian organization, even as orderlies.[41]

Given the intense need for medical personnel during the Great War, however, the Russian Red Cross was forced to reevaluate this policy and began to make exceptions to the religious requirements. Early in the war the main administration of the Russian Red Cross approved the admittance of Jewish nursing personnel, but the provision designated that each application made by such Jewish applicants be individually reviewed and approved by the administration.[42] A number of these requests were approved, especially if the woman requesting designation as a sister of mercy already had substantial training and experience. The case of T. I. Deul', who requested to become an official sister of mercy in November 1915, provides a illustrative example. Deul' had completed nursing courses under the auspices of the Vilnius Hospital Jewish Community and had worked in the capacity of a nurse assigned to a field hospital by the All-Russian Union of Towns.[43] Thus, while the Russian Red Cross did allow some Jewish women to become nurses, this requirement of individual review of each Jewish applicant would provide a serious impediment to real religious integration. And as late as 1916, Jewish medics were still being prohibited from enlisting in the Red Cross per the original statutes of the organization.[44] Moreover, all Russian sisters of the Red Cross would continue to be consecrated by an official of the Orthodox Church when entering active service, despite their beliefs. Thus, although it would have been tremendously beneficial for the Red Cross to be transformed from a private, religious establishment to a public, civil society organization in order to successfully meet the needs of wartime Russia, its authorities resisted this kind of modernization.

The source of this kind of bureaucratic obfuscation and hesitation on the part of the Red Cross to accept Jewish women into the ranks of wartime nurses stems from deep-seated suspicion of Jews by Russian authorities (and the general population). Anti-Semitism has a long and violent history in Russia, but during the war it took on the added dimension of treason. Jews of the Russian empire were found primarily living in the lands of Poland, Lithuania, Ukraine, and Belarus, concentrated as a result of the laws of the Russian empire that had, since the time of

Catherine the Great, restricted them to living in the area known as the Pale of Settlement (although nearly three hundred thousand Jews actually lived outside of the Pale, many in large cities of the empire). These regions became hotly contested during the war and in fact were directly within the area deemed the front. There was tremendous anxiety about the Jewish populations in these regions as potential spies and traitors, thought to have little reason to be loyal to a Russian empire that had treated them extremely poorly over the last several centuries, and thus incentivized to help the enemy achieve victory and take control of those lands, with the hopes that their treatment would be better under German or Austrian overlords. Moreover, Jews were closely associated with revolutionary movements and radical socialism, and authorities feared that Jewish nurses would be able to use their positions to gain access to the soldiering masses in order to spread revolutionary propaganda and defeatist ideas.[45] As Eric Lohr explains, the Jews were deemed "unreliable," particularly by the Russian military leadership. The fear of Jews on the part of Russian authorities led to the deportation and expulsion of large numbers of Jews, with estimates ranging from half a million to a million, from the Russian empire.[46]

Considering the difficulties Jews faced in the anti-Semitic atmosphere of the Russian empire, it might be somewhat surprising that so many Jewish women desired to serve a nation that did not accord them basic civil rights or respectful treatment. However, many Russian Jews believed that carrying out wartime service would prove their devotion to the state and afford them greater protection and rights in return for their sacrifices. Nursing was clearly seen as a means by which Jewish women could demonstrate their civic virtue. Thousands of Jewish women appealed to the Red Cross requesting permission to become sisters of mercy, but, as indicated previously, while some were admitted, the organization continued to insist that each application made by Jewish women be individually reviewed by the main administration. This requirement made the process of accepting such women painfully slow. Moreover, although women accepted into the ranks of the Red Cross and assigned to nursing communities during the war were considered "civil sisters," on completion of their training they were consecrated in a religious ceremony conducted by a Russian Orthodox priest.[47] Although it was difficult for Jewish women to serve directly as part of the communities of the Red Cross with the designation "sister of mercy" (and thus they were denied the accompanying prestige and compensation), they could serve as "volunteer sisters" and as part of the other civilian organizations that provided medical service during the war, such as the Union of Zemstvos and the Union of Towns.

Despite these obstacles and the general mistrust with which they were viewed, Jewish nurses played extremely important roles in providing medical service for numerous victims of the war. In many of the Russian empire's cities with substantial Jewish populations, members of the local community used their resources to establish medical treatment facilities, in which Jewish nurses, as well as other medical personnel, were often the primary, if not exclusive, caregivers to both Jewish and gentile patients. There were several medical facilities established in Moscow, including the Moscow City Infirmary, built by the city's Jewish community; another was constructed through the patronage of the Jewish Women's Circle.[48] Moscow also was the location of the Belov factory infirmary, where Jewish medical personnel primarily treated Jewish patients and even operated a kosher kitchen.[49] The Petrograd Jewish community also established several medical facilities, including an infirmary set up by the Petrograd Circle of Jewish Intelligentsia.[50] In Kiev, local Jewish sugar magnate Israel Borisovich Babushkin and his wife donated the funds to establish a hospital, named in their honor, with one hundred beds and staffed entirely by Jewish medical personnel. In that same city, M. B. and S. I. Gal'perin donated ten thousand rubles to the Red Cross Military Hospital of Kiev.[51] Jewish nursing personnel also served in another facility in Kiev, the M. I. Zaitsev Infirmary. The Council of Spiritual Direction of the Synagogue and House of Prayer of Odessa sponsored the training of Jewish nursing personnel in that city.[52] The Orenburg Jewish community established its own infirmary, which was not only staffed with Jewish nurses but also included in its ranks a Jewish woman doctor.[53] In the Jewish community infirmary in Vitebsk, numerous Jewish nurses cared for wounded and ill soldiers and civilians. In Mitava the Jewish community set up an infirmary staffed with Jewish nurses.[54] The town of Sedlets operated a Jewish infirmary, as did that of Kamenets. In Smolensk a hospital was established through the support of the local Jewish women's society and was staffed exclusively by Jewish medical personnel, doctors, and volunteer sisters, as well as Jewish brothers of mercy who served on the night shift.[55]

Jewish nurses also proved especially useful in regions of the Russian empire heavily populated by Jews, such as Poland, which was also a primary area of conflict on the eastern front. There, they were vitally important to providing assistance not only to the soldiers fighting in the region but also to the local population, who suffered from epidemic diseases, food shortages, homelessness, and other problems of social dislocation caused by a war being fought essentially in their backyards. Jewish hospitals also existed in these regions and were used for the treatment of both Jews and gentiles, combatant and civilian. When the region was occupied by the Germans during the Great Retreat of 1915, these sisters became extremely important for the treatment of Russian prisoners of war now in German hands, as well as continuing to provide assistance to the civilians now under German control.[56]

Although Russian society maintained a strong strain of anti-Semitism, whereby Jews were viewed with a great deal of suspicion and often treated with malice, some instances demonstrate that soldiers were not disturbed when treated by Jewish nurses. Many of the peasant soldiers who were cared for by Jewish nurses held these women in high regard and were unconcerned with their religious affiliations. I. S. Grigor'ev, a correspondent of the popular Petrograd newspaper *Den'*, visited the Vilnius Jewish Community Infirmary and found a cache of letters from soldiers expressing fond sentiments toward the Jewish nurses on staff there. One soldier, Dmitrii Prokopovich, wrote:

> Greetings dear little sisters, I bow low before you and send you wishes from my soul for all that is good in the world and that God should grant you all that you desire in your lives, my dearest little sisters, I miss you very much. I will remember you for as long as I live and ask you dear sisters to write letters to me, I will be grateful to you for my entire life dear sisters, who I have promised to bring sweets to, I miss you very much and every day that goes by hope that all with you is happy, I ask you to write me at my address and send something to remember, until then, farewell.

Another, a junior noncommissioned officer named Vasilii Mikhailovich Lavrinovich, similarly had high commendations for the Jewish nurses who provided him with medical care while he was recovering in this facility. In statements strikingly reminiscent of the biblical passage describing Christ in Matthew 25:31, he wrote of the sisters, "I kiss you one thousand times and am ever grateful to you that when I was hungry, you fed me and when I was thirsty you gave me drink, when I was naked you clothed me. . . . You saved me from the terrible plight of death and thus I will never forget such sisters."[57]

Muslim women, despite the fact that they existed in large numbers in the Caucasian and Central Asian regions of the empire, seem to have presented less of a problem. Few records indicate that Muslim women attempted to join the ranks of the Russian Red Cross or other organizations providing medical service during the war. Here too, the fact that one of Russia's enemies in the war, the Ottoman empire, was predominantly Muslim contributed to the notion of unreliability and potential disloyalty.

Although nationality and religion as indicators of loyalty to the empire were highly significant, the voluntary nature of nursing meant that, for most, some form of patriotism was a primary impetus for service. As with many men who enlisted in the armed services, many women were affected by the desire to contribute to the national crisis. However, as opposed to blind fidelity to the tsar and his government, this was manifested more often as love for Russia as a country and the *narod* (the people).[58] Most women who joined medical services commented on their desire to "do their part" in the war effort and believed that medical service was the best way for them to do so, as it was consistent with what they perceived to be normative gender roles and characteristics of Russian women. For these women, war was not an exclusively male arena off-limits to them as a result of their gender. They believed nursing to be an entirely appropriate wartime activity for women. They would not kill or destroy; rather, they would mend and heal. As one female reporter noted, in wartime women must—in fact, are predisposed to—fulfill a role "that men are unable to do."[59] Vanda Stepanova similarly expressed her desire to enter nursing courses so that she could be "useful."[60] Aleksandra Tolstaia remarked, "I could not sit at home, I had to participate in the general crisis." Her mother, as well as the Tolstoyans who remained loyal followers of her father's pacifism, tried to talk her out of her desire to become a sister of mercy. "Why do you want to go to war?" her mother asked. "Your father was against war, and you want to take part in it?" Aleksandra responded that she did not believe her father would be against her helping the ill and wounded. Even before her father's death in 1910, she had an interest in medicine. She had studied anatomy and physiology and helped their family physician establish a clinic for the peasants who lived on their estate, Iasnaia Poliana, and in the surrounding area. Despite her significant reservations, Tolstaia's mother relented and allowed her daughter to enlist. "Mother was unhappy," Aleksandra recalled, but recognized there was little she could do. "Well, I have told you my opinion," she chided, "but I know that it is useless. You always do as you please."[61]

For many women, such as Tat'iana Aleksinskaia, entering medical service in wartime Russia meant choosing to give up comfortable lives as expatriates. Countess Ol'ga Putiatina, granddaughter of Admiral Evfimii Putiatin, whose family had relocated to England prior to the war, immediately entered the Anglo-Russian hospital, serving as a translator for the British medical staff in Petrograd. Putiatina, who had been born in Russia but lived most of her life in Great Britain, felt herself to be Russian at heart and deeply wanted to help her native country. However, she found the work in the Anglo-Russian hospital unrewarding, as she was relegated primarily to translating and other administrative duties. Instead, she longed to be of more direct service to her Russian compatriots in a medical capacity. As a result, she secured a transfer to the Russian Red Cross.[62] Mary Britnieva, holding dual citizenship in Britain and Russia, could easily have returned to the former to serve safely behind the lines in home front facilities. The desire to contribute to the war effort was a strong motivating factor among non-Russian nationals who joined the Russian medical services as well. Florence Farmborough could have returned to her native England as opposed to working with flying columns on the eastern front. Violetta Thurstan, another Englishwoman serving with a Russian Red Cross flying column, remarked that as women, "we should rise to the occasion and do the utmost that was expected of us."[63]

Many of the women who enlisted as nurses and served during the Great War in Russia had religious motivations consistent with notions of Christian charity and ethos. Russian Orthodoxy strongly promoted notions of service and self-sacrifice consistent with nursing. Many believed it was their Christian duty to engage in the care of wounded men. Nurses such as N. Chelakova indicated that the spiritual component of their mission was extremely important. She rejected advice given to her at the outbreak of the war to serve in well-equipped rear units of the Red Cross in favor of more "primitive" facilities at the front, which she was convinced would indicate greater "faith in Jesus."[64] Indeed, some were actually members of the clergy, including novices and nuns who were part of the Orthodox monastic tradition but trained as nurses and served in the communities of the Red Cross during the war.

Even women who rejected nationalism and its call to war found themselves working as nurses for the benefit of the soldiers, who were often their fathers, brothers, husbands, or other male loved ones. There were those whose politics were even more radical than socialists such as Aleksinskaia and whose antiwar stance was well established even after many others were swept up in patriotic fervor. Bolshevik leader Vladimir Lenin's younger sister, Maria Ul'ianova, served as a sister of mercy on a hospital train for the duration of the conflict. Despite her brother's vitriolic stance against the war and her own status as a dedicated Bolshevik, she entered the war effort, at least partially in order to divert the attentions of the tsarist political police from her radical activities. Like Aleksinskaia, however, as she served, she found that she was dedicated to the peasant soldier.[65]

There were also those with more personal motivations for enlisting in medical service. However, these were not always seen as exclusively selfish, as in the cases of those women who enlisted in medical services in order to escape personal sorrow. A nurse on Aleksinskaia's train had joined "in the hope of finding oblivion and relief from her sorrow; she had lost her son, whom she had loved passionately, and her husband, who not the only man she loved, but a real friend and comrade."[66] Lidiia Zakharova was so depressed by her husband's conscription that she felt compelled to leave her two young sons to join the Red Cross. "After my husband's departure, both my bed and my heart were empty. I needed energetic activity, many things to do, movement and fatigue, so that somehow at night I could fall asleep and forget myself." She further remarked, "Returning to the children turned out to be 'horrible': The oldest asked about papa, and the youngest looked just like him." These statements are striking in the face of normative values of womanhood of early twentieth-century Russian society that emphasized, even venerated, the role of mother. Her remarks seem to indicate that caring for her two young sons did not provide her with emotional fulfillment, but in her work as a sister of mercy, she "found a refuge from my depression."[67] Here, however, she framed her decision around the notion of serving others, the soldiers, which made the leaving of her young children palatable. Enlistment in nursing service offered the possibility of restoring purpose and meaning to the lives of women who failed to find this in peacetime life. Tolstaia lamented that she had felt an emptiness and lack of purpose ever since her father's death in 1910. In going to the front as a wartime nurse she recalled that she "wanted to forget myself, I wanted great feats, heroic actions. Political events were passing by, without touching me!"[68]

RUSSIAN WARTIME NURSING AND FEMINISM

Participation in the war had further political meaning for many women who became nurses in that they were infused with the desire to prove their worth as citizens. In so doing, they hoped to accomplish long-sought-after rights and equality. The connection between wartime nursing and the Russian women's movement is an important one, both in terms of how feminism motivated women to serve in medical capacities and in terms of the support for such services by the women's movement. Many Russian women, especially progressives and members of organizations seeking to expand women's roles in public life, were highly supportive of female wartime nursing. Even those who previously had expressed staunchly pacifist attitudes could embrace nursing for its life-giving rather than violent and destructive aims. The war-era women's journals presented medical service as the most effective way for women to demonstrate their usefulness to the nation during the conflict, with the hopes of being rewarded with rights of participation in the polity. Women's organizations such as the Mutual Philanthropic Society and the League for Women's Equality were quick to express their support for women's enlistment in wartime medical service, seeking to "present themselves as responsible citizens who recognized their obligations as well as their rights."[69]

Indeed, a number of prominent feminists were themselves medical professionals. The editors of the journal *Zhenskoe Delo* ("Women's Cause"), the organ of the League for Women's Equality, led by Dr. Poliksena Shishkina-Iavein, appealed to the "daughters of Russia" to join the war effort: "We women have to unite: and each of us, forgetting personal misfortune and suffering, must come out of the narrow confines of the family and devote all our energy, intellect, and knowledge to our country. This is our obligation to the fatherland, and this will give us the right to participate as the equals of men in the new life of a victorious Russia."[70] Through her journal *Zhenskii Vestnik* (Women's Herald), physician Maria Pokrovskaia, head of the Women's Progressive Party, proclaimed that when "men go to war, women exert all their force with work to ease and care for those suffering and to lessen the consequences of war on the country."[71]

Progressive women seeking to expand women's rights and opportunities viewed wartime nursing as an excellent opportunity to demonstrate their usefulness to society, and therefore many such women enlisted in the Red Cross and its subordinate organizations during the war. Aleksinskaia, who was assigned to the hospital train, called it a "feminist train" because of its predominantly female staff. Aleksinskaia was very proud of this and attributed progressive ideas to all of the female members of her unit. For them, wartime nursing was a way to be useful not possible for them in peacetime conditions. She describes them as "mostly Russian intellectuals who can find no satisfaction in their ordinary life in the provincial corners of our immense Russia, and are seeking an outlet for their moral energy and their social aspirations." In an allusion to the *narodniki* (groups of politically radicalized young people who went into the countryside in an effort to "enlighten the masses" regarding their oppression under the tsarist system and encourage them to advocate for socialism) of the 1870s, Aleksinskaia remarked, "the war has the same attraction for them as the struggles and sufferings of the people used to have."[72]

Some men even viewed the contribution made by women in wartime nursing as an action deserving of national recognition in the form of greater rights. V. V. Brusianin proclaimed, "Now we cannot count how many Russian women are taking direct part in the war on the same level as men. In the war a huge cadre of sisters of mercy and women doctors are working in hospitals and field infirmaries hand to hand with men. The activities of these women will be taken into account after the war, and no one now doubts the necessity of their self-sacrificing work."[73]

CLASS AND NURSING EXPERIENCE

As determinants of experience, issues of class and social status are equally important in understanding wartime nursing in Russia during the First World War. True, for some women, wartime nursing presented an opportunity for class equalization, or at least they perceived it as such, removing the impediments of social interaction and behavior imposed on them by their status. Nurses often commented on how their modest Red Cross uniforms effectively erased individual (as well as sexual) identity and any markers that would indicate social origin. Although it is unlikely that high-profile sisters such as the empress or the grand duchesses were able to move about incognito, wartime nursing did allow some women from elite backgrounds to operate in ways and engage in activities that likely would have been impossible in their peacetime lives. The Grand Duchess Maria Pavlovna (first cousin of the tsar) remarked, "Almost no one knew me. . . . We all lived the same life and had the same interests." She worked hard to assimilate with the nurses with whom she served, explaining that when she arrived at a new hospital, she immediately set to work in order to prove to the other nurses that she was no different from them. "I armed myself with a wet rag, tucked up my skirts, and washed and scrubbed floors and furniture."[74] Although we may question the extent to which the grand duchess was truly unrecognizable, the sentiment of camaraderie seems sincere on her part. Moreover, her experiences of living and working in close proximity to those of nonprivileged sectors of Russian society was something unique to the atmosphere created by the war, providing a kind of social mingling that otherwise likely would have been improbable, if not impossible. A number of the activities in which sisters of mercy engaged, at least to some degree, contributed to the leveling of social differences. The extensive physical labor that wartime medical service required was something those of the upper classes would not have performed in normal peacetime conditions. Although one may question the extent to which Grand Duchess Maria Pavlovna was successful in convincing the other nurses that she was just like them, one can safely assume that cleaning floors would not have been part of her usual daily routine. And while such activities were at first difficult for such women to successfully complete, they managed, and even became accustomed to them over the course of the war. Meriel Buchanan, daughter of the British ambassador, remarked that although many of the elite women who volunteered in the hospitals had never done the kind of hard work associated with nursing before, they stuck with it and continued to serve.[75]

While certainly as a sister of mercy the grand duchess may have shared certain wartime experiences with commoners, by no means should we assume that such experiences effectively erased the vast chasm of social difference that existed between her, as a member of the royal family, and the average peasant. Moreover, although nursing could act as a social leveler in some instances, in many others class and social status still played significant roles in shaping nurses' wartime experiences. In many cases, a nurse's position in society, in addition to her gender, seemed to be most significant in terms of determining the place and type of service for most of Russia's wartime nurses. Sisters with aristocratic pedigrees and valuable social or political networks did not usually perform their service under the most adverse conditions (unless they so desired). Well-connected members of the nobility seemed to be able to choose when and where they served and could use their influence to obtain choice assignments, secure leaves when desired, and transfer to other medical establishments if they found their placement unsatisfactory. Sisters of mercy with the right associations could ensure that they were assigned to stationary hospitals in the rear, in places where they continued to have ready access to the comforts of life. Their accommodations, even when at the front, were often considerably better, usually in commandeered buildings and homes in towns and villages, or permanent structures that served as hospitals. In their free time, nurses from Russia's social elite associated mostly with men of the officer corps, and some even went to theater performances and other urban forms of entertainment. Even in their work, nurses from Russia's upper classes could operate in a social sphere similar to peacetime, providing medical service primarily for officers, and coming into contact with soldiers from the peasantry and working classes only when absolutely necessary. Some privileged women served exclusively in hospitals for officers. In medical facilities that treated both officers and soldiers, those without rank were usually separated from those of the officer corps, and the latter were often provided with superior housing (for example, beds with spring mattresses for officers as opposed to cots with straw for soldiers). That Russian wartime nursing preserved many of the social divisions present in peacetime society should not be surprising, however, considering the highly stratified nature of late imperial society.

The records of women's wartime nursing reveal the influences of class privilege quite clearly. The wife of the chief of Russian general staff, General Gurko, used her connections to be placed in the divisional hospital of her choice, and insisted on being assigned to facilities wherein she was the only sister of mercy. She did not explain the reason for such a request (perhaps she did not wish to "compete" with other women), but her position in society ensured that it was fulfilled.[76] N. Chelakova benefited from highly placed connections as well. She and her fellow nurses were deeply disappointed by their assignment to an infectious disease hospital in the rear rather than to a frontline establishment for the treatment of wounded soldiers. One among them, her friend Liliia's aunt, Sister N., described by Chelakova as a "socialite lady," appealed to a well-placed personal acquaintance in the main administration of the Russian Red Cross. The successful appeal granted them a transfer to a military hospital near the front, located in the Ivangorod train station. After the Germans withdrew from the area and the fighting subsided in the region, very few wounded arrived at the facility for treatment. Chelakova and her companions became bored. Once again, Sister N. appealed to her connection in the Red Cross administration, who immediately secured a transfer for herself and her niece Liliia. The two women were assigned to a hospital train, and as they departed, they promised to do something similar for Chelakova and her remaining companion, Anya.[77] Transferred to a hospital near Warsaw, Sofia Bocharskaia and the members of her unit soon became frustrated because they found there was little work to be done there. When asked to be sent to a part of the front where they would be needed, they were met with indifference from medical authorities who, she reported, did not have "the time or the inclination to attend to us." Finally, as a "special favor" to the head of their unit, a prince, they were given the chance to transfer to a village where they were assured there would be wounded to attend to. They packed up their equipment and supplies, including a very large mirror belonging to the chief doctor's wife, which she absolutely insisted on taking everywhere they went.[78] Despite her designation as a wartime sister and limited training and experience, Aleksandra Tolstaia secured a place in a Union of Zemstvo mobile medical unit formed in 1916 and exclusively composed of Red Cross staff nurses (i.e., permanent members of nursing communities), intended to serve on the Turkish front. Her acceptance was accomplished solely through the intervention of the organizers of the unit, two highly placed members of the Union of Zemstvos, Tikhon Polner and Sergei Glebov, with whom she had long been personally acquainted.[79]

Conditions of service were also affected by class and social status, and those with elite associations could secure comfort even in the hardship and depravation of war. Noble sister Mary Britnieva's unit was housed in Teresino Palace, the lavish country seat of Prince Drutsky-Lubetsky, which had been converted into a hospital for officers during the war.[80] Meals for these women of the elite were equivalent to those of the officer corps; in fact, they usually dined with the officers (many of whom were their relatives and acquaintances from the circles of Russian high society). Sofia Bocharskaia described dinners of roasted chicken, wine, brandy, coffee, and chocolate; time spent on long rides on horseback through the countryside with flirty officers; and even an afternoon relaxing on the yacht of one of her noble cousins.[81] In fact, her memoir of the war reads more like a romantic adventure than an account of the trials of war. Vanda Stepanova was given a "cozy little room" of her own, complete with a camp bed with a "soft mattress," a camp chair, writing table, and wash basin. She shared meals with the officers of her unit, and she often had access to cakes, chocolate, candies, liquors, wine, fruits, and other items that would be considered delicacies in the wartime economy. She too went on picnics in the countryside and had free time for games and other forms of entertainment. When she was transferred to a facility where there was little work, she spent much of her time with her horse, Klara, taking long rides in the countryside with an officer escort.[82] Tat'iana Varnek was put up in a lavish palace in the town of Iaslo, in the Carpathians, and she and a fellow sister of mercy shared a "beautiful, large bedroom with red doors." The head of the hospital to which Varnek was transferred later in 1915, Countess Bobrinskaia, lived in her own well-appointed apartments attached to the medical facility and had access to her own automobile, her own chauffeur, and her own lackey. Everyone was afraid of the countess, whom they addressed by her aristocratic title rather than as "sister." Varnek commented that "the countess did not do any actual work, but saw everything and held everything in her hands."[83] Varnek's description contrasts sharply with that of S. Ansky, who was briefly assigned to this unit and described the countess and all of the other titled medical personnel serving under her as those who "behaved very simply acting as bureaucrats and merchants, eating the same food as the rank and file with the same wooden spoons."[84] Chelakova recalled sitting in the well-apportioned private railway car of a high-ranking official of the Russian Red Cross passing through Ivangorod on a visit to the battlefields, where they sipped tea and ate cakes and other sweets, and "sat and chatted as if it were a Petersburg social call."[85]

Women of high social standing were also protected from criticism of their work (or even from working too hard). Tatiana Aleksinskaia related an episode in which the commandant of a bath train became distressed on noticing that the ambulance train that had stopped alongside his seemed to lack any doctors or nurses overseeing the orderlies and attending to the wounded. "I made inquiries," he said, "and I found a nurse and told her that the orderlies ought not be allowed to work without someone in charge. She was annoyed, and a doctor jumped down from a carriage and shouted: 'How dare you be so rude to Nurse Z——?' Then it was explained that the lady was a very important personage." The commandant was infuriated at his inability to reprimand the woman for failure to carry out her duties as a result of her status. Clearly he valued merit and hard work over social significance. "But how was I to know that?" he complained. "All nurses are the same to me. An important personage! If she does her work well, I am at her feet. If not . . . "[86]

It was not merely membership in Russia's nobility that afforded sisters of mercy special treatment. Khristina Semina, as the wife of a regimental chief doctor, was allowed to operate as a free agent, often in situations where other women would have not been given the same privilege. She insisted on being able to enter units when she wanted to and to leave when she so desired. As indicated in the previous chapter, Semina was allowed to choose the place of her service, live in her husband's military quarters, accompany him when transporting wounded at the front, and even remain with the army even when other civilian personnel were forbidden to do so. Her status allowed her to come and go as she pleased and to work when and where she desired, regardless of where the greatest need for her services might have been.[87]

Not all women had such freedom, however, and even those from Russia's elite sometimes found it difficult to control the circumstances of their service. A particular problem stemmed from the fact that the trustees or patronesses of Red Cross sister of mercy communities were often titled women of the aristocracy who wielded considerable influence in Russian society and therefore over the women who became nurses in their *obshchiny*. Doctors, nurses, and even high-ranking officials of the Red Cross often found themselves powerless in the face of the will of these women. Bored with her position in a hospital in Kiev, where she had no friends or relatives, Tat'iana Varnek (who came from an aristocratic Saint Petersburg family and served with one of the most prestigious nursing communities of that city, the Kaufman *obshchina*) asked the head of her unit, Countess Bobrinskaia, for a transfer to the front. The countess replied that the authority to make such a decision did not rest with her but with the *obshchina*. However, when she appealed to the baroness who was the trustee of the *obshchina* (most likely Baroness V. I. Ikskul), she was refused. Varnek then asked her well-connected father to intervene with the request that if she could not be sent to the front, could she at least be sent to a hospital in Petrograd where she could be closer to her family? Her father appealed to the senior sister of the community, who promised to take up the matter with the baroness. But once again, the baroness refused and Varnek was forced to remain in Kiev. When the baroness arrived in Kiev to inspect the hospital, Countess Bobrinskaia convinced her to give Varnek an audience. After waiting more than an hour, she was finally allowed to see the baroness. She entered the room to find the baroness "lying on a wide bed, completely wrapped up in gypsy shawls." She did not allow the young nurse to utter a single word but instead chastised her for a long time and then sent her away. The young nurse was so offended and outraged at such treatment that on her next day off she went to see the chief authority of the Red Cross on the southwestern front, Senator Boris Ivanitskii, an extremely high-placed figure in the Russian government, who also served on the tsar's state council. The senator received her well, listened carefully to her story, and assured her that she was in the right. She asked him to dispatch her to Petrograd. He told her that with any other unit, he could do so, but with regard to the Kaufman *obshchina* he could do nothing. He told Varnek that he could issue the appropriate documents giving her the right to travel, but that the baroness was so powerful that at the very first station she would be arrested and sent back. He apologized, explaining that even he did not have the power to fight such a formidable woman.[88]

Despite being beholden to those in socially and politically superior positions, women of the nobility shared little with those of lower social ranks unless they so desired. As a result, in a number of ways, their experiences contrast sharply with those of nurses from the lower gentry and middle strata, the professional classes, and the merchantry.[89] Even for those fortunate enough to come from backgrounds of wealth and education, lower social standing and lack of powerful connections meant they were usually deprived of the ability to affect the terms of their service. Possession of a significant level of material comfort in their peacetime domestic lives secured through economic means did not shield many from facing hardships and deprivations at the front. They usually lived in tents or huts, ate the military provisions of soldiers or whatever limited food was available, and had limited access to even small luxuries. This is not to say that conditions in rear hospitals were always ideal, either. Shortages of personnel and high numbers of sick and wounded often meant that nurses in those facilities had to work long hours under difficult conditions. But in many cases, when their shifts were over, they could return to their homes or other fairly comfortable accommodations. This was not the case for sisters of mercy serving in frontline establishments, particularly in mobile medical units. As part of frontline units, a number of Russia's wartime nurses operated under very dangerous conditions. Even those stationed in field hospitals miles from the frontline positions were not safe, as aerial bombardments frequently hit medical establishments.[90] While there were instances when medical facilities in the rear were threatened with bombardment, especially those located in the quickly fluctuating lines of the Russian western front in Poland and Ukraine, for the most part, service in these hospitals was considerably safer and more comfortable.

Those such as Florence Farmborough and her fellow nurses assigned to the *letuchka* (flying column) in which she served along the Russian western front endured severe extremes of temperature and frequent shortages of food. They were housed in makeshift accommodations in the open air, usually tents, but because the canvas lacked protection from the elements, her unit learned to quickly construct temporary wooden structures, which they greatly preferred. The food available to her unit was irregular in both quality and quantity. Farmborough described how at times the unit was reduced to eating *sukharki,* "odd scraps of black bread in various sizes, baked or dried hard, and guaranteed to last for years. They were, indeed, as hard as stones. . . . Sometimes, the only way of demolishing them was to soak them in tea or water, until they became a 'sop.' . . . 'Crumbs from the rich man's table,' we called them jokingly and, indeed, they often looked like partly demolished, cast-off scraps." When they were able to secure fresh bread or a few potatoes, she and her fellow nurses were overjoyed.[91] Lidiia Zakharova faced similar conditions with regard to food and accommodations. Several months into her service, she was thrilled to learn that her unit was being transferred from a mobile field hospital on the front lines to a village, which brought the promise of accommodations "in a closed-in building under a roof" and the chance to sleep "on something much softer than the raw, cold ground."[92]

The discrepancies in conditions between rear and front medical facilities were often felt by the sisters themselves, which sometimes led to antagonism between nurses. Those serving with frontline units questioned the extent to which women attached to rear medical establishments were "real" nurses. This kind of animosity often mirrored that between the highly trained professional nurses in British medical services and the amateur nurses of the VADs. British volunteer nurses often were tasked with carrying out the most difficult and unseemly work of wartime medical service, but that which required the least skill.[93] In the Russian case, like the disdain of professional nurses for VADs, such tension often stemmed from what was perceived as insufficient training and seriousness about nursing. In fact, there was a belief that volunteers had merely joined the Red Cross or other medical organizations as a result of the prestige associated with being a sister of mercy. Russian staff nurses, those who had been members of the sisters of mercy communities prior to the war and who had completed much more comprehensive and lengthy training (usually from one to two years), often questioned the ability of the volunteers who joined during the war and received significantly abridged training, never experiencing the hardships associated with nursing service. When Tat'iana Varnek and her fellow sisters arrived at the mobile field hospital to which they were assigned, they soon found that the senior nurse, a staff sister named Bol'shakova, barely tolerated them, as they had only volunteered for service when the war began and received shortened training. On their arrival at the unit, Varnek reported that "she immediately hissed: 'What do I need these "volunteers" for? If they had just sent me two staff sisters, it would have been better.'" The senior nurse had so little confidence in the medical capabilities of the "volunteers" that she even refused to allow them to dress the wounds of the men in the field hospital, despite the fact that none were serious cases.[94]

Social status and class combined with the front/rear divide in creating tensions between staff sisters and volunteer wartime nurses. The antagonism between Bol'shakova and the volunteer nurses in her unit was particularly heightened by class difference, as the head nurse hailed from the peasantry while the wartime volunteers were members of the privileged elite. Varnek, for her part, made no effort to hide her disdain for the senior sister, describing Bol'shakova as a "nasty, loose *baba*"[95] and finding it "incomprehensible" that she could have been a member of the prestigious Kaufman *obshchina*, the majority of whose ranks were filled by the elite women of Saint Petersburg (including the tsar's first cousin, the Grand Duchess Maria Pavlovna). In retaliation for her maltreatment of the volunteers, the latter took great delight in vexing the senior sister by sitting around the dining table and gossiping about Saint Petersburg high society. "We noticed that this infuriated Bol'shakova and we purposely poured oil on the fire, frequently making up the most unbelievable names and titles, sprinkled with French phrases, which she did not understand. She would get into such an unbelievable rage and shout 'oh, them counts and princes!'"[96]

Similarly, Aleksandra Tolstaia experienced strained relations reflecting class antagonisms with the professional woman doctor charged to her unit. "Look what kind of 'worker woman' they have sent me," the doctor complained about Tolstaia. "Without protection, she would have never ended up here. What does she know? A countess, an aristocrat!" Conscious of this, Tolstaia worked hard to avoid being "laughed at for her worthlessness" and called a "white-gloved aristocrat." Antagonisms worked both ways, however, as Tolstaia expressed no lost love for her superior, whom she characterized as a "swarthy, wizened, it seemed to me, by malice, socialist with a cigarette constantly dangling from her mouth."[97] The conflicts did not just exist between women. Brother of mercy Dmitrii Furmanov (future revolutionary writer of the famed Civil War novel *Chapaev*) similarly had little respect for the aristocratic women who served as sisters of mercy in his hospital train on the Turkish front. He complained bitterly about two of the nurses in his unit that he labeled "sister-ladies," who never lifted a finger to do any work but instead acted as if they were there "to take the waters, as if in a resort." Furmanov was particularly irked about their attitude of superiority, their complete lack of understanding of the "nobility and sanctity" of the medical work, and the fact that all day they chased their servants around to cater to their "nasty and ridiculous needs." He reported a great "triumph" when he and the other male nurses succeeded in getting them expelled from the unit.[98]

The division of labor with regard to nursing assignments did not always fall neatly according to the demarcations of Russian imperial social structure. The war allowed women to cross class lines and operate outside normative boundaries of Russian society. Moreover, location of service was highly significant. In particular, in Russia frontline nurses, regardless of their social status, did the hardest and most dangerous work. Although some women from the upper classes often served in better conditions as a result of their social status, others members of Russia's elite did not shy away from the hardships of wartime medical service on the front or use their social standing to secure less dangerous or more comfortable surroundings. Ol'ga Aleksandrovna (Tsar Nicholas II's sister) wore the uniform of a common sister of mercy, shared humble quarters with her fellow nurses, and worked long hours, often depriving herself of sleep to care for the wounded.[99] Some elite women even requested assignment to units that operated very close to the frontline fighting, including mobile field hospitals, hospital trains, field dressing stations, and flying detachments. When she found her work in the divisional hospital unsatisfying, General Gurko's wife secured transfer to the nearest bandaging station along the front lines. Her preference for working closer to the battlefields would ultimately cost her her life. After the Revolution of 1917 forced her into exile, she was killed by a German shell dropped on her station while serving with the French army.[100]

Moreover, upper-class status was not always an advantage for sisters of mercy. Men who understood the rigors of wartime medical service were not convinced that noblewomen were up to the task of carrying out nursing duties in conditions of war. Semina's husband begged his wife not to enter service in wartime nursing because he assumed the work would be much too difficult for her to bear considering her noble upbringing.[101] Aleksandra Tolstaia appealed directly to Prince Georgi L'vov, head of the All-Russian Union of Zemstvos, to be assigned to a unit at the front after her disappointment with her original assignment in a rear hospital. But the prince initially laughed at Tolstaia's request to be sent to a frontline unit. "You at the front?" he scoffed. "If you want such responsible work, I can tell you straight off: you are not suited to it. You are impractical, inexperienced." Tolstaia was angered and offended by his mockery. "How do you have the right to think that I am not capable of working?" She had to wait several months, proving herself in rear medical service, before she would finally secure permission to join a hospital train on the northwestern front.[102]

In some cases elite social status clearly impeded nurses' abilities to carry out the duties associated with their service. In particular, performance of manual labor tasks was often difficult for upper- and middle-class women who had never done such work, or any kind of work, for that matter. The supervisor of medical units on the northern front, Dr. S. K. Solov'ev, complained that while many women from privileged backgrounds had received adequate medical training, they were often unable to perform more menial duties required of nursing staff (and assigned to them because they were women) such as cleaning and cooking.[103] Meriel Buchanan commented that "the hospitals were full of girls who had probably never known how to make a bed before the war." She remembered "one of the spoilt beauties of Petrograd society . . . standing irresolute before a particularly unappetizing old beggar with sores on his legs," completely at a loss for what to do when ordered by the senior nurse to wash him.[104] When assigned the task of acquiring the food provisions for the field hospital in which she was working, Khristina Semina balked, explaining to the chief doctor that she had no experience with such things and rarely ever had seen raw meat.[105] Sofia Bocharskaia, when ordered by the doctor in charge of her unit to clean the operating room floor, had little idea how to accomplish this task. She attempted to emulate what she had seen the peasant women in her country house do when scrubbing the floors, remembering that they "lifted up their skirts very high, and did something with a pail of hot water." Unfortunately, she "failed to recall what they did next" and so after lifting her own skirts and pouring water all over the floor, she was at a loss about how to proceed. She was rescued by an officer who, on seeing her engaged in what he considered to be an inappropriate activity for someone of her status, sent a group of peasant soldiers in to finish the job, while the two of them went for a leisurely stroll around the village.[106] Aleksandra Tolstaia was also initially flustered when ordered to clean all the floors, windows, doors, and tables in her operating theater. Determined to prove her usefulness and dispel her chief doctor's misgivings, however, she completed the job herself.[107]

To some extent, however, sisters of mercy were something of a class unto themselves, entrance into their ranks often conferring privileged status on the wearer of the nursing uniform. The position afforded them abilities and rights that were restricted or even denied to the majority of the civilian population. Associations of sisters of mercy with the social elites of Russia were present in the minds of many who came into contact with them, regardless of whether the nurses themselves actually hailed from the upper classes. Indicating the distinction made between sisters of mercy and average women, the priest of the hospital where Bocharskaia was serving scolded the chief doctor's servant for asking the nurses if they wanted some wine "to drink." Sisters, he chided the servant, "do not drink, they refresh themselves."[108] Sister B. Radonich recalled "with pride" how she and her fellow sisters were allowed to move freely around train stations and towns when their transport unit traveled from place to place, while civilian women were denied access to the station and the platform when military trains came through.[109] The issue of mobility given to wearers of sisters of mercy uniforms would become problematic, however, as some were believed to be abusing the privilege for personal gain, and others, unauthorized to don nurses' garb, used the clothing to give them undetected movement.

CONCLUSIONS

Tat'iana Aleksinskaia continued to serve the Russian wounded as part of her hospital train until mid-1916, when she returned to France to rejoin her husband. During her service, she had, despite her original ambivalence about the war, become convinced that the Russian soldiers supported the war after working with the wounded for several months. As a result, she became "a firm champion of the war 'to the finish,'" believing that this was what the majority of the Russian population desired: "to defend themselves and to conquer." Along the way, however, she experienced a number of hardships and witnessed the large-scale slaughter of thousands of Russian lives in the war. Nonetheless, she continued to insist on the necessity of continuing the conflict, even portraying the politically leveling effects of the war, which she argued had united reactionary and revolutionary in a common cause of justice. Near the end of her memoir of the war, she wrote about meeting an officer who, when her train was filled and had no more room for wounded, suggested that they be placed on the train of a famous reactionary (who Aleksinskaia identifies merely as "P—tsh," but most likely was Vladimir Purishkevich, staunch monarchist and assassin of the infamous Grigorii Rasputin), which was coming behind theirs. She said she needed some authority to do this, to which the officer replied that she had his authority: he was "P—tsh" himself. She marveled at how the war had brought together those from opposing political views—she a socialist and this man, who addressed her warmly as "sister," a reactionary. "This was the fierce reactionary and instigator of pogroms, and I am 'sister' to him!" she recalled. "Only the war could produce such results. The German social-democrats are my 'enemies,' and I, a Russian socialist, have become a 'sister' to P—tsh!"[110]

The varied experiences of Russia's sisters of mercy indicate that the war meant many different things to women, depending on a variety of factors and circumstances. In many cases, social status remained the primary determinant of experience, particularly with regard to the place, character, and type of service to which sisters of mercy were assigned. For a number of the elites of Russia, ties of patronage and connections continued to define and delimit experience, privileging members of the elite over nonelites. Social status remained a potent force even with the disruptions caused by the war; for many nurses, wartime experience was structured along traditional lines of social division as in their prewar lives. Thus, sisters of mercy from Russia's upper social strata could, if so desired, continue to live in distinctly separate spheres and behave in ways consistent with prewar norms for the elite. While many encountered numerous challenges presented by the war, privilege remained an important component of their lives, and their wartime experiences often proved much less difficult than those without the influence afforded by social position. For wartime nurses who were members of Russia's nonprivileged orders, for those without connections to or protection from the highly placed and influential, the war experience presented great danger and difficulty. These women were unable to use their status to negotiate for better conditions, attesting to the resistance of structures and less social upheaval. In fact, despite the chaos of the crisis, it seemed the traditional social order, with its distinctions between the dominant and subordinate classes, and particularly, with its heavy emphasis on the importance of personal connections based on status, was retained to a significant extent. The experiences of Russia's sisters of mercy indicate that although the war led to important social and cultural convulsions, the old order, to its own detriment, was highly resilient.

Concomitantly, Russia's sisters of mercy of World War I indicate the ways that traditional social and cultural boundaries became increasingly porous during the war, allowing increased interaction and maneuverability between categories. For a number of women, even some members of Russia's elite, the war proved to be an opportunity to cast off the restrictions of gender, class, and status. In some cases, it becomes clear that these categories were somewhat flexible and underwent change during the period of the war, accelerating a process that had already begun before the outbreak of hostilities. Sisters of mercy were required to face situations and engage in behaviors that would have been considered inappropriate and even off-limits to them in prewar Russian society. They performed tasks clearly outside of the expectations and limitations of action not only for their gender but also for their social positions. Wartime nursing allowed women to mingle with a variety of subjects of the Russian empire, similarly transcending traditional boundaries and operating in ways that contrasted sharply with their prewar lives. As such, the war did much to upset the old imperial social order and chip away at separations. Thus, ultimately, the experiences of Russia's women wartime nurses muddied conceptions of gender, status, and class, further demonstrating the dynamism created by war in late imperial Russian society. And, as shall be revealed in the next several chapters, the experiences of female nursing personnel share much with those of male combat personnel, further blurring the lines that divide by gender.

These experiences reveal the tremendous difficulties facing the country as a result of the failures of the tsarist system to cope with the challenges of a changing, modernizing world in general and the strain of total war specifically. The successful prosecution of the war required the participation of both men and women, of all classes, in public roles, roles that many Russian authorities found difficult to accept but were forced to rely on as a result of the exigencies of war. Even within the disruptive context of total war, many continued to hold strict expectations of behavior, especially for women, while simultaneously women were being asked to perform functions that clearly lay outside their purview in peacetime conditions. Many women themselves, however, were increasingly attempting to move beyond these confines, to find places in the public sphere, to contribute to national interests, and to shape and define those interests through their own agency.

4

BLURRED BOUNDARIES: GENDER AND RUSSIAN WARTIME NURSING EXPERIENCE

FLORENCE FARMBOROUGH: BRITISH EXPATRIATE TURNED RUSSIAN SISTER

In the summer of 1914, twenty-seven-year-old Englishwoman Florence Farmborough was living in Moscow, working as a governess and tutor for the family of Doctor Pavel Usov. She had been in Russia since 1908 and had come to love her adopted country, its language, and its people. When war broke out in August, Farmborough decided that instead of returning to Great Britain to serve in her homeland's war effort, she would remain in Russia and enlist in medical services there. Her employer used his connections as a renowned heart surgeon to place Farmborough and his own daughters as volunteer aids in a local hospital run by Princess (Tatiana?) Golitsyna. Farmborough was "elated beyond words" that she was able to be of use, but she had a deeper desire: "to be accepted as a nurse in a Red Cross front line unit!" That, for her, had "become more than a wish," and it developed into one she expressed as "a longing which I know has to be gratified." But when she shared this idea with others, she was met with considerable resistance from many who assumed she would be unable to withstand the extremely demanding conditions that front-line nurses faced. Moreover, only women who had received appropriate training under the Red Cross or one of its subordinate organizations and had earned the designation of "sister of mercy" were allowed to work at the front. She therefore resolved to become a "real" sister.[1]

Farmborough spent six months training in the Moscow hospital, working in both the medical and surgical sections of the facility, and attending three-hour courses in the evenings after she completed her shift. Although it was exhausting, she successfully completed the courses and passed her examinations, earning the title of "Red Cross

Sister of Mercy." She and her cohorts were consecrated in what Farmborough described as a "beautiful and moving" ceremony conducted by a Russian Orthodox priest. Although an Anglican, she was allowed to be blessed and conferred with the Red Cross insignia. Doctor Usov and his wife refused to allow their daughters to go to the front, fearing it would be too difficult and dangerous for them. But Farmborough insisted, so the doctor arranged an interview for her with the commander of the Tenth Field Surgical Unit of the All-Russian Union of Zemstvos. She was accepted as a surgical nurse. The unit consisted of two *letuchky* (flying columns) that were used to retreive wounded soldiers along the front lines. Each *letuchka* was staffed with a commanding officer and his assistant in charge of supplies, four surgical sisters, one "housekeeping" sister, two doctors, a feldsher, four male nurses, and about thirty orderlies. They were equipped with about two dozen light, two-wheeled horse-drawn carts covered with canvas hoods, along with grooms and drivers. Farmborough's transport also had two automobiles. At the beginning of March 1915, the unit was dispatched to the Russian western front in East Galicia. Farmborough was attached to the First Flying Column, which was stationed in the Polish town of Gorlice (Gorlitse as it was called in Russian). They set up a small field hospital in town but traveled throughout the front to pick up wounded.[2]

Farmborough had only been at the front for a little over a month when the Germans launched a massive attack on Gorlice. This was her first direct experience under enemy fire, but she had to continue working despite the dangerous conditions. Her description is vivid:

> The roar of the rival cannons grew increasingly intense. Rockets and projectors were at work. Patches of lurid, red light glowed here and there where fires had been kindled by shells. Our house [the hospital] shook to its very foundations, its windows rattling and quivering in their hinges. Death was very busy, his hands full of victims. Then the wounded began to arrive. We started work in acute earnest. At first we could cope; then were overwhelmed by their numbers. They came in their hundreds, from all directions; some able to walk, others crawling, dragging themselves along the ground. We worked day and night. And still they came! And the thunder of the guns never ceased. Soon their deadly shells were exploding around our Unit; for hours on end, the horror and confusion continued. We had no rest and were worn out with the intensity and

> immensity of the work. . . . And all the time the bombardment of Gorlitse was continuing with brutal ferocity.[3]

NURSING AS ANTIDOTE TO THE MASCULINE "MYTH OF WAR"

Although Farmborough herself was not a native Russian, her experiences as a sister of mercy were fairly typical of frontline nurses who served Russia's wounded and ill during the war. They not only reveal the significance of women's medical service to our understanding of the war but also expose the fallacy of the notion of war as a distinctly male experience. This chapter[4] seeks to demonstrate, through the particular experiences of Russian wartime nursing during the First World War, that the lines of distinction based on gender cannot be drawn so clearly, and that while gender was highly significant in shaping wartime nursing experience, it did so in ways that were not always consistent with traditional notions of masculinity and femininity. In fact, Russian women's wartime nursing experiences share many of the features of the male war experience, even in its mythological form. Moreover, despite the overwhelming focus of most studies of wartime experience on male actions in planning and carrying out operations on the battlefields, they demonstrate clearly the extent to which combat is not the defining feature of warfare. As literary scholar Margaret Higonnet has argued, "'combat' is not the sum total of 'war,'" and "the assumption that female populations stood *outside* the line of fire is also false."[5] Nurses' writings challenge us to "reconsider the symbolic separation of the civilian zone from the militarized zone, so often identified with the distinction between women's sphere and men's sphere."[6]

To better understand how Russian wartime nursing demonstrates a blurring of gender dichotomies, one must see it within the context of Russia and the war on the eastern front. As indicated previously, this was a very different kind of war experience than the stagnant trench-bound conflict of the western front. This is not to discount the dangerous and difficult work performed by women in medical services in other nations. The women who became nurses for the other belligerents during this conflict also endured conditions that in many ways were similar to those of combatants. They faced fatigue, extremes of heat and cold, exposure to disease, vermin infestation, filth, and lack of hygiene, as well as being constantly surrounded by death and dying. In particular, nurses who served in France (both those who served France but also those of British and American medical units stationed there), where heavy fighting took place, experienced tremendous hardships. Often overwhelmed with high numbers of casualties, nurses worked for days on end with little, if any, rest or even nourishment. They weathered extreme cold, particularly through the winter of 1917–1918, when temperatures dropped to record lows. Many lived in tents or other temporary accommodations and rarely had the opportunity to bathe. Often they had no light in their tents for fear they would be spotted by the enemy. Some nurses were occasionally sent with medical teams to dressing stations or field hospitals closer to the front lines.[7] More than a few were exposed to enemy shelling.[8]

But nursing was somewhat different in Russia compared to the Western Allied nations and even the Central Powers. This was largely a result of the much greater tendency for Russian sisters to serve very close to the fighting, which, although prohibited officially as in all other countries, was routinely practiced as a matter of necessity. Coupled with a strong desire on the part of the nurses themselves to serve at the front, this meant that a great number of Russian sisters of mercy actually carried out their work at the forward positions. Furthermore, gender relations and behaviors in Russia were also distinct in a number of significant ways from those in the West. Most notably, in this comparative context, the ideology of domesticity, while certainly present to some extent in Russian culture, had not developed along the same lines as it had in the West. In particular, notions of female physical weakness and incapacity had not been inculcated in Russian values, especially in peasant society.[9] Such factors did not go unnoticed even by contemporary observers. English nurse Violetta Thurstan, after about a year serving in Russian medical facilities, made a point of distinguishing between British and Russian practices with regard to the roles of men and women in the war. She discussed how the British, as a result of a "chivalrous point of view," believed women "must be sheltered from danger or discomfort as far as possible" and thus did not allow women to work near the firing lines. In Russia, however, she commented, "there is a comradeship between men and women" not present in her native land. As a result, she argued, "Russian men seem to realize how much women appreciate being allowed to share, in ever such a small measure, the discomfort and hardships of the men. Thus it comes about that in Russia, sisters are allowed to work as a matter of course quite close to the firing line in a way that would not be possible, or perhaps even desirable, on the Western front." In fact, while she understood the perspective of her compatriots, Thurstan herself "as a woman" could not "help preferring the Russian plan," even though it meant that many nurses lost their lives in service, "having died of shell and bomb wounds and from asphyxiating gases."[10] Although she overstates the degree of gender equality in Russia, Thurston reflects significant differences in attitudes about women there, where notions of gender were more ambivalent than those in the West.

This argument is not suggesting that wartime nursing and combat were or are identical. It is certainly true that in a number of important ways, women as nurses remained distinctly different and apart from men as soldiers, most notably in their divergent missions of healing and killing, respectively. Moreover, there is no denying that wartime nursing was gendered specifically as feminine in early twentieth-century society. Indeed, it is important to remember that just as soldiering was highly "masculinized," by its connection to behaviors and activities that contemporaries associated with men, such as heroism, courage, and aggressiveness, so too was nursing highly "feminized," associated with essentialist characteristics seen as biological features possessed by women, including caring, nurturing, preserving life, and self-sacrifice. Nursing culture was thus largely understood as a distinctly feminine one, and women were seen as particularly well suited to carrying out the tasks associated with nursing care. Most of the women who became sisters of mercy in Russia during the First World War, and the men with whom they served, as well as most of Russian society, shared this view. They specifically enlisted in medical services because they believed it to be an entirely appropriate, feminine activity. Dominant culture indicated that while men went to fight and kill, women were supposed to heal and comfort. The writings of many of Russia's wartime nurses and those who observed them reflect these attitudes.

Yet, while some women entered nursing service without any contemplation of gender transgression, and may have continued to understand their activities as sisters of mercy within this feminized context, particularly those who carried out their service in rear facilities, others clearly saw the gendered implications of their actions in the "male" war zone, either from the start or as the result of undergoing significant transformative processes that led them away from these conventional gendered notions. Confronted with the realities of the war, the women who became nurses in Russia entered a much more nebulous terrain with regard to gender, both consciously and unconsciously. Indeed, for a number of women who served at the front, the experience was at the very least gender neutralizing, while for some it was distinctly "masculinizing."

ECHOES OF COMBAT EXPERIENCE

The ways in which the wartime nursing experience shared elements of the male combat experience can be seen in a number of different aspects of women's medical service. This is reflected both in what women wrote about their nursing experiences and in the actual conditions they faced and events they endured during the war. Clearly, the former was shaped by the latter, but it is significant that women chose to represent their war experiences in ways similar to male forms of recollection. Whether the women writers were conscious of it or not, most of the models for war writing available to them were records left behind by men. Moreover, male writings were seen as "real" or "true" war stories, to be emulated in order to produce a more "authentic" product. But women's wartime writings were not merely imitative, lacking any unique perspective influenced by gender. Female medical personal often wrote about aspects of the war that were not seen in male writings, and women expressed ideas about similar phenomena in ways considerably different from male reflections. But despite such difference, which was often gendered, it is possible to discern strong congruence in female nursing and male combat experiences.

Parallels with male combat experiences become clear from the moment women enlisted in medical service. Although sisters of mercy were not conscripted into service like the vast majority of men who became soldiers during the war, the motivations that impelled women to go to war share important features with the experience of male volunteers and even some male draftees. Moved by the patriotic upswell that occurred in the heady early days of the war, women as well as men offered to serve "For Faith, Tsar, and Fatherland." Some women felt guilty for being able to remain safely behind the lines as a result of their sexual exclusion from military conscription. When asked why she enlisted, a sister named Sofia serving with Florence Farmborough's unit explained, "I came to the Front because I felt that I had to come. War seemed too far away in Moscow and I wanted to help where help was most needed. I wanted to share in the hardship, the suffering." Farmborough herself was infected with a patriotic desire to serve Russia, despite the fact it was not her native land.[11] Against her husband's admonitions, Khristina Semina felt she could not remain safely at home when so many were suffering.[12] Even those already devoting their lives to the care of others saw the war as taking precedent over their regular duties. Sister Feoktista Nikandrovna Slepchenko, who had been a sister of mercy for many years and had served in the Russo-Japanese War, left her position as a nurse in a leper colony in Iakutsk to join the war effort, remarking, "There were no chains that could hold me in the colony."[13] Such sentiments were similarly expressed by men who were not conscripted, who also experienced guilt in remaining safely at home while others went off to fight and die for their country. Indeed, social pressure was applied to both men and women to serve the nation in its time of crisis. As indicated previously, Semina attempted to shame her brother-in-law for his overt draft evasion.[14] And as with women, men opposed to the violence of war and to the imperial cause also felt the need to make their loyalty to the Russian people known. Leonid Andrusov, a radical who stood firmly against the tsarist government and its perceived warmongering, joined his fellow students in a protest against ending draft exemptions. Nonetheless, he and the other young men felt the need to draft a statement in which they proclaimed their willingness to "lay down our lives" for the motherland. Andrusov enlisted as a medic in order to serve his country without participating in the act of killing.[15] Hundreds of Russian Mennonites, opposed to participating in violent action, similarly joined medical services during the Great War.

Women expressed other motivations for going to war as well. Like numerous young men who became soldiers in 1914, many of the women who enlisted as nurses during World War I held romanticized conceptions of war and saw it as an opportunity for adventure. This was a common impetus for young men to enlist, especially in countries with volunteer militaries. As George Mosse contends, for many men the war presented "an escape from the restraint of bourgeois life, giving purpose to purposeless lives, was described as a festival—that is an event exhilarating through its exceptionality, standing outside and above the daily routine."[16] Samuel Hynes points to numerous instances in the war narratives of British soldiers who felt compelled to join up not only out of patriotic motivations but also in search of excitement and adventure.[17] Nurses often shared these emotions and desires. Violetta Thurstan was thrilled by the prospect of "going right into the thick of things."[18] Sister

N. Chelakova appealed to her local Red Cross society immediately on the outbreak of the war, requesting to be sent "right to the action on the front lines."[19] In fact, as indicated previously, many women conceived only of frontline service as "true" wartime nursing. Although there were numerous medical facilities established in the rear, safely located in cities and towns that were far from the battlefields and military action, a great many women who volunteered as nurses expressed little interest in serving on the home front. As detailed in chapter 2, the desire to be assigned to frontline medical units was so prevalent that it presented a real problem for Russian medical authorities, who needed women to staff rear hospitals as well as field infirmaries. The notion that the combat zone was a male preserve that should be off-limits to women was never expressed by female medical personnel, despite futile attempts to keep them away from the fighting on the part of male military personnel.

For women, however, the opportunity to go to war presented something even more salient in terms of freedom and independence, as a chance to free themselves from the constrained lives of women in early twentieth-century society. The possibility of living without direct supervision of parents and other authority figures attracted a number of women to nurses' training courses. In particular, because wartime nursing came with a salary, it offered women the opportunity to shake their financial dependence on their families and make their own decisions about their lives. A number of Vanda Stepanova's friends urged her to enlist so that they could escape familial control. "You will make money and you won't depend on your parents," they told her.[20] The uniform of the sister of mercy accorded the wearer with considerable freedom of movement that would have been difficult for young women in early twentieth-century society.

Once in service women as nurses found that gendered boundaries were rather porous. This was especially true as a result of the highly motile nature of the war on the eastern front. Maintaining the barrier between front and rear, between combat and noncombat zones, between active and passive, proved to be virtually impossible for wartime medical services. Thus, Russian nurses were likely to serve very close to the fighting and were subjected to conditions similar to those of combatants. Sisters of mercy were exposed to serious deprivations and extreme danger associated with combat life; they experienced shortages of supplies and food, extremes of weather and temperature, constant fatigue, vermin infestations, and infection with contagious and epidemic diseases. Medical facilities, despite their display of the international symbol of the Red Cross to indicate their noncombatant status and thus their protection under the statutes of the Geneva Convention, were often subject to enemy fire and bombing. Mobile medical units in particular faced very dangerous conditions, because they established dressing stations close to the forward positions in order to carry out triage for wounded as quickly as possible. Nurses were often sent to the trenches and the battlefields to attend to wounded men, usually after the fighting had ceased, but even then, they often drew enemy fire.

The danger that Russian sisters of mercy faced in performing their duties is readily evident in the recorded memories of nurses' experiences. Tat'iana Aleskinskaia wrote that "booming of the guns never ceases." Her hospital train was targeted for bombing by enemy aircraft on several occasions. During one instance, a bomb completely destroyed the hut where the medical personnel had set up a dressing station; during another, a bomb fell a few feet from the train and injured several medical personnel.[21] N. Chelakova remembered that from her hospital, located in the barracks of the railway station at Ivangorod, the sounds of war were clearly heard. "Day and night we listened to the unending fire of the cannons, reminding us that the enemy was extremely near. . . . The constant boom of weapons got closer and louder, then somehow faded and became quieter, but never grew completely silent. At night, the sky was lit up by the burning woods and the entire horizon was on fire."[22] Lidiia Zakharova's mobile hospital unit was subject to heavy artillery fire and bombing on numerous occasions as well. The explosion of shells and whizzing of bullets rattled and even broke the windows of the peasant houses her unit was using as makeshift hospital rooms.[23] Farmborough's unit was shelled multiple times. She recalled one episode when she awoke in the middle of the night to the thundering sound of explosions. She and her fellow sisters ran downstairs from the room where they had been sleeping just as a shell hit and caused the house to "rock as in an earthquake; a crash of timber splitting, falling; a cascade of broken glass spilling from a height."[24] Sofia Bocharskaia and her unit sat for days listening to the rumbling of the guns.

> We began to hear the sound of heavy artillery. At first one deep, rumbling discharge . . . then another, and each seemed an individual death. They came more quickly, the sound overlapping. It went on like a storm that lasted day and night. We became

> oppressed, and the cold seemed more intense. We were never warm except in our sleeping bags. . . . For days, the earthen floor shook with the reverberation of the guns, the windows rattled.[25]

When nurses were required to carry out medical service directly in the forward positions, even in the trenches, and went into no-man's-land to retrieve wounded soldiers, they risked being shot at by enemy troops. Many became casualties themselves, wounded or killed because they were required to carry out their duties despite close proximity to the fighting. While serving as a nurse in an automobile detachment, Countess Shuvalova (Ekaterina Feodorovna Vol'f) broke her right arm as the result of an automobile accident. Sister of mercy Slushina was wounded by a bomb that fell on her unit located on the southwestern front.[26] A young nurse who had been serving in a frontline dressing station was brought into Bocharskaia's hospital for treatment after being struck by a bullet that shot through a loophole in the lines of earth in front of the trenches. The bullet lodged in her spine and paralyzed her.[27] Of course, enemy fire did not discriminate based on sex. Male medical personnel were also exposed to great danger and were wounded and even killed in the performance of their duties. Although the greatest danger came when they risked their lives carrying men from the trenches and the battlefields, they were also exposed to enemy fire at other times.

A survey of contemporary press reports clearly indicates the extent to which women performed medical duties under combat conditions. Numerous nurses were awarded medals of bravery for carrying out their duties "under heavy enemy fire," "in deadly danger," "in the midst of battle," and "in conditions of clear threat to their own lives."[28] Such examples indicate that Russia's female nurses were capable of carrying out the same kind of "heroic deeds" as men. Although many Russian military authorities insisted on the fundamental masculinity of military life, it seems clear that others accepted the idea that both men and women could display, and indeed were valued for demonstrating, heroism and other military ethics. This is most clearly demonstrated by the praise garnered by women who became soldiers during the war, but it also becomes readily evident in a number of wartime sources of Russian patriotic culture representing nurses.[29] While depictions of nurses as passive sources of comfort and solace to active male combatants were the standard, prowar sources also often portrayed nurses as active, frontline participants rescuing men in need. This was especially true with regard to images of nurses serving at the front, as opposed to those serving in the rear, and corresponded with the gendered conceptualizations of the front as masculine and the rear as feminine. Women who served as nurses on the front were often featured in more active and masculine terms, as valiant, strong, composed figures.

In his memoirs about the war experience, General Aleksei Brusilov took special note of the stellar performance of the nurses he encountered, even when under direct attack. Recalling one instance when the medical facility he was visiting was bombed, he remarked on the nurses' abilities to go about their duties without interruption:

> I should like to say a word about the nurses. The little groups of them that day had rejoiced my heart by their coolness and self-possession when the bomb fell. . . . I consider it my duty to history to put on record the unremitting, devoted and heroic services rendered by the enormous majority of them, who would not allow enemy bombs to distract them from their painful and exhausting duties as they bent over our blood-stained, suffering soldiers. How many of them, too, were wounded or killed![30]

The Russian patriotic press in particular emphasized both the immense value of services provided by these women and their undertaking of acts of great courage and self-sacrifice to treat the wounded. The term "hero" was often employed in describing such sisters of mercy. Articles in wartime periodicals featured the actions of women who put their own lives at great risk in order to attend to wounded men, displaying great strength and fortitude in extremely dangerous conditions. In fact, the story of the heroic nurse who "endured enemy fire without regard to her own life" in order to attend to the needs of the soldiers was a standard trope in the Russian press.[31] Sister Ksenia Bondarenko was awarded several military honors after her consistent efforts in bandaging the wounds of men on the battlefield. After seeing the commanding officer of her unit badly wounded, she rushed to him, lifted him up onto her shoulders, and carried him more than two kilometers to the nearest dressing station.[32] Sister N. Chelakova recalled how after their participation in the treatment of wounded during the Battle of Ivangorod, during which her military hospital came under direct enemy fire and aerial bombardment, she and her fellow nurses were awarded Saint George's medals, fourth class, which they immediately pinned to their jackets. One of her companions was from a military family, well versed in military regulations, and was quick to point out to the nurses that the medals entitled them to military pensions of one ruble per month, just like male Saint George's cavaliers.[33] Despite the active roles undertaken by these women, contemporary sources tended to emphasize the nurses' passive ability to endure hardship and danger, thus differentiating them from male combat feats.[34] Even stories about women soldiers rarely included any mention of active killing on their part, emphasizing instead their willingness to sacrifice themselves for the good of the nation.[35] Regardless, female nurses were awarded military honors for their actions in medical service. As Joshua Sanborn points out, crucial to this kind of praise was the fact that it was "shared by both women and men who were recognized for fulfilling the military ethic of 'selflessness' (*samootverzhenie*)."[36]

Although nurses serving in the forward positions shared more experiences with men in combat, even those nurses stationed in field hospitals miles from the frontline positions were not safe. Despite the established conventions of war that dictated that civilian and medical establishments were not to be targeted, aerial bombardments frequently hit medical facilities even far behind the lines. Nurses treating soldiers suffering after gas attacks were sickened and even died because the men carried gas on their clothing. Epidemic diseases did not spare female medical personnel, many of whom died after becoming infected with typhus, cholera, typhoid fever, dysentery, and other highly contagious diseases contracted from their patients. The rate of infection among medical personnel was extremely high as a result of poor sanitary conditions and close contact between patients and medical service providers. The journal of the Russian Red Cross, *The Red Cross Herald* (*Vestnik Krasnago Kresta*), as well as the main administration of the Red Cross, regularly reported illness and death among nursing personnel.[37] Both Tat'iana Varnek and her close friend Ksenia Ispolatova contracted typhus while treating soldiers ill with the disease early in 1917.[38] Florence Farmborough developed typhoid fever in August 1916, but after months of treatment and recuperation, she was able to rejoin her unit at the front in December of that year.[39] Lidiia Zakharova contracted pleurisy in late 1915, which effectively took her out of medical service for the rest of the war.[40]

There were so many sisters of mercy who fell ill early in the war that the Red Cross began to establish special hospitals dedicated to the treatment and recovery of nurses. The need for such facilities arose as a result of the fact that all other medical establishments were so full of wounded and ill soldiers that there was no place for sick nurses. By January 1915 several such hospitals had been established, including one in Warsaw with one hundred beds and another in Vilnius with fifty beds. There were also several facilities set up in Petrograd.[41] These efforts, however, did not stop nurses from being infected. In mid-1916 Aleksandra Tolstaia watched helplessly as the members of her unit stationed in Van (in eastern Turkey) fell ill with typhus one by one, from the doctors to the nurses and orderlies. Frustrated by the inability to stop the ravages of the disease and the lack of sufficient food and supplies to treat the sick, she sought out the commanding general of the Van region where she was serving. The general, however, refused to admit her to his quarters, afraid that she would infect him, and instead would only converse with her through his window.[42]

Female nurses were also vulnerable to enemy capture, despite international conventions against taking medical personnel as prisoners of war. While some sisters of mercy were only held for short periods of time, others faced lengthy captivities in the hands of German or Austrian military authorities. Their treatment was not always in line with the humane standards established by the Geneva Convention, and their captors often forced them to go without food and other necessities. Sister of mercy B. Radonich served less than a month at the front before being taken prisoner by the Germans. She and the three other nurses assigned to her unit were held for more than four months in enemy hands. Radonich kept a diary during the entire period of captivity, carefully recording their experiences.[43] While Radonich indicated that she and her fellow nurses were not harmed, even if their needs were often neglected (they were often deprived of food and denied medical attention when they became ill), she was much more disturbed by the horrible treatment of the Russian soldiers who were in German captivity, and by the fact that the Germans refused to allow them to provide care for the ill and wounded among them, who were barely fed enough to survive.

Frontline nurses also shared the same kinds of depravations and harsh conditions of life in a war zone that men often underwent as soldiers. As indicated in chapter 3, they often lived in makeshift accommodations such as tents with little in the way of creature comforts, exposed to the elements. Some even expressed the idea that women were more capable of enduring the demanding conditions of field life. Quite surprisingly, Countess Ol'ga Putiatina, who had never known any discomfort in her civilian life, remarked that she quite enjoyed living in a tent, even noting that "the airy nights in tents keep us all fit." In fact, she lamented when her unit was transferred to more permanent indoor structures: "It is sad to have left our dear camp and be in rooms but 'thems our orders' because our menfolk don't care for tents."[44]

Even women used to much more luxurious accommodations made sacrifices and adjustments to frontline life. Grand Duchess Ol'ga Aleksandrovna (youngest sister of Tsar Nicholas II), unlike many of her royal and aristocratic counterparts who served in rear medical facilities and experienced little disruption of their standards of living, went to the front and served in a military hospital that lacked many basic necessities, including sufficient bathing facilities. The grand duchess was, however, able to use her position to occasionally escape the deprivations of the war zone by visiting her brother-in-law "Sandro" (Grand Duke Alexander Mikhailovich, who was married to her eldest sister) on his private military train, where she was able to have tea and bathe.[45]

Scarcities of basic necessities plagued both medical workers and combat troops. Food was often in short supply, and problems of distribution further exacerbated this problem. Soldiers' letters home are full of complaints about food, this being a primary concern (giving teeth to the old adage, "an army runs on its stomach"). As one soldier dictated to Lidiia Zakharova in a letter to his wife, "with regard to food, of course, it is bad—so many days we sit in the trenches without anything hot, only some dry crusts and raw cabbage, because it is forbidden to light fires in the trenches. However, this is military life."[46] Farmborough related a similar situation in her flying column. "There were times," she recalled, "when our *sukharki* meant all in all to us." On one occasion, the unit was overjoyed when they received word that a bakery had been persuaded to supply them with fresh bread. They waited all day, "hungry, angry, tired and wet through, for the weather had no pity on us," but the bread never appeared. They finally were given one *pud* (roughly equivalent to 36 pounds) to feed the entire unit. The bread was given to the rank and file (the soldiers who served as orderlies, drivers, and other auxiliary personnel), while the medical staff "had to be content with potatoes." But considering the conditions, Farmborough exclaimed, "We were more than content! We boiled some, roasted others in the hot ashes of our fire and, then, under shelter of the overhanging trees . . . we lay down on the damp earth and dozed."[47]

The pace of life for wartime nurses at the front was also reminiscent of experiences of the men in the trenches. Soldiers often remarked that much of their time was spent in inactivity, awaiting the next skirmish or battle. Military nursing in the forward positions was also often characterized by long periods of inaction, frequently punctuated by intense bursts of activity, during and immediately following significant military engagements. When this occurred, wartime nurses found themselves treating hundreds of patients in what seemed to be a never-ending stream of mutilated bodies. These sessions could last for days, and nurses usually worked consistently through them until the wounded men stopped flowing into their units. Nurses needed to demonstrate tremendous endurance during these periods. They worked for hours on end without pausing to eat or sleep. Tat'iana Varnek, when transferred with her unit to the Carpathians in mid-1915 where heavy fighting was occurring, remembered having to work thirty-six-hour shifts as a result of the shortage of nurses in her field hospital. Three nurses treated more than one hundred heavily wounded men, and they alternated performing night duty after completing their day shifts every three days.[48] Even when they did rest for short periods, they often found these little respites were not useful. Lidiia Zakharova discovered this the hard way, after her first night at the front:

> Only by morning, with an aching head and worn-out legs, did I doze off for an hour in a corner of the tent, and this short rest served as a graphic lesson for me, demonstrating that at war one must forget legitimate, everyday, narrow-minded life rules, such as that at night one must lay down to sleep and that after work it is necessary to rest in order to restore one's lost energy. At war, one must remain at one's post while one's legs do not collapse out of fatigue, and that a short, restless nap only makes one less lively and weaker.[49]

Khristina Semina also commented on the effects of fatigue:

> Clean, young, girls, bubbling with life, left home, and after one year these were pale, nervous women. Many began to smoke, so as not to fall asleep on their feet. Often they did not sleep for two or three nights in a row, when a battle was going on and wounded were brought into the hospital in a continuous stream. There was already no space, no beds, not even on the floor. And the wounded continued to be brought in and brought in, without end. . . . You only heard—"sister! sister!"—coming from all sides. . . . You did not

> know where to go, who to offer help to first! Your legs still moved. Your head was spinning. Your back hurt. . . . But you could not sit or rest. You had to go help those who were suffering.[50]

Sleep deprivation was one of the most common results of these periods of constant activity for frontline nurses. Zakharova noted these effects. "Sleeplessness made itself felt. Consciousness of double-vision: while the hands were doing some familiar task, the other part of the brain . . . was carried off into fantasy."[51] After spending an entire day and night treating patients on a hospital train, Chelakova returned to her accommodations in the military hospital in Ivangorod in a state of complete exhaustion, fell into her bed fully clothed, and slept feverishly for more than twenty-four hours. Despite the fact that she was supposed to report for duty in the hospital ward early the next morning, her nursing comrades were so worried about her health that they covered for her, allowing her to sleep off her fever and recover.[52]

Yet, as for soldiers in the trenches, constant action was not the norm. Like combat, medical service was also characterized by periods of waiting and boredom, when nurses had few patients and few duties to perform. During such lulls, nurses, like soldiers, became restless, even malaised, wondering what purpose they were serving. Zakharova's mobile hospital experienced downtime between battles, and even after being moved to new locations to serve in areas deemed to need medical service, she and the members of her unit often sat around for days with little to do. Chelakova, on arriving at the infectious disease hospital to which she was first assigned, found the facility completely empty of patients, leaving her and the three other nurses dispatched with her with nothing to do but sit outside the facility and wait. Later, while serving in the military hospital in Ivangorod, she once again found herself with little to do once the battles had ceased and the Germans had withdrawn from the area. She recalled that after the German withdrawal, she felt despondent: "The war, with its heroism and self-sacrifice had left us behind. We remained in the barracks with empty beds. All of the brightness we had experienced and the feeling that we were taking part in something grandiose, disappeared with the departure of the soldiers, and Ivangorod once again became a small, dirty station . . . standing forlornly under the winter sky, among black puddles of melting snow."[53] Bocharskaia complained that her unit was often idle and she had to beg the medical authorities to send them to an area of the front where wounded men needed attention.[54]

Aleksinskaia remarked that during the periods after all the wounded carried by her train had been delivered to local hospitals, she too felt bored.[55] Nurses had to balance these periods with those of intense, seemingly endless work. Male medical workers similarly complained when there was insufficient work to keep them busy. Dmitri Furmanov recalled periods when "there was nothing to do. The dropping of hands, the ceasing of thoughts of work, has a mournful effect on the soul."[56]

Perhaps most surprisingly, male combatants and female medical personnel actually share some commonalities with regard to the violence of war, despite the fact that nursing and soldiering seem to be distinctly set apart by the binary opposition of their missions. Men in trenches and on battlefields have as their purpose the intentional infliction of violence on the bodies of others, which seems worlds away from the nurse's mission of providing care and medical treatment to the ill and wounded. However, violence is not exclusive to the vocation of soldiering and to its associative masculinity. True, nurses were not called on to kill, rather to cure, but to argue that they were not expected to inflict violence on human bodies is not entirely accurate. Often the act of providing lifesaving treatment involved participation in the cutting of flesh, the amputation of limbs, the removal of organs, the boring of holes into live beings, and not infrequently without the benefit of proper sterilization or anesthetic. Nurses themselves often commented on how such actions seemed brutal and violent. During her first experience assisting in surgery to remove the shattered leg of a soldier, Sofia Bocharskaia had such a reaction. "A frantic protest rose in me that to do such a thing to a man's leg was butchery," she remarked. "It was unnatural. The flesh looked firm and healthy. You could not turn a human body into a dreadful, lopped fragment of a man."[57]

Women's wartime nursing echoed other, more positive (whether real or imagined) aspects of male combatant war experiences. In particular, women in wartime nursing service often spoke of forming close personal connections with other members of their units. These relationships were forged by the extreme circumstances in which they were placed, wherein they endured hardships and worked together to achieve a common goal. This camaraderie was portrayed as cutting across national as well as class lines, and as such was highly reflective of elements of the male myth of war experience that emphasized social leveling and the creation of national unity.[58] In the last years of tsarist rule, military theorists had promoted the idea that soldiers needed to feel closely, even emotionally connected to one another in order to be willing to kill and die for one another. They did so most frequently by invoking the theme of the nation as a family, encouraging the creation of a "band of brothers" among troops, officers and soldiers alike, cutting across class lines. Intellectual Ia. Okunev, despite the large educational and social chasm that existed between himself and his fellow soldiers, remembered his war experience as one in which "we somehow became simpler, we merged. We organically grew together, soul to soul, body to body, with the golden-bearded *muzhiks* [peasant men] striding side by side with us on Austrian soil. . . . In our soul it became spacious and clean because the usual labels and formulas for things, ideas and feelings were no longer there."[59] Similarly, they strove for the construction of a unified, multinational army (reflecting the multinational character of the Russian empire). As Joshua Sanborn explains, "Russia was the mother and soldiers were 'fellow brothers.' The idea propagandized by the military leadership that soldiers were fellow brothers caught on well before the February Revolution put the word fraternity on everyone's lips."[60] As soldier Vladimir Paduchev commented, "[Being] in constant proximity to the enemy, with equal chances for life and death, brought individuals together into a tight and friendly family. The content of living relationships was suffused by equality and friendship."[61]

In this formulation of the imperial family, the women who became nurses were literally the "sisters," giving adding national significance to their duty. It was through their medical service that they could be part of this national family, which would inspire the same feelings of "loyalty, closeness, and above all, unity"[62] intended for male soldiers. Like combat, wartime medical service also fostered cohesiveness between individuals from various nationalities living in the Russian empire. Entering the ranks of medical service allowed women from diverse social and national backgrounds to work, live, and socialize together. In many cases, this would have been unlikely, if not impossible, in civilian life. The shared living conditions, the dangers, the deprivations, and closeness to death led to the creation of close ties among female medical personnel. Some even developed personal relationships that cut across the lines of social stratification. Chelakova expressed such sentiments, commenting on the social diversity of her military hospital, where she claimed doctors and nurses from the social elite served harmoniously with peasant orderlies.[63] Varnek, despite her aristocratic pedigree, remarked similarly that she had formed friendships with the peasant orderlies in one of the hospitals to which she was assigned. She spoke of their mutual affection and trust, even to the point that the orderlies would come to her for advice.[64] Sisters of mercy spoke of feelings of camaraderie with fellow nurses similar to the kind of male bonding often attributed to soldiers. Farmborough wrote about the fellowship she witnessed between the wounded in the rear hospital where she served before being sent to the front: "There is a remarkable camaraderie among them: White Russian [Belarussians] mingles in the most friendly fashion with Ukrainian; Caucasians with soldiers from the Urals; Tatars with Cossacks."[65] Britnieva spoke of close relationships with the fellow nurses in her unit, despite their differences in national origin (Russian, Baltic, Italian, and English). Writing about her experiences years after the war, Britnieva commented about her relationship with her fellow sisters of mercy, "this friendship has lasted to this day; even though we are all scattered now."[66] Lidiia Zakharova, being evacuated to the interior after falling ill with pleurisy, exchanged bittersweet farewells with her fellow medical personnel. As her ambulance pulled away, she said through her tears, "No, I will not forget you, dear Aleksei Petrovich, [the head doctor], Ol'ga Aleksandrovna [the senior nurse], dear gentle Nikolai Nikolaevich [one of the medics], and all the rest of the dear sisters. . . . I will not forget even one day, one hour, spent with you. I can save all the valuable treasures, which I found through valuable work, deprivation, and sleepless nights."[67] Chelakova remembered fondly her military hospital "family," which was composed of Russians, Poles, Jews, and Ukrainians. She commented that "all of us, doctors, nurses, and orderlies, gathered together from different ends of the country and from different environments (backgrounds), as if to create a colorful pattern of national customs and foundations, beliefs and devotions, that constitute all of the diverse conditions of existence. Soon we became like one big, friendly family."[68] Grand Duchess Maria Pavlovna commented, "The nurse's uniform brought me close to those who wore khaki."[69] Grand Duchess Ol'ga Aleksandrovna commented that she and her fellow nurses developed very tight friendships. In the evenings, if and when they had any free time, they would occasionally all "pile in bed together" and spend hours on end "conversing comfortably in rare pleasure."[70] In a statement that is reminiscent of many male sentiments that emphasized the close relationships forged by war, English expatriate Violetta Thurstan commented, "War would be the most glorious game in the world if it were not for the killing and wounding. In it one tastes the joys of comradeship to the full, the taking and giving, and helping and being helped in a way that would be impossible to conceive in the ordinary world."[71]

In many ways, as it was for the men in combat from varying social, national, and political backgrounds thrust together forcibly by the circumstances of conscription, this kind of social melding, and even the notion of camaraderie in the trenches, was mythological. Male soldiers did not always feel true connections with their fellow combatants. The "brothers-in-arms" notion has been challenged by a number of scholars who have discovered a very different vein running through the writings of soldiers of the Great War.[72] As historians such as Karen Petrone have indicated, the feelings of closeness and familial surrogacy were promoted vertically rather than horizontally to reflect tsarist social structures, with commanders as substitute father figures rather than fraternal equals to their soldier charges. Petrone has found that some Russian soldiers expressed considerable antipathy toward their officers and even their fellow combatants at times. Nor were the markers of nationality removed by wartime service, and many members of non-Russian nationalities continued to be ostracized and persecuted, even within the context of the Russian military. And as indicated in chapter 3, social status was still a powerful determinant of experience and greatly influenced the ways that nurses served and were treated, often causing rifts between nurses that could not be overcome even in the context of the war. Thus, we need to take the statements by the women who served as nurses regarding the camaraderie they claimed to experience with some reservation. Nonetheless, whether real or imagined, this kind of bonding was one expressed by nurses and soldiers, men and women alike.

TRANSFORMATIVE EXPERIENCES: APPEARANCES

Perhaps one of the most obvious blurrings of gender boundaries came in the form of the outward appearances of the women who performed wartime nursing service. At first glance, the visual representation of nurses seems entirely consistent with normative values of femininity. The uniform of the sister of mercy consisted of traditional elements of female clothing: a long dress, a smock covering the dress, a head kerchief. These were items that only women would wear. Moreover, their dress, as well as the title of "sister," was specifically reminiscent of that of a particular kind of woman: a nun, even the Virgin Mary herself. This is the most prominent image associated with Russian sisters of mercy (in fact, of nurses from nearly all the belligerents), as depicted in figure 4.1.

While maintaining such attire while working in rear hospitals and other medical facilities away from the forward positions may have been unproblematic, a number of women in medical service at the front found their work easier when they abandoned what were considered to be other normative feminine characteristics and attributes of their physical appearance. Long, loose dresses and women's shoes were not ideal for carrying out service at the front, where nurses faced the extremes of weather and the ever-present mud of the forward positions. They needed protection from the elements and the ability to move about freely under difficult conditions. As a result, many women adapted their clothing to suit their circumstances. Most commonly, they adopted high leather soldiers' boots and very masculine-looking leather jackets (those reminiscent of the early Soviet commissars). Some communities of sisters even recommended that nurses acquire these items before leaving for the front. A few went so far as to abandon their dresses in favor of trousers. Numerous photographs of nurses at the front, such as the one depicted in figure 4.2, attest to this very different visual impression from the saintly, white-hooded sister of mercy of conventional wisdom. In early 1915 the popular journal *Niva* published a picture of a sister of mercy who was awarded a Saint George's medal for carrying out difficult work under enemy fire on the front lines. The young woman was dressed in pants, a leather jacket, high boots, and a Cossack hat, sitting on horseback. The only indication of her status as a nurse is the white armband with the Red Cross insignia emblazoned on it. Otherwise, she looks distinctly masculine in her dress and pose.[73] The cover photo on Florence Farmborough's memoir of her experiences with the Russian Red Cross features her in leather jacket, pants, hat, and high boots—again, with the white armband decorated with a red cross the only indication of her status as a nurse.[74]

Changing one's outward appearance often had internal effects on wartime nurses. In general, the war was a transformative experience for many women. Lidiia Zakharova commented that when she arrived at the front, she felt as if she had been "swallowed up" in a new life, "carried away in a powerful stream," as if the war was changing her into an entirely different being. The process initiated a specific gender transformation in

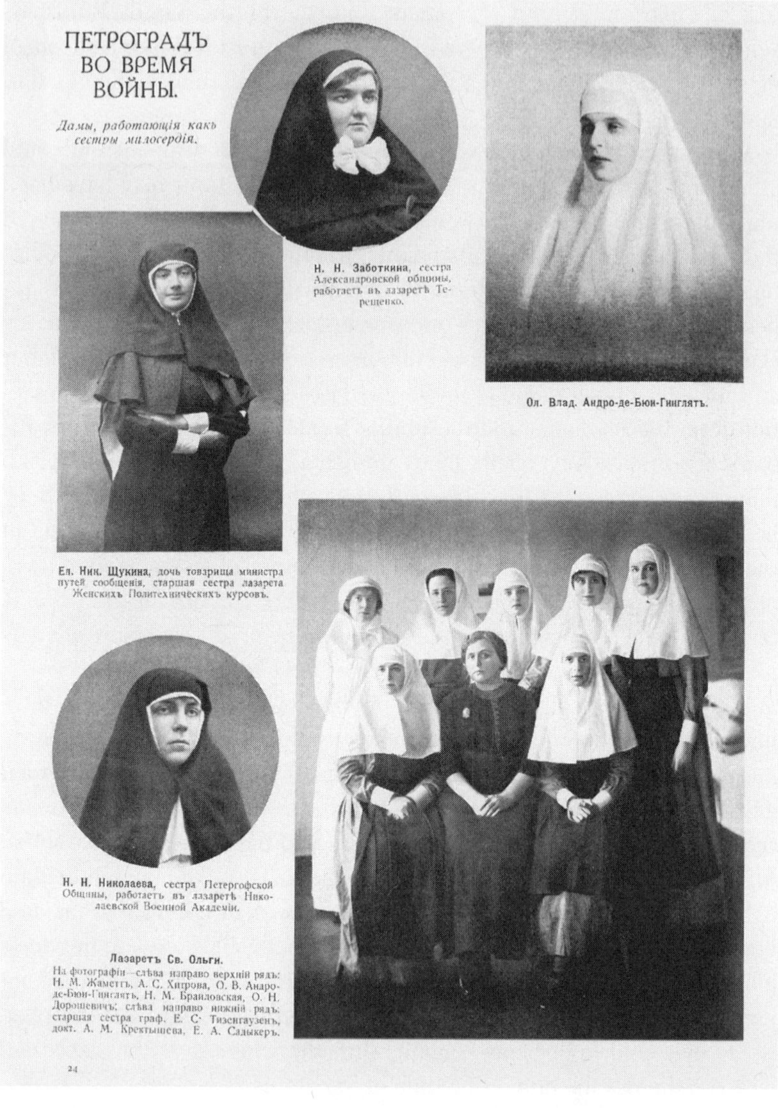

ПЕТРОГРАДЪ ВО ВРЕМЯ ВОЙНЫ.

Дамы, работающія какъ сестры милосердія.

Н. Н. Заботкина, сестра Александровской общины, работаетъ въ лазаретѣ Терещенко.

Ол. Влад. Андро-де-Бюи-Гинглятъ.

Ел. Ник. Щукина, дочь товарища министра путей сообщенія, старшая сестра лазарета Женскихъ Политехническихъ курсовъ.

Н. Н. Николаева, сестра Петергофской Общины, работаетъ въ лазаретѣ Николаевской Военной Академіи.

Лазаретъ Св. Ольги.

На фотографіи—слѣва направо верхній рядъ: Н. М. Жаметтъ, А. С. Хитрова, О. В. Андро-де-Бюи-Гинглятъ, Н. М. Брайловская, О. Н. Дорошевичъ; слѣва направо нижній рядъ: старшая сестра граф. Е. С. Тизенгаузенъ, докт. А. М. Кректышева, Е. А. Садыкеръ.

24

Figure 4.1. The traditional uniform of the Russian sister of mercy. "Petrograd vo vremia voiny" [Petrograd during the war], *Stolitsa i usadba*, February 15, 1915, 24.

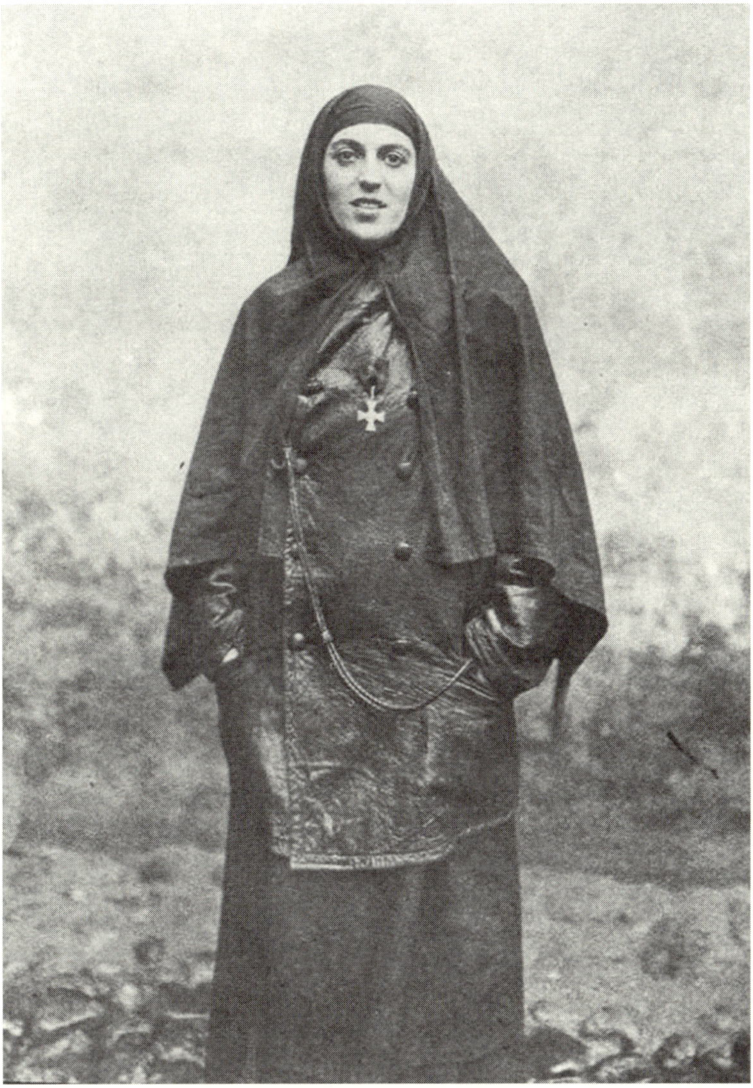

Figure 4.2. Wartime nurses often opted for more practical clothing, such as sturdy leather jackets and high men's boots, in order to better endure the conditions of war. An unknown sister of mercy in leather jacket, awarded a St. George's cross. http://www.pravmir.ru/georgievskie-kavaleryi-velikoy-voynyi/.

her, and she commented that over time "there remained in me less and less of the feminine." Her change, like that of other women in war service, took on physical manifestations, and she remarked that she felt more comfortable in her role after purchasing a man's leather coat. She also felt very fortunate to acquire a pair of what she called "excellent men's boots," which she remarked came in handy on a number of occasions when she was trudging through the deep, sticky mud that characterized much of the front.[75]

The physical transformations caused by the experience of war, particularly the loss of associative characteristics of female beauty, were not always intentional or welcomed by nursing personnel, however. Ol'ga Putiatina complained in a letter to her mother that as a result of working in the field, she "had turned brown."[76] Farmborough lamented the effects of service at the front on her appearance. "We looked at our hands; they were rough, reddened, scratched and weatherbeaten; our boots were clumsy, shapeless, lumbering; our black leather coats, torn, scraped and discoloured; and our faces! Ah! Surely our faces had suffered the most! . . . We knew without being told, or shown, that our faces were bronzed, freckled, lined by lack of sleep and hardened by the endless effort to endure discomfort and to alleviate pain."[77]

For Aleksandra Tolstaia, the change in her appearance was attributed to her long absence from the "civilized world," from the comforts of "automobiles, electricity, [and] good restaurants." After merely a month with her mobile unit, she commented that she had been "completely weaned from civilization and no longer paid any attention to my appearance. Indeed, this would have been impossible to do during campaigns." The skin on her face was flaking off as a result of extended exposure to sun and wind. Instead of wearing the long dress uniform of a sister of mercy, for easier travel by horseback she had adopted Caucasian dress, including undergarments and trousers that had become greasy, gray, and soaked in horses' sweat. She also sported high boots and a black sheepskin hat with a white hood, worn in defense against the beating sun. Although she realized that for practical reasons, this transformation was necessary, nonetheless, she bemoaned that "truly, I was a scary sight." Tolstaia even carried a revolver with her at all times as she traveled through the Caucuses and eastern Turkey, despite her mission as a medical worker.[78]

TRANSFORMATIVE EXPERIENCES: BEHAVIORS

The war also gave some nurses the opportunity, or forced them, to act in other ways clearly outside normative behaviors for women. Rather than adopting purely passive and supportive roles, as secondary background figures to the primary male heroes of the war, many women engaged in activities that were active and even aggressive at times. They took on leadership positions and gave orders to others, including men. They carried out significant organizational roles and undertook important decisions. They sometimes even engaged in military action, including combat. In a number of ways, frontline service imposed a level of "masculinization" on wartime nurses.

The conditions of war, especially at the front, were such that women who became wartime nurses often displayed characteristics and behaviors that would have been problematic for them in normal peacetime conditions. Khristina Semina recalled that nurses were encouraged to smoke as much as possible to allow them to stay awake during long shifts. If a doctor noticed that a nurse was showing signs of extreme fatigue, he would often give her a cigarette. This was despite the fact that, according to Semina, most of these women had never touched a cigarette before in their lives. Even her own husband, who had argued vehemently against Khristina's participation in arduous medical service, came to encourage this behavior in his genteel wife.[79] Although not completely uncommon for women, smoking carried with it significant gendered associations in early twentieth-century Russia (and elsewhere), as it was a trait specifically associated with masculinity, and particularly the military. For women, it conveyed a certain cultural taboo, and female smokers were attacked for lack of womanliness.[80] As such, smoking was inconsistent with the conventional feminized image of the nurse, but its practice by wartime nurses reflected the more fluid gender space of the front lines.

Wartime nurses acted in ways clearly outside their gendered peacetime experiences when, in certain circumstances, they were placed in positions of leadership. Russian sisters of mercy were supervised by senior or head nurses, who had extensive authority over the women, and men in the form of orderlies, in their charge. Although Red Cross regulations dictated that senior nurses be appointed exclusively from staff sisters (i.e., professional trained nurses who had been part of the Red Cross societies prior to the outbreak of war, in contrast to the wartime sisters who enlisted after), aristocratic women without such designation were often found in these positions. The exigencies of personnel shortages dictated that nurses without sufficient experience be appointed as head nurses, while others used their "social positions and their connections in society" to secure senior nurse status.[81] For example, the Grand Duchess Maria Pavlovna, despite her youth and limited training and experience, was made head nurse of a rear hospital in Pskov in October 1914.[82] In other instances, deficiencies of personnel and poor organization sometimes required women to step into roles of command designated for men. When male doctors or other personnel were killed or unavailable, sisters of mercy sometimes ended up leading flying or other mobile medical detachments at the front.

While female authority in the domestic realm was significant in Russian society, such authority would have been highly improbable in the public sphere in normal peacetime conditions. Yet, as head and senior nurses, women found themselves in the position of giving orders rather than following them, sometimes for the first time in their lives, and sometimes even with authority over men. For many, such experiences were exhilarating and liberating for women who had previously lived restricted lives. Most interestingly, one encounters these comments among women of the upper classes, who, in a number of ways, had less freedom of action and less ability to operate in the public sphere than their working-class and peasant counterparts.[83] Grand Duchess Maria Pavlovna experienced difficulty adjusting to a role that demanded that she give, rather than receive, orders and make important decisions regarding the hospital's administration. She remarked, "I had since childhood been taught submission and obedience. It was easy and perfectly natural for me to carry out orders; but I could not, did not know how to, give any."[84]

Despite reservations about women's authority, the shortage of medical personnel coupled with the great need for qualified doctors meant that women often took on leadership roles. This included a number of female doctors who were placed in charge of medical units and had authority over men. Tat'iana Aleksinskaia served under a chief woman doctor, who not only had authority over all the other doctors in the unit, some of whom were men, but also commanded forty male orderlies assigned to their hospital train.[85] Aleksandra Tol'staia was also commanded by a female doctor who oversaw the operations of her hospital train. Not all men were opposed to female leadership; the senior doctor of the military hospital to which Chelakova was assigned was so impressed with the way that the head nurse of the unit handled her position that he gave her additional duties. She was put in charge of the management of all the medical personnel in the hospital and assisted in all surgeries.[86] Clearly, this doctor did not have a problem with a woman supervising male personnel, since there were four other doctors assigned to the hospitals, plus a large number of male orderlies.

The women who went farthest outside the traditional gender boundaries were the sisters who became active in combat activities. Some actually entered nursing only in order to get to the front and then, when the opportunity presented itself, exchanged their sister of mercy uniforms for soldiers' garb in order to become combatants. A number of these women had attempted to enlist in military capacities but had been turned away as a result of the imperial Russian law that prohibited women from combat service. Accomplished pilot E. P. Samsonova resorted to nursing only after her numerous requests to become a military pilot were turned down by the Russian military authorities. She did not last long in this capacity, finding nursing to be unsatisfying, and instead became a military driver at the front.[87] Farmborough mentioned encountering at the front women who had enlisted as nurses but, once they arrived at the forward positions, shed their nursing attire, shaved their heads, and donned soldiers' uniforms. Aleksinskaia similarly noted a volunteer in her hospital train who joined the medical services only in order to get close enough to the front to slip into the ranks of a combat unit.[88] Other women ended up serving as nurses after being discovered in the ranks of combat units, disguised as men, and were sent to nursing communities for medical training.[89]

Some nurses entered combat less deliberately, as was the case with Rimma Ivanova. Ivanova's story is illustrative of not only how Russia's wartime nurses sometimes broke with convention to act in ways clearly outside traditional notions of femininity but also the ambiguity with which women's active roles in war were regarded in Russian society. On the outbreak of the war, Ivanova enrolled in nursing training courses in her hometown of Stavropol'. After completing the courses, she was sent to a local hospital. But she wanted to be closer to the front, so, despite the exhortations of her parents to remain safely in the rear, in January 1915 she left to join the 83rd Samur Infantry Regiment. Initially, she did so disguised as a male medic, using the pseudonym Ivan Mikhailovich Ivanov. Apparently, this disguise did not last (although it is unclear why), because soon after she was back in the nurse's uniform as Rimma Mikhailovna Ivanova. She spent six months with this unit, attending to wounded men on the battlefield. While in this capacity, she earned two military (noncombat) medals, third and fourth degree, for her bravery. According to Stavropol' archivist Elena Gromova, however, what Ivanova cherished most was the "tender brotherly love of the officers and soldiers" whom she served. She wrote home proudly stating that she needed to be at the front, because "here they do not look at me as a woman, but see me as a sister of mercy, deserving of greater respect."[90]

Ivanova returned home in July 1915 but remained there only briefly, returning to the front in August to serve with the 105th Orenburg Infantry Regiment alongside her brother, a junior doctor in the unit. Apparently, her brother tried to convince her to stay in the regimental hospital, but she insisted on going to the front. She was attached to the tenth company of this unit and served directly on the front lines. Despite the great danger to which she exposed herself in this capacity, she successfully pulled more than six hundred wounded men from the battlefield. On September 9, 1915, Ivanova was in the trenches bandaging wounded soldiers when she realized that all the officers had been killed or wounded and the unit was left without command personnel. She took it upon herself to lead the troops on the attack. Her efforts were successful and the unit broke through to the enemy trenches, but she was wounded in the fray and died shortly after the attack.

The men of her unit were so moved by her actions and by her death that they successfully petitioned the tsar to grant her a Saint George's Cross for her bravery. The order was one usually only given to combatants (the last woman who received such a military award was Nadezhda Durova, a woman who had fought in the Napoleonic Wars of the early nineteenth century, disguised as a man). But while the Russians lauded Ivanova's actions, they were protested by the German Red Cross, which cited the international convention requiring the neutrality of medical personnel and complained that as a nurse, it was not "fitting to carry out military feats." The case was brought before the International Committee of the Red Cross in Geneva, but the office did not agree with the Germans' conclusions and it was dismissed. Ivanova retained the posthumous award and became a legend in Russia.[91]

CONCLUSIONS

In August 1916 Farmborough fell ill with typhoid fever just before her *letuchka* was ordered to move to another position. After examining her, the doctors forbade her from traveling with the unit and instead ordered her to be sent to a base hospital far behind the lines. She was distraught. "I wept bitterly and protested vehemently, but tears and protests were of no avail. So this was the end; a miserable, humiliating end to all my longed-for Red Cross work. I lay helpless in my bed, torn by misery and fever." She was transferred by means of a horse-drawn cart, which made her feel guilty, believing she did not deserve the same comforts afforded to wounded soldiers. Despite her serious illness, she longed to return to the front and hated the thought that "work was going on without me."[92] After a month at the base hospital, Farmborough was sent to a sanatorium in the Crimea to complete her recuperation. During that time, her hair, which had been falling out in large clumps, was shaved completely to allow new growth. This was a very disturbing experience for the young woman, despite the fact that she had earlier admitted how "rough" she had come to look as a result of her field experience. She took to wearing her nurse's veil at all times to hide her bald head. When she finally had made a full recovery, she used her remaining leave time to return to the Moscow home of her Russian employer, Doctor Usov, who had recently suffered a heart attack. After several weeks there, her leave was up and she happily rejoined her unit at the front in December 1916. Her hair had still not grown back, so she kept it covered whenever she was in male company, only allowing her fellow sisters to see her without her veil. She served with the unit through 1917, observing from afar the events of the revolution that brought down the tsarist government in February/March, when little military action was taking place. But beginning in mid-June 1917, with a new offensive launched by the Provisional Government, her work intensified once again when scores of wounded and dying men were brought into her unit for treatment.

As with many memories of war, Farmborough's reminiscences are full of commentary about the tremendous strain of war on those who came into contact with its destructiveness. They also frequently point to the shared experiences of those in wartime service, regardless of gender. Thus, an examination of the services performed by Russia's nurses demonstrates the problems with the common assumption that medical positions were less dangerous and better suited to "weaker" women than other wartime activities such as combat. Their writings indicate clearly that Russian nurses did not merely stand by the bedsides of the wounded as a passive source of comfort and solace to the active male combatants. They were sometimes required to perform tasks clearly outside the conventional purview of early twentieth-century female roles. They acted in dynamic, forceful, and sometimes even aggressive ways. Women's wartime nursing activity also obscured the separation between gendered conceptions of public and private spheres. They operated outside of the protected domestic realm in distinctly public service. Although performing functions that were considered normatively feminine, they were carrying them out in what was considered the most masculine of spaces: the war front. Thus, the nurses disrupted traditional notions of caring and nurturing, of motherhood itself, by taking it out of its domestic context. In a number of significant ways, they defy categorization, confound traditional notions of gender, and indicate the fluidity of gender roles and behaviors created by the war. As such, these experiences challenge us to think about war in ways outside of strictly gendered conceptions.

5

PSYCHOLOGICAL WARFARE

LIDIIA ZAKHAROVA: WIFE AND MOTHER TURNED SISTER

Lidiia Zakharova recalled that the evening she departed Petrograd for the front was warm and clear, with a light breeze. She stood on the railway platform with doctors, orderlies, and other nurses, all waiting to board the train that would take them into the war zone. As she watched the large, white head kerchiefs of the sisters "flapping like the wings of butterflies flying under the glass roof of the station," she was unable to imagine "this terrible and ominous thing called war." Once on board the train, she and her fellow medical personnel passed the time on the long journey being amused by the humorous stories of one of the doctors in their unit. Occasionally, Zakharova lapsed into daydreams, envisioning the recent summer months she and her two young sons had spent on the golden beaches of Estonia. These pleasant thoughts were brutally interrupted by her memory of the call to war, which had forced her husband to leave the family vacation prematurely to join the fighting. She remembered seeing him off at the train station, surrounded by hundreds of others similarly bidding farewell to their loved ones, "crying, all wishing to go, demanding, angry, praying." Feeling unsettled and empty after he left, she had decided to enlist in nursing services and go to the front herself.[1]

After going as far as they could by train, Zakharova and her unit continued to their destination by horse cart. The farther they went, the more desolate the places became, most of the inhabitants of the villages and towns having fled the advance of the war. Travel became increasingly difficult. The cart bumped along roads that had recently been shelled or torn apart by large numbers of marching troops dragging their weapons, ammunition, field kitchens, and other equipment and supplies along with them, the remnants of which were often strewn along the road. They also encountered lightly wounded soldiers, recently bandaged at a nearby dressing station, who appeared to Zakharova as "strange human figures, grey, dusty, as if burned in the fire of war . . . walking slowly and obediently, without lifting their heads, a few of them stopping by the edge of the road to allow our convoy to go by, and following them with long, indifferent looks." Behind them were the transports carrying the seriously wounded, who "lay motionless in uncomfortable positions, with their eyes closed and faces pale." Soon after, Zakharova and her traveling companions saw their first corpse. It was a German infantryman, lying on the side of the road with his legs tucked up under him. "Instinctively, I tried to lie to myself to get myself to believe that he wasn't dead, just asleep or drunk," she recalled. The lie did not work well, and she glanced at the nurse sitting beside her to gauge her reaction: "Sister Mosina sat straight and looked ahead with an unblinking stare. Her eyebrows were knitted, her lips tight, and her kind young face showed suffering of many years." The doctor traveling with them, Aleksei Petrovich S., sensing their emotional distress, tried to comfort them. "It is nothing, nothing, sisters, hold on to your nerves. At first it is terrible, but then you get used to it." Initially, this was of little consolation. "We tried to smile, but the sound of a live human voice had an unsettling effect," Zakharova remembered. Over time, they became accustomed to such sights and were even able to channel their emotions into more constructive responses. "Little by little, the terrible feeling dispersed, and the sight of blood and suffering no longer caused fainthearted weakness, but rather burning, sharp desire to heal and help." When the field hospital to which she was assigned, the final destination of their journey, came into view, Zakharova was somewhat heartened by the prospect of getting to work.

> Far away on the edge of a small wood, in relief against the dark leaves, a tall pole with the flag of the red cross flying from it could be seen. . . . I was engulfed by a feeling of deep emotion and the desire to bow my head before the beautiful banner of mercy, under the canopy of which I was getting ready to fight, as a small, insignificant private in a great army.[2]

Arriving at the hospital, Zakharova and her unit quickly went to work unpacking and setting up their dressing station. The potential to be useful in the war effort continued to buoy her spirits; "I quickly came to the realization that from this moment I was not that previous woman, who lived, suffered and enjoyed up to this minute, that something else had begun, that I did not even have my previous name, I was 'sister,' a new person with a name that came before all other interests, sadness and happiness." Despite her newfound sense of purpose and direction, the effects of carrying out medical service among the wounded were harrowing. After the first twenty-four hours of work, during which Zakharova had been so overwhelmed with patients that she had had no time to rest or even to eat, she felt emotionally raw, so much so that the sound of a soldier's voice expressing concern for her well-being caused her to burst into tears. Once again, the doctor tried to reassure her and fortify her for continued work. "'Stand firm, sister,' said Doctor S., 'this is only the beginning . . . ' He did not finish his thought."[3]

COPING MECHANISMS

Women who served Russia as nurses during the Great War not only shared many of the external and physical experiences of war with men who fought; they endured similar emotional and psychological effects. Although for some the impact of the war was too great a burden psychologically, leading to breakdowns and serious mental disorders, most nurses managed to cope, employing a variety of different means to function effectively under extremely trying conditions. They grew accustomed to seeing the disastrous effects of modern weapons on human bodies, to hearing constant cries of pain, to being exposed to violence, mutilation, death, and dying. They adjusted to the sounds of bombs and shells exploding, to the point where they often no longer registered them as menacing or even heard them at all. And perhaps most significant to the gendered nature of wartime nursing, in order to continue to perform their duties, many sisters of mercy shut off their emotions, at least partially or temporarily. A number of Russia's wartime nurses indicated that emotional care and support was not always possible or practical in carrying out their medical duties. The vast numbers of wounded being treated, the high death toll, the rapid pace at which nurses were required to work, the limited amount of time they spent with each patient, and the dangerous conditions under which they labored meant that nurses could not, and in many instances found it easier not to, form bonds with or even express sentiment toward their charges.

Examining the psychological impact of wartime nursing is immensely instructive in indicating the extent to which separation of gender roles and of masculinity and femininity proved difficult, if not impossible, in the chaotic upheaval of the conflict. It is particularly important in the context of early twentieth-century notions of nursing as an appropriate activity for women, which were largely based on essentialist assumptions about female emotionality and nurturance. In fact, while the duties of Russia's sisters of mercy primarily concerned providing treatment and comfort for wounded and ill soldiers, many believed that comforting the troops psychologically was a vital aspect of their work, perhaps even more significant than the medical services they provided. The extremely high mortality rate for wounded soldiers coupled with the rapid and insufficient training volunteer nurses received often meant that these women could do little more for wounded soldiers than provide them solace before inevitable death. The ability of women to provide compassion and healing in the midst of destruction and death was considered particularly valuable and uniquely feminine. Men and women alike, military and civilian, spoke of the positive psychological, even "spiritual" impact that the mere presence of women had on the wounded and dying soldiers. As one Russian journalist commented, in the role of caring nurturers, sisters of mercy were seen as not only healing wounds but "uplifting souls."[4] This was considered to be woman's special role, consistent with the passive and supportive one she was supposed to maintain in early twentieth-century society and with what was considered to be her most important function in society: mothering. Indeed, this was often held in higher regard even than the scientific value of medicine. Sofia Bocharskaia's head doctor expressed this view when he became overwhelmed with the numbers of seriously wounded men for whom he could do little. When approached by a sister of mercy asking how to proceed with treatment of seemingly hopeless cases, he responded, "How do I know how to make a man live? I'm not God. You should know better than I, you should *feel* it with your heart."[5] Many nurses themselves saw their role as primarily to provide care and comfort for wounded men, while the more technical components of medical treatment were to be left to doctors. When the senior doctor of her military hospital asked N. Chelakova to take on the role of surgical assistant, she flatly refused, stating that she had become a sister of mercy "in order to care for suffering people, not to service inanimate objects such as knives and forceps."[6] So important was the caring and nurturing aspect of wartime nursing that the women acting in this capacity were sometimes referred to as "sisters of comfort," a term that placed emphasis on their ability to provide emotional solace to wounded men. Although this term would take on a pejorative meaning over the course of the war, indicative of suspicions surrounding female nurses' sexual behavior, in this context it resonated with essentialist ideas of feminine nurturing ability.[7]

The realities of the war were that it inflicted tremendous damage on human minds as well as bodies, and medical personnel were especially affected by the conflict in this way. As Christina Hallett has indicated, "nurses were among the first to realise the true meaning of the First World War: the extent of the destruction that could be wreaked by industrial warfare; the fragility of the human body and mind in the face of its chaos."[8] Confronted with these effects, nurses were often forced to abandon emotional and psychological comforting mechanisms. The brutality of the conflict often convinced female nurses to "harden their hearts" in order to function effectively. A number of sisters indicated in their writings that they had to shut off the sympathetic and empathetic aspects of their psyches to continue working in the conditions of war. This was certainly not unique to Russian sisters of mercy. Nurses across the continent, faced with the dehumanizing effects of modern warfare, the frequent death of patients, and the speed at which they had to treat casualties, often did the same in order to handle, in the words of Margaret Higonnet, "the dilemmas faced in frontline nursing, where self-control and technical efficiency conflict with emotional involvement and the threat of hysteria."[9] Grand Duchess Ol'ga Aleksandrovna wrote that after witnessing the first ten men in her care die of their wounds, she "cried for each of them." As the war dragged on, however, she found herself unable to shed tears for so many lost lives.[10] This kind of emotional reaction could not be sustained as the death toll crept ever higher. Sofia Bocharskaia admitted that the first few times she saw the mangled bodies of wounded soldiers she was "overcome with revulsion." Entering a factory that had turned into a hospital in Poland, she recalled that she "felt dizzy as the smell of death came to me from the mortuary." But she soon became accustomed to such sights and odors and they rarely affected her thereafter. She explained, "The bodies of the men came in like heavy burdens that seemed to weigh us down, until we worked mechanically, growing more oppressed with fatigue, and after a while we only felt conscious that we wanted rest." Later in the war, she acknowledged that the only way she could continue to be effective in her duties was to completely suppress any emotion. She worried that if she did not, her fate would be similar to those who had succumbed to what was perceived as weakness. "Two sisters had already broken down, what if I should be the next?" she worried. "I must not think or feel. I worked without looking at the men . . . only safe in blankness."[11]

Witnessing the brutality inflicted on bodies by modern weapons made indelible impressions on the women who nursed them. Their experiences were shaped by the various sensory and often shocking perceptions with which they were confronted. Aleksandra Tolstaia remembered a wounded man who was brought onto the hospital train on which she worked on the northwestern front. "A shell had almost completely torn away both of his buttocks. Apparently, he had not been brought immediately from the battlefield. A terrible stench emanated from his wound. In place of his buttocks, there were two gaping dirty-grey wounds. Something swarmed within them, and bending over him, I saw . . . worms!" She cleaned and dressed the wound but was haunted by the sight and the smell, which lingered in her memory and affected her ability to sleep and eat for a long time after.[12] Nurses had to overcome feelings of revulsion at seeing mangled bodies in order to work effectively. Florence Farmborough was surprised at how quickly she adjusted to the gruesome sights around her: "We are very raw recruits, and it is not surprising that we sometimes wince, even shrink into the background, when an unusually ugly wound is bared for dressing, or when a man's cry of anguish follows an awkward attempt to alleviate an excruciating pain, it is, however, astonishing how quickly even a raw recruit can grow accustomed, though never hardened, to the sight and sound of constant suffering."[13] Commenting on the frequency of head wounds among the seriously injured, she later remarked, "At one time I had thought it a most terrible thing to have a man's brains bespattering my hands and white overall; but . . . I grew accustomed to it." As time went on, Farmborough even became convinced of the necessity for nurses to ignore the desperate cries of pain and fear emanating from wounded soldiers, to walk away from hopeless cases in order to tend to those who had a chance of survival, and to leave behind immobile patients during unplanned retreats, despite their begging exhortations. On another occasion, she came across a soldier lying in the corner of a makeshift hospital room, covered in blood and breathing very heavily. She knelt down beside him and began to tear away his clothing, revealing a horrible sight: "a pulp, a mere mass of smashed body from the ribs downward; the stomach and abdomen were completely crushed and his left leg was hanging to the pulped body by only a few shreds of flesh. . . . The soldier's dull eyes were still looking at me and his lips moved, but no words came." Realizing that there was nothing that could be done to save this man, and despite the fact that he was still alive and conscious, Farmborough gathered her composure and moved on the next patient. "What it cost me to turn away without aiding him, I cannot describe, but we could not waste time and material on hopeless cases, and there were so many others . . . waiting . . . waiting . . . " After a few months at the front, one of her fellow Russian sisters lamented, "I would never have believed that I could grow indifferent to pain and grief. In another year's time, if the war still continues, what shall we be feeling if we feel numb now?"[14] Violetta Thurstan similarly wrote about how she and her fellow nurses had to adjust to living with the horrors of war all around them, even to be able to eat despite the conditions:

> About four in the morning there was a little lull and some one made tea. I wonder what people in England would have thought if they had seen us at that meal. We had it in the stuffy dressing-room where we had been working without a stop for sixteen hours with tightly closed windows, and every smell that can be imagined pervading it, the floor covered with mud, blood and debris of dressings wherever there were not stretchers on which were men who had just been operated upon. . . . Two dead soldiers lay at our feet—it was not safe just at that moment to take them out and bury them. People would probably ask how we *could* eat under those conditions. I don't know how we could either, but we *did* and were thankful for it, for immediately after another rush began.[15]

Under these drastic circumstances, abandonment of characteristics of traditional "femininity" was encouraged. Writing anonymously in the *Red Cross Herald,* a sister of mercy commented that on her acceptance into the Red Cross, she and her fellow nurses were told to "forget that you are women, forget that you have personal desires, sorrows or joys." Only then, she maintained, would they be of any significant use.[16] Doctors echoed these ideas for practical reasons, wherein nurses' time was precious and could not be "wasted" on cases that had little chance of survival. Some even became impatient when nurses wanted to linger over dying patients and provide some solace for them in their last moments. As Farmborough sat with a fatally wounded man, she was called away by the doctor, who needed her to attend to another patient. She refused to leave the side of the dying man, who clenched her hand tightly with cold, clammy fingers, begging her to stay. "'Don't go, don't go,' he gasped piteously, 'don't leave me in the dark,'" Farmborough recalled him imploring, while her head doctor called to her insistently. "His irate voice sounded: '*Sestra,* we are waiting.' 'Alexander Mikhailovich,' I urged, 'it will be very soon.' 'There is nothing for you to do here,' he replied roughly. . . . And still more roughly: 'Have the goodness to come *at once.*' His words were final and he turned away."[17] Mary Britnieva also recalled that male doctors were very critical of nurses who became emotionally attached to patients. When told that a young nurse cried profusely after the death of a soldier in her care, the head doctor in her unit retorted, "If all the nurses are going to weep like this over every death-case, we shall be drowned. Once they have come to the War they must learn to control their emotions. Otherwise they can't work."[18]

Zakharova similarly commented on the ways she was forced to suppress emotion in order to carry out her duties. She remarked that she reached a point at which being surrounded by dead, mangled bodies no longer had an emotional effect on her. Like a "sponge that could no longer absorb water," she described having reached the limit of the human mind's ability to process the horrors around it.[19] Zakharova's comments regarding the emotional effects of witnessing the horrors of war are particularly poignant, especially in comparison to the impact of combat experiences on male soldiers, something that did not go unnoticed by the nurse herself. While on the road traveling from one mobile unit to another, she encountered a young officer sitting in a dark corner of a small shop. He told Zakharova of his "baptism in fire," wherein he was hit in the neck by an enemy shell that exploded behind his back. He had not thought his wound serious, so he did not leave the trenches to seek medical attention. Yet the effect of the blow soon became apparent. As he spoke, she noticed that his face contorted into surprising, seemingly disingenuous smirks. At first she was annoyed, as his facial expression in no way matched the words he was speaking, "making it seem as if he was engaged in some kind of strange game." But then she realized this was the result of the contusion, which she surmised "must have hit the part of his brain or nervous system that controlled the muscles of his face, causing an imbalance between his brain activity and external reflexes." He referred to himself as "*L'homme qui rit,*" in allusion to Victor Hugo's novel about a young boy whose face had been disfigured into a permanent, horrific-looking smile. The image of the young officer's face, distorted in an awkward, unsettling grimace, haunted Zakharova, not because she was horrified by it but because it had aroused intense interest and curiosity in her rather than sympathy or sorrow. She worried that she too was suffering some kind of "mental imbalance." On being transferred to a new location at the front very close to the fighting, Zakharova, along with her unit, endured heavy enemy shelling. She found herself strangely unafraid. Listening to the sounds of explosions all around her, she remarked: "Suddenly, the awareness of close and imminent danger, glaringly, clearly, and palpably appeared in my brain, but surprisingly, it brought on a feeling of curiosity, not terror or agony. What was this strange departure from conventional logic? Unexpectedly, the memory of '*l'homme qui rit*' arose in my mind. . . . Was this not an analogous impairment of emotional balance that was happening to me?" Zakharova did not have much time to contemplate this, however, as the activities she was engaged in took all of her emotional and physical strength. Later, she found herself thinking about the contused officer again, as wounded soldiers coming into her field hospital recounted horrific stories of a particularly bloody battle on the banks of a river. Once again, she was surprised when their stories did not make her shudder.[20]

These examples present a stark contrast to the conventional notions concerning the value of nursing and the realities of wartime medical service. The characteristics of emotionality in normative femininity so prized in nursing often had to be cast aside when women were faced with the realities of modern warfare. Abandonment, at least temporarily, of such characteristics and behaviors was widely recognized as a survival trait for wartime medical personnel. Indeed, the anonymous nurse who advised others to "forget that you are women" recognized that this "proved to be a paradox: love without love, mercy—without mercy."[21] The qualities that made a woman best suited for wartime medical service thus seemed to fly directly in the face of the conventional associations of nursing with caring and nurturing and the view that the "love and mercy" female nurses extended to wounded men was as, if not more, important than the medical care they provided.

It can be argued that this shutting off of emotions was a "masculinizing" experience, necessary for women to function in the male sphere of war, where there was little place for "feminine" characteristics. Emotional control and even coldness has traditionally been gendered as masculine. The sentiments expressed by wartime nurses echo the effects of war often reported by male combatants, who, exposed to ever-present death and destruction, similarly closed themselves off emotionally as a psychological coping mechanism. German officer Ernst Jünger remarked that although initially encountering the corpses of fallen soldiers was very unsettling, they became so familiar that the sight of them no longer elicited any emotional response. He explained, "We were so accustomed to the horrible that if we came on a dead body anywhere on a fire step or in a ditch we gave it no more than a passing thought and recognized it as we would a stone or a tree."[22] I would argue, however, that such a process is more accurately understood as a dehumanizing, rather than gendered, experience of transformation. In fact, it has long been argued that in order to bring oneself to kill, soldiers had to see their enemies as less than human; so too did nurses need to see their patients as parts of bodies rather than whole human beings, or nameless, faceless bodies without individual identities, in order to cope with their physical destruction and death. Indeed, the personal advice of the anonymous Red Cross nurse quoted above to other women who wanted to become "genuine" sisters of mercy was to "forget that you are people."[23]

Simultaneously, the emotional and psychological support and comfort that women as nurses were supposed to provide—indeed, even the very emotionality attributed to them as natural, essential traits of their gender—were not at all limited to female medical personnel. Brother of mercy Dmitrii Furmanov commented on his interactions with wounded soldiers in his care, which often included soothing their fears and anxieties as well as their pain. One evening, while on night duty, Furmanov came across a young soldier who was sobbing. "Why are you crying?" he asked. "My arm hurts, it aches all over, I cannot sleep," the wounded man answered. He was extremely anxious and unsettled. Examining the wound, which had penetrated through his shoulder, Furmanov proceeded to reassure the young man that everything would be all right. After administering pain medication, he sat with the patient until he was able to fall asleep. Furmanov also remembered that he and the other male medical personnel "shed many tears" when a sister of mercy of whom they had grown quite fond died from a serious illness she had contracted at the front.[24]

WAR AS "SPECTACLE"

Another important way that men in combat handled the horrors of war and the constant fear of death was by emotionally distancing themselves not just from other people but also from their immediate surroundings, especially those that were most directly threatening. While male soldiers usually did not have the option of physically removing themselves from combat (except through authorized retreat or unauthorized desertion), they could, and often did, emotionally and psychologically separate themselves by portraying the war as a "spectacle" they were observing, rather than something in which they were directly participating. Viewing the war as "spectacle" became another important coping mechanism employed by both male soldiers and female nurses in order to endure the intense psychological and emotional disruptions and trauma caused by the war. As Christopher Schultz has noted in reference to soldiers in the trenches on the western front,

> When speaking of "distance," one is often referring to the term in a spatial or temporal sense. In another sense, however, the term refers to a psycho-social separation in which one creates distance through the enacting of an imaginatively conceived and detached experiential space. There does not need to be any significant, empirically measurable separation, only the *perception* (actively constructed or not) of distance between the self and the event being perceived. . . . With modest regularity the combatants do speak of their consciously enacted separation from the events around them and thus, as will be argued, they become spectators of war rather than fundamentally implicated participants. By extension, war becomes a spectacle to the observing party.[25]

Russia's sisters of mercy also attempted to endure the deeply disturbing aspects of their war experiences by separating or distancing themselves from them emotionally. In fact, this idea of "war as spectacle" may be even more applicable to women's experiences in the war. Although the experiences of female wartime nursing, particularly at the front, mirrored those of male combatants in a number of very significant ways, it is important to note that a physical separation existed between female nurses and male soldiers in many everyday situations of the war. While the men engaged in combat were the regular participants in the conflict, women as nurses were often only occasional visitors to combat zones, especially the women who served in medical facilities located in the rear. Yet even the women who became frontline nurses were not usually constantly present in the trenches and on the battlefields. Most often, they were sent there after the major fighting of a battle had ceased to attend to wounded men. In some instances, they could visit the battlefields as civilian observers, as if they were spectators in some gruesome sport. This idea of war as something like an "attraction" becomes very clear when reading the memoirs of some nurses who arranged to "tour" the battlefields and the trenches. Sisters sometimes went to the forward positions to attend to the wounded, and they could "visit" the battlefields when they wanted some excitement or even entertainment, but very few carried out the majority of their service in the combat zone. In fact, nurses sometimes related their experiences in war as witnessing a "spectacle" from which they were psychologically or emotionally separated. Some viewed the trenches and battlefields in a completely detached (and unrealistic) way, as a place that promised the excitement of a dramatic theater scene. Chelakova seems to have held something of this notion from the very moment of her enlistment, insisting on bringing her camera with her to the front to document her "adventure." Almost immediately after arriving at her first place of assignment, the hospital at the Brest-Litovsk Fort, she began snapping pictures of the facility and of the fortress itself. Her actions raised the suspicions of the soldiers on guard duty outside its walls, who initially took her for a spy, and forbade any further photography in the vicinity of the military structure. Transferred to service in the military hospital at Ivangorod, Chelakova expressed a strong desire to see a "real field of battle," which she imagined in hyperromanticized terms. "In my imagination it was like a scene from the play by Rostan[d], *The Eaglet*. The battlefield under a moonlit sky, on the ground lay bodies of dead grenadiers, which suddenly came to life at the sound of the Marseillaise."[26] Farmborough similarly brought her camera with her when she joined the Russian Red Cross, taking multiple pictures of her experiences. She often "visited" troops at the front and photographed them in their encampments. She had wounded men and medical personnel pose in various positions and included numerous examples of these constructed shots in her memoir of the war.[27]

Nurses spoke of "visiting" the trenches to observe, even when they were sent to carry out medical work. Zakharova wrote that one evening she "had the chance to see the German trenches up close." She described the dugouts in great detail, especially how neatly and accurately they were laid out in a system of labyrinths, very comfortably apportioned, especially the officer quarters, which were filled with furnishings and other items stolen from the villages they had "joyfully" burned to the ground. In one of the trenches she even noticed a child's high chair. Her "visit" occurred after a bloody episode in the war, leaving the trenches full of the dead. Seemingly unfazed by the horrors she witnessed, she described the corpses in a very detached manner, noting their positions, some lying on their backs, others with their faces to the ground, with their arms and legs entangled with one another. "Many sat in positions like living people, looking out over the parapet or at the back wall of the trench. The strangest ones were those who had not fallen after they died, but remained standing, shoulder to shoulder, with their rifles in their hands and their glassy eyes open, with the peacefulness of not hearing the evil cries of the ravens flying above their heads."[28] Violetta Thurstan and some other members of her unit went to see the trenches near Radzivilov (Radyvyliv in present-day Ukraine), carrying out this "visit" during a skirmish with the Germans. Despite the danger that surrounded her, Thurstan described the experience as if she was watching an exhilarating adventure:

> We went through the wood silently in single file, taking care that if possible not even a twig should crackle under our feet, till we came to the very front trenches at the edge of the wood. We crouched down and watched for some time. Everything was brilliantly illuminated by the moonlight, and we had to be very careful not to show ourselves. A very fierce German attack was going on, and the bullets were pattering like hail on the trees all around us. We could see nothing for some time but the smoke of the rifles—We stayed a while talking, and then crawled along to visit one of the men's dugouts, a German bullet just missing us as we passed, and burying itself in a tree.[29]

Thurstan was able to distance herself from feeling fear in spite of the danger of the shells exploding close to their position. She remarked, "One felt rather like a disinterested spectator at a far-off dream. It was probably partly due to want of sleep; one's hands did the work, but one's mind was mercifully numbed."[30] Sisters of mercy also expressed experiences of emotional distancing in terms of dreams and dreamlike states. Chelakova described the relief she felt after bringing the wounded she had been treating on a hospital train to the medical facility where they would receive further care: "It seemed to me that I had been awakened from a terrible nightmare, having experienced the feeling of deep relief and at the same time terrible heaviness of my soul."[31]

A WAR ON THE PSYCHE

Although many wartime nurses were able to find ways to cope with the horrors they witnessed and experienced, others often found it difficult to handle the heavy psychological toll the war exacted on them. Like those of combat, the conditions in which they lived and the events that they endured often weighed very heavily on the minds of women in nursing service. A number of Russia's sisters of mercy suffered from mental and emotional disorders, many of which can be compared to those that afflicted male participants in the conflict. Indeed, an examination of the psychological effects of participation in wartime medical services on women is particularly useful in dispelling the notion that such activities were less demanding, dangerous, or damaging than combat, as well as indicating the limitations of a purely masculine notion of war. The importance of examining the trauma of war on noncombatants, especially women who served in medical capacities, has been argued by scholars such as Margaret Higonnet, who has demonstrated the traumatic aspects of nursing as reflected by women who served in the West. Higonnet argues that an investigation of the trauma experienced by nurses is essential in allowing us to revise the canon that "entailed a gendering of trauma" in which it "became a privileged, masculine form of testimony about the complex meaning of war."[32]

World War I is often noted among scholars as the first major conflict in which the psychological impact of war received significant attention—mostly because of the incapacitation of thousands of men who participated in combat as a result of debilitating mental conditions that rendered them unable to continue fighting. Physicians and mental health professionals had to treat men with no discernible physical ailments or limitations, but whose emotional and mental states made them no longer fit for military service. Thus, there was a concerted effort to find the causes of such mental illnesses and cure them, so that these men would once again be useful to their nations on the battlefields.[33] In Russia, although the nature of the fighting was much more mobile and fluid than that of the static trench warfare of the West, the kinds of psychological effects experienced by soldiers were similar. In particular, the term "shell shock" entered the parlance with regard to mental trauma suffered by combatants, although in Russia this condition was more commonly referred to as "military contusion" or "traumatic neurosis."[34] As historian of Russian military psychiatry Paul Wanke explains, "The soldiers' order to attack across barren killing fields clashed with the desire for self-preservation. The result, for some, was mental collapse."[35] This, coupled with the feelings of lack of control, of "being led to the slaughter," deeply affected the psyches of many men. But these were not the only factors that caused mental distress and trauma among men at the front. The sights and sounds of war were also very difficult for some to accommodate, a particular effect of the conditions of modern warfare. By World War I, Russian mental health officials had come to recognize this concept and, in contrast to many Western practitioners, did not attribute psychological disorders to weaknesses in character or personality, or to preexisting mental illness, but rather to the unique stresses and horrors of industrial warfare. In fact, Russia was the first nation to employ military psychiatrists in an attempt to treat soldiers suffering from debilitating mental disorders.[36]

In examining British cases of shell shock, scholars such as Elaine Showalter have posited gender as primary in the psychological impact of the war. Showalter and others have argued that men suffered from hysteria as a result of a crisis of masculinity brought about by mechanized trench warfare. In such a formulation, it was impossible for many men to display the definitive masculine characteristics of heroism and stoicism because the conditions of industrialized warfare turned them into passive victims, unable to control their conditions, faced only with the terror of death. Showalter asserts that "the Great War feminized its conscripts by taking away their sense of control."[37] Laurinda Stryker has challenged this interpretation, however, by pointing to the fact that in this argument, it was the conditions of the war that caused mental breakdown—conditions that even Showalter herself admits would affect anyone, regardless of gender.[38] The case of Russia's wartime nurses supports this challenge, as women suffered from similar kinds of mental trauma brought on by the experience of the war. Female medical personnel also became disillusioned and suffered from the kind of mental distresses often associated with the soldiers of the Great War. Fear of death was coupled with revulsion at the effects of mechanized warfare on human beings.

Furthermore, as Laura Phillips has noted, in Russia psychological trauma of soldiers was not always conceived of as emasculating or feminizing, rejecting the binary of able male/disabled female. Rather, "physicians and patients in Russia often *preserved* the masculinity of mentally-ill soldiers."[39] Irina Sirotkina's scholarship supports such a view, demonstrating that Russian psychiatric practices during the war were less brutal than those employed in the West because most Russian mental health professionals believed the causes of mental illnesses during the war were largely the result of external conditions rather than internal failings. "Russian psychiatrists, for various reasons, rejected the identification, widespread in the West, of traumatic neurosis with hysteria, which made shell shock a shameful disease and a sign of weak will bordering on cowardice and malingering," she asserts. Instead, they focused on the ways that the specific conditions and experiences of the war served to cause or exacerbate mental disorder. And although initially the general consensus among Russian military psychiatrists was that traumatic neurosis was caused by physical injury incurred in the brain by exploding shells, by the time of the First World War, many had already come to conclude that mental illness could occur even when shells fell too far away from soldiers to cause any bodily harm, and even when soldiers had not experienced shelling. Thus, it was not even the direct participation or wounding in combat that resulted in such trauma. Rather, as Sirotkina argues, it was widely recognized that "the brutality of the war is the main cause of psychiatric casualties."[40] One can easily infer that women serving in medical capacities could be affected in similar ways, leading to mental disorders among nurses as well.

This assumption can be seen directly through the practice of military psychiatry in Russia during the war. Military psychiatrist Dr. S. A. Preobrazhenskii insisted on including medical personnel in his study of the psychological illnesses affecting those participating in the war, which he argued deserved equal attention to that of combatants. Preobrazhenskii noted that involvement in medical services was extremely difficult work, which had "significantly negative effects on both the moral and physical constitutions of those engaged therein, and could not be discounted from weakening neuropsychiatric stability." He and his colleagues studied the conditions of medical personnel who had been serving at the front but were removed from service and evacuated to the rear for treatment of specifically psychological disorders. He reported cases of sisters (as well as brothers and other male medical personnel) of mercy suffering from "manic depressive psychosis," "hysteria," "psycho-polyneuritis," and "neurotic constitutions." The prevailing disorder that Preobrazhenskii observed among nursing personnel was nervous agitation. Although he noted that some of the women had suffered from symptoms prior to the war, these conditions began to manifest themselves after the patients had been overworked and were suffering from exhaustion, resulting from the fulfillment of their duties in the combat zone. Some of the nurses, after rest and treatment, were returned to their duties in the theater of war, only to suffer from relapses brought on by the conditions of their service. He noted similar conditions, particularly manic depressive disorders, among medics, often induced by their involvement in carrying corpses from the battlefield.[41] Such disorders, as well as the other psychological effects described by nurses, closely resemble those of male soldiers.

Preobrazhenskii included detailed notes about individual case studies he conducted with nurses in his treatment. One sister had suffered an attack of hysteria after working very long shifts without sleep. She recovered from this episode and was sent back to the front, only to return to the hospital after three weeks, following extreme weight loss and another episode of nervous agitation brought on by sleepless night duty. During this attack, she had become aggressive, screaming until she had become hoarse. Another nurse developed psychological illness generated by physical stresses. She was diagnosed with psycho-polyneuritis, which manifested itself after she had fallen through a hole in the ice and developed a very high fever. She became severely emaciated and weak in her extremities, and she developed nausea, blood in her urine, hyperalgesia, and paresthesia. The illness affected her personality as well, making her "cantankerous" and "capricious," and causing her to suffer from memory loss. Preobrazhenskii also treated a wartime sister of mercy who had left her post in an infectious disease unit on her own accord and returned to her Petrograd *obshchina* with the hopes of being reassigned. However, when she arrived, she was clearly manifesting signs of neuritis, then she "accidentally" drank mercuric chloride, which was highly poisonous. The doctor's placement of the word "accidentally" in quotation marks seems to indicate that he believed this to be a deliberate suicide attempt. She was diagnosed with manic-depressive psychosis. A wartime sister with a history of prewar depression relapsed into this condition after carrying out strenuous work at the front, refusing to eat for eight straight days; she was also diagnosed with manic-depressive psychosis. Another young woman who had become a nurse when the war began was assigned to service in a reserve field hospital in Russian Poland. There, as a result of the hardships she endured as part of her work, she came to suffer from delusions of persecution by the local Jewish population, and in her delirium she developed the notion that she personally was entrusted with the task of "saving" Poland. After two months of treatment, her delusions began to dissipate, but she required another seven months of treatment before she could be returned to work.[42]

Even for those who did not suffer from mental breakdown, many of the women who became nurses in Russia also described the war as an experience of significant trauma. Violetta Thurstan described the field hospital in which she worked briefly near Lodz in traumatic terms. "It was more like hell than anything I can imagine," she recalled. "The never-ending processions of groaning men being brought in on those horrible blood-soaked stretchers, suffering unimagined tortures, the filth, the cold, the stench, the hunger, the vermin, and the squalor of it all . . . was almost enough to make even Satan weep.[43] The effect of seeing men's bodies ripped apart by bullets and shells in particular was very traumatic. Sofia Bocharskaia was taken aback by her first exposure to open wounds: "my head turned dizzily at sight of the shattered flesh."[44] Chelakova was repelled by the dehumanizing effects of combat on encountering her first group of wounded, crammed into the cars of a freight train, lying on the dirty, blood-soaked floor of the dark, dank, fetid wagons. "Very recently, perhaps yesterday or even that very morning, they all had been strong, healthy, fully alive," she mused regretfully. "But now they lay in this freight car like carcasses of animals after the slaughter. It was impossible to determine individual faces from among this mass of mangled humanity, from among the bandaged heads, arms, legs, from the smell of clotted blood, sweat, and pus, from their pain and misery."[45] Tat'iana Aleksinskaia, who was accustomed to caring for men after they had passed through initial treatment at frontline medical aid stations before being dispatched to her hospital train, was aghast when she was sent to the front lines to pick up the wounded coming directly off the battlefield. "Most of them had no dressing at all. Some had been bandaged up by themselves, or their comrades," she remarked. "Their wounds were horrible to look upon . . . full of blood and mud; and fragments of cloth were clotted up with the coagulated blood."[46]

The wounds inflicted by industrial arms were often more than early twentieth-century medical practices could mend. This, coupled with lengthy waits before surgery and unsanitary conditions that often led to infection, resulted in many wounded limbs that had to be removed rather than repaired. Participating in the numerous amputations performed during this war took a significant mental toll on wartime nurses. As indicated in the previous chapter, Bocharskaia found it difficult to accept amputation as a medical treatment, viewing it as inflicting additional violence on an already damaged body. As she listened to the doctor cavalierly whistle a waltz while cutting through a soldier's limb, "angry pulses beat all through" her. She glanced down at the stump that remained after the leg was sawn off and "was overwhelmed with revulsion."[47] Aleksandra Tolstaia commented that she too had difficultly growing accustomed to the experience of assisting in surgical amputations. She was unnerved by the feeling of holding the leg or the arm of a wounded soldier during amputation, wherein suddenly, after the limb was removed, "one felt a dead mass. A part of a human body remained in one's hands." Her acrimony was directed at the Turks, however, whom she accused of using exploding "dum-dum" bullets, which expanded on impact and thus made the injuries they inflicted much more damaging and severe.[48] Farmborough was deeply affected by the experience of seeing amputated limbs piled up in a shed outside of her field hospital. "I had not been in that shed before and I turned away hastily; I went to our room, drank some water and swallowed two aspirins; the choking feeling disappeared and I was myself again," she wrote. She was unable to recover quickly from the sight, remembering that "my thoughts would not adjust themselves so easily: after the war, what would happen to these limbless men. . . . I began to wonder how long my physical strength would hold out under the heavy burden of these never-ending sorrows."[49]

Witnessing the effects of gas attacks also had traumatic effects on wartime nurses. Mary Britnieva described a haunting scene in a field, where soldiers who had been exposed to gas and were laid out for emergency treatment convulsed and gasped, attempting to cling to life. Despite writing a number of years after the war, she could not shake the memory of that sight:

> The ghastliness of what we saw is beyond description, the memory of it making me shudder to this day. They lay on their backs mostly, their upturned faces terribly swollen and livid—some almost blue—choking and coughing, their bloodshot eyes protruding, unable to

> utter a word, yet fully conscious, only their eyes and their occasional spasmodic feeble movements proclaiming the supreme agony that they were enduring. Some were even coughing up pieces of their lungs that the cruel gas had disintegrated in their living bodies.[50]

Her language was eerily reminiscent of Wilfred Owen's poetry (which she indeed may have read), which depicted the effects of gas on soldiers in the poem "Dulce et Decorum Est":

> If in some smothering dreams you too could . . .
> watch the white eyes writhing in his face . . .
> If you could hear . . . the blood
> Come gargling from the froth-corrupted lungs . . . [51]

The horror of this visual image, Britnieva commented, continued to haunt her many years after the war. But even worse for the young nurse was the fact that she and the other medical personnel could do nothing to assist these dying men: "We felt utterly helpless, there was no remedy, we were powerless. . . . The realization of our helplessness was almost unbearable."[52]

Feelings of useless, powerlessness, and guilt over poor performance were expressed by a number of wartime nurses. Sisters of mercy often commented that when they were idle, without wounded to care for, or when they were forbidden from attending to wounded on the battlefields because of the extreme danger of enemy fire, they too had such thoughts. Tat'iana Varnek remembered experiencing guilt and anger when her unit was transferred to a location along the front where there were no wounded to be treated, knowing that in other areas a great need for their services existed while they sat being useless where they were. The negative emotional response even had a deleterious effect on her relationship with her fellow nurses, so much so that she began to quarrel with her best friend, Ksenia Ispolatova (whose uncle was Aleksandr Aleksandrovich Il'in, chairman of the main administration of the Russian Society of the Red Cross).[53] Chelakova could not shake this feeling of helplessness, as well as the image of the wounded men, for a long time after her first experience providing medical service on a train full of soldiers. "Before my eyes all the time were the immobile lying figures in the darkness of the wagon, with unspoken agony in their eyes—people for whom so little could be done," she remarked. She tended to men with gaping wounds, punctured lungs, smashed skulls, ruptured stomachs, and shattered limbs. She hurried from bed to bed as the wounded called out to her in desperate pain and agony, begging for water, for medicine, for anything to ease their suffering. There were many she could do little, if anything, to help, and they died before her eyes.[54]

Scholar Santanu Das has suggested that these types of expressions of helplessness can be characterized as a gendered "impotence of sympathy," unique to women's writings and women's experiences in war. Das argues that, "called upon to serve the shattered remnants of the body, the subjectivity of the nurse is doubly eroded—first, through the gap with the male trench experience, and second, through the sheer magnitude of suffering, an experience that can never be owned by women either historically or ontologically."[55] Despite using both the poetry of Wilfred Owen and the memoirs of Mary Britnieva, Das overlooks the striking similarity of their comments about gas attacks and fails to acknowledge the fact that both female medical workers and male soldiers experienced these kinds of reactions. Moreover, it was particularly the effects of gas attacks that inspired these feelings of helplessness, which were shared by both men and women who saw the suffering and horrific damage caused by this chemical agent. Men such as military doctor L. M. Vasilevskii and journalist Stanley Washburn both describe the inability to help soldiers who had inhaled gas.[56] As Margaret Higonnet's research into the effects of war indicates, the lines of gender demarcation fall away as medical workers "not only dealt with soldiers' physical and psychological traumas, but were themselves exposed to situations that triggered breakdowns similar to those experienced by combatants." Soldiers faced feelings of guilt, remorse, impotency, and lack of usefulness as they watched helplessly while their comrades in arms were wounded or killed, when they could not get medical attention, and languished and even died before their eyes. Soldiers also experienced guilt when they survived while others did not, or when they came out of the war unscathed while others' bodies were permanently mutilated, or when they were wounded and sent home for good, leaving others behind to continue fighting. Higonnet also found that in treating soldiers suffering from mental distress, "doctor after doctor remarked that the devastating "'sight of dead comrades' or 'the sight and sound of his lacerated comrades' was sufficient to arouse morbid agitation, nervous breakdown, with paralysis, cramps, or even delirium."[57] Men also felt a distinct lack of individual agency in this war, with its heavily technological emphases and the use of trenches, which led men to believe that they were unable to control their circumstances. Indeed, some even describe themselves as passive victims rather than active participants in the conflict. According to Samuel Hynes, "soldiers came to war believing that individual wills would have a role there, that what a man did—his decisions—would affect whether he lived or died. The new weapons of war challenged that conviction; they made death accidental." Hynes points to the comments of British historian C. R. M. F. Crutwell, who fought in the war in the trenches at Ypres, with regard to gas attacks, to explain: "In the face of gas, without protection, individuality was annihilated; the soldier in the trench became a mere passive recipient of torture and death. . . . Nearly every soldier becomes a fatalist. . . . If the very air which he breathes is poison, his chance is gone: he is merely a destined victim for the slaughter."[58]

Lack of control over one's fate often led to intense fear, which is one of the most potent causes of mental trauma cited by military psychologists, with potentially debilitating effects. Fear had traditionally been suppressed among soldiers, but by World War I it was an emotion increasingly articulated by men at war for a number of reasons. According to historian Jan Plamper, the most important of these was the rise of mechanized warfare. He explains,

> since this expansion coincided with the modernization of warfare, it was connected with an increase in the real psychological stress that modern war produces. Modern war exposes soldiers to drastically longer periods of rifle and machine gun shooting, shelling, and air bombardment. It makes the source of the attack difficult to locate. Trench warfare, a major feature of World War I, immobilizes soldiers, thus incapacitating the reflex to flee from the source of danger; by contrast, a premodern open battlefield and one-on-one bayonet combat offered the—shame-free—option of forward attack as an outlet for fight-or-flight reactions. . . . All of these factors amount to a real and significant increase in psychological stress that had to spill over into the ways soldiers felt—and sometimes wrote—about what they endured.[59]

Ernst Jünger wrote about how this fear affected him as well as his men, who often mistook an innocent noise for an incoming shell. These sensations were caused by an extreme fear, which Jünger describes as "something that would accompany us all through the war, the habit of jumping at any sudden and unexpected noise. Whether it was a train clattering past, a book falling to the floor, or a shout in the night—on each occasion, the heart would stop with mortal dread."[60] Russian accounts also indicated that fear was pervasive and that bravery and courage did not come naturally to soldiers. Those such as Dmitrii Os'kin indicated that he and his comrades needed alcohol, often in copious quantities, to motivate them to attack the enemy.[61] Others found the fear too great to be soothed by vodka, fleeing the battlefields instead. Some even decided that becoming a prisoner of war was preferable to being led to the slaughter "like cattle," such as platoon commander V. Dmitriev, who, along with his entire unit, surrendered to the Austrians. This act was inspired by fear for their lives, which was significantly enhanced by a severe shortage of ammunition.[62]

Such fear, however, was not limited to men in the trenches. Medical personnel also experienced intense fright when faced with bombardment, artillery fire, and death. Like their male counterparts, female nurses serving in the forward positions experienced similar fear, and they expressed it in ways that resembled male emotional responses. As indicated previously, Russian medical units were stationed very close to the actual fighting and subject to the dangerous conditions of warfare. Zakharova commented that although she eventually became accustomed to the sounds of booming cannons and exploding shells, at first she would instinctively cross herself each time she heard these terrifying sounds.[63] Khristina Semina recalled a feeling of terror the closer her transport got to the front as she traveled from Kars to Sarykamysh (present-day Sarıkamış, Turkey), where a battle was raging between the Russian and Turkish armies. She felt increasingly depressed and had the terrible feeling that there was no going back, as if she was being enveloped in something like pond scum.[64] Ol'ga Putiatina wrote to her family about the experience of working in the Anglo-Russian hospital in Petrograd (which was far behind the front lines) when it was hit by the blast of an explosion on September 6, 1916. She told them that while no one was injured and only the windows were shattered, "we all or nearly all found ourselves groveling on the bandage-room floor in a most undignified way—the result of combined shock of the air and noise and instinct for self-preservation." But it was not just the medical personnel who suffered from this intense fear. "Some of our poor patients were frightened out of their wits," emitting "the most bewildering and piteous cries all around."[65] Chelakova described how everyone in her military hospital, soldiers and medical personnel, men and women alike, froze with fear as a German airplane bombarded them:

> The aircraft was now immediately above the barracks [in which the hospital was housed], even though the roof was painted with a large red cross. There was a large explosion and a column of black smoke went up over the fence. "Lay Down! Lay Down!" someone yelled. But people just stood there, still, as if they had been turned to stone, with their eyes fixed on the airplane, like magnets. Another explosion—and again, another column of smoke rose above from the earth, like a black cloud. . . . This was followed by two more explosions. One bomb fell on a cart with two horses, tied up to the fence. The soldier standing next to it was killed immediately. And yet, still no one stirred. A deathly silence prevailed. Another several minutes went by. The German aircraft turned and began to flee. A sigh of relief, like a gust of wind, came over the crowd, and every hand made the sign of the cross. "Thanks be to God, it has passed!"[66]

These reactions resemble those of a soldier who expressed feeling a kind of paralysis in the trenches:

> I want to walk away, but can't lift my leg; it's as if someone grabbed my ankle. I can't look left, can't look right—I'm afraid. Fear of death has taken hold of me, has overwhelmed my heart, and no fear is more brutal than this kind of fear. It's as though someone poured cold snow under your skin; your jaw starts chattering, and your blood stops flowing in your veins: it has frozen. I wanted to aim with my rifle, but it was so damn heavy, like a *pud;* I wanted to scream, but I could only rattle like an animal, I wanted to pull the trigger, but I couldn't.[67]

Nurses also experienced trauma as a result of their frequent encounters with dead and dying soldiers. In addition to the experience described in the opening vignette when she saw her first dead body, Zakharova recalled her intense fear in several other instances when she had been sent to the battlefields to help collect wounded soldiers. On one occasion, she was separated from her unit and became lost in the dark. She attempted to make her way through the field strewn with dead bodies, but the feeling of the corpses under her feet caused her to shriek in terror. Later, on a foggy day while retrieving wounded men from the bank of a river, she stumbled over the head of a dead German, and again she found herself screaming "desperately and loudly," in such a way that she did not even recognize her own voice. At first, she was immobilized by her fear, but the sound of her scream had attracted the attention of a nearby medic, who rushed to her, asking if she was all right. The sound of his voice broke her temporary paralysis.[68] Chelakova recalled her first experience seeing dead bodies on a freight train full of wounded soldiers early in the war. As she moved through the wagon attending to the wounded, she heard a voice. "'Sister, this one is already . . . ' Someone pointed to his neighbor. With great difficultly, the orderly removed the dead body from the wagon. A cold horror filled my heart."[69] Mary Britnieva reported encountering the corpses of fatally wounded soldiers in a dugout, which were "terrible to behold." She recalled with horror the "five frozen bodies, they lay in their trench-coats. . . . They were all in different crouching positions and it looked as if they had all crawled to one place. . . . Field-mice had made a nest in the head of one."[70]

Seeing dead bodies caused similar emotional distress for soldiers. For the vast majority of men who served in combat during the First World War, this was a particularly transformative experience. Because most were civilians who had been conscripted or had volunteered, the war was something worlds apart from their everyday lives. The same was true for nurses. Samuel Hynes's assertion that "the first sight of the dead is a fundamental part of the soldiers' tale, being as it is the extreme case of war's unfamiliarity for civilian soldiers," could easily be rewritten with the words "soldiers" replaced by "nurses." Jünger recalled his experience seeing dead men for the first time: "And now at our first glance of horror we had a feeling that is difficult to describe. It was too entirely unfamiliar. We looked at all these dead with dislocated limbs, distorted faces, and the hideous colors of decay, as though we walked in a dream through a garden full of strange plants, and we could not realize at first what we had all round us."[71] These comments very much resemble those of Lidiia Zakharova, quoted in the opening vignette of this chapter, regarding her first experience seeing the dead.

This notion that the war was something totally different, strange, and separate from peacetime life, or even from the lives of those back home living through but not directly participating in war, is something that is often argued as a defining experience for soldiers. Yet again, this idea can also be applied to the experiences of women who served as nurses. A number of Russian sisters of mercy commented on how the war had taken them away from the concerns of civilian life. Farmborough actually came to yearn for her wartime life, which she contrasted to the idleness and lack of purpose in domesticity. After a short leave in Moscow where she was able to spend time with friends and enjoy all of the comforts of home, she recalled that "it palled quickly" and she was soon "counting the days which were left before my return to the Front." She found it difficult to enjoy the things that had previously made her content. "There was something lacking in the serenity of home-life. Gradually, it was borne to me that to be happy while the world was unhappy, to laugh while the world was in pain, was incongruous; in fact, impossible."[72] Similarly, male medical workers experienced such transformations. Furmanov commented on how the realization of the gravity of his duties in caring for the wounded men of Russia's armed forces affected him. "I even saw my own face from this perspective—it was serious, focused, infused with a single thought about the importance of the very task. There was not even a smile on this face, it was so severe, serious, zealous in silent peace."[73]

While nurses shared the terror of being shelled or bombed, hit by bullets or in other ways killed or wounded under attack, like soldiers, in order to perform their duties they had to suppress their fears and continue to work under dangerous conditions. In some cases, they did so even when soldiers did not. When a German airplane was heard flying above her military hospital, Chelakova reported that many of the soldiers there for treatment reacted with panic. They ran out of the hospital seeking to hide themselves anywhere they could, screaming and pushing each other in their rush to protect themselves.[74] Farmborough related an episode when the medical personnel stood fast while the soldiers shrunk away in fear. On one occasion, she was bandaging a badly wounded soldier, "when an angry hiss was heard, grew louder and louder, and then the explosion! The roar was deafening, the room shook and there were frightening noises of splintering, slicing masonry and of glass breaking and falling. A great silence followed, but the room continued to shake and tremble; or was it, perhaps, our own limbs? The soldier in front of me was still shaking with ague." Farmborough tried to calmly continue with her work, but the soldier was spooked, and as soon as she turned her back on him to get some fresh bandages, he fled, despite the fact that the wound in his back was large enough for the nurse to put her hand into and his lung had been pierced. "In his half-bandaged condition he had run off, not caring for aught else and possessed with the one wild desire to escape to a safer place." A number of other wounded soldiers in the field hospital behaved similarly, and "many of those whom we had thought too weak to move had, under this violent shock, been imbued with supernatural strength, as it were, had arisen and crawled away out into the night."[75]

Intense fear often led to the inability to perform on the battlefield or in the field hospital. These individuals were often diagnosed with mental conditions and sent to the rear for psychological treatment. Mental distress manifested itself in a variety of different ways, but most cases were not gender specific: both male soldiers and female medical workers suffered from the inability to speak or move, visual and auditory hallucinations, and/or severe depression. Dr. Preobrazhenskii reported on numerous cases of male medical workers, including feldshers, brothers of mercy, and orderlies, who exhibited various mental disorders brought on by their wartime medical service. He highlighted an example of a male feldsher serving in a military medical unit who began to experience inexplicable fear. His fright was so intense that he lost consciousness for several days. When he regained consciousness, he was "highly suggestible" and suffered from "hypochondriacal syndrome," as well as a loss of physical reflexes. He was diagnosed with "psychoasthenia," an outdated term for a psychological disorder characterized by obsessions, phobias, or compulsions.[76] Such effects were similar to those experienced by combatants as well. Catherine Merridale has detailed the ways war trauma affected male soldiers. One specialist treating soldiers noted the psychological impact of technological warfare on soldiers, particularly among the infantry, who were subject to frequent artillery fire. "The symptoms he observed included hallucinations: 'some believe they are still swatting Germans like flies.' One soldier could repeat nothing but the words, 'Oh Lord, save the Tsar and Russia.'"[77] Aleksinskaia recalled a soldier on her train who had been wounded for a third time and, close to death, was experiencing hallucinations as his fever rose. "All night long he was haunted by bad dreams," she recalled. "In his delirium he fought the Germans, shouted, leaped from his bed, and hurled himself at his neighbors; the orderlies kept him back: he took them for enemies."[78] Not only direct exposure to the fighting brought on such symptoms; disease had similar effects. An Armenian soldier infected with typhus imagined that his fellow ward mates, as well as his nurse, Aleksandra Tolstaia, were enemies attempting to kill him, and he attacked them in a hallucinatory rage.[79]

Thus, it should not be surprising that wartime nurses exhibited similar psychological reactions to their experiences. Sofia Bocharskaia related how one young sister named Lala suffered from "hallucinations of amputated arms and legs that took on a life of their own, and when she slept, they moved about the room." Another nurse in Bocharskaia's hospital, Shura, experienced a nervous breakdown in March 1916, when she became convinced that all of the men in her care had died. The other nurses tried to convince her that the men still lived, making her feel their heartbeats, but to no avail. "Pulses prove nothing," the emotionally shattered young woman said, "everyone dies." When a new round of wounded came in to be prepped for surgery, she tried to prevent the doctor from operating. "Don't, don't, they will die anyway," she pleaded, as "she wrung her hands and wandered about listlessly murmuring of death."[80] Lidiia Zakharova described how she, suffering from a fever brought on by lack of sleep and the onset of pleurisy, seemed to view everything through the fog of smoke. She hallucinated that the patients being brought into her mobile unit were the friends and acquaintances she had made over the last several months while serving as a nurse. But when she asked them how they ended up at her station, instead of their faces, she saw the "strange eyes of the grey figures of soldiers" looking back at her. Even after being evacuated to a rear hospital for treatment, for several weeks she suffered from feverish delusions, visions of the horrors she had experienced at the front. Images and sounds of "crawling wounded men, blood, distorted sick faces, shots, soul-chilling shots" filled her mind, sometimes even during the day when her fever would subside. In a statement that reveals her own awareness of how similar these experiences were to those of men in combat, Zakharova commented that they fostered in her an "increasing, emotional longing for home, like that of the soldiers' [war] weariness."[81]

Despite the fact that women and men seemed to experience fear in similar ways, there were those who believed that such a reaction was the result of gender—in fact, of biological sex. Princess Kati Dadeshkeliani, who served in the Great War disguised as a man, felt as if she could never overcome what she believed to be the physical and mental limitations of biological female traits. When the war broke out, Dadeshkeliani cut her hair short, donned a soldier's uniform, and enlisted as Djamal Dadeshkeliani in order to escape the personal sorrow she had recently experienced as a result of the death of her father and sister. She was assigned to the Fourth Squadron of the Tatar Regiment, which was part of the Grand Duke Mikhail's so-called Savage Division. Dadeshkeliani's social status (as a member of the Georgian aristocracy) and expertise with horses allowed "him" to become an officer of the cavalry, assigned to carry out the duties of a military courier. In this position, she was required to undertake very risky journeys under heavy enemy fire in order to deliver important military messages to command personnel. But despite the danger associated with this assignment, Dadeshkeliani became bored with the work and requested a transfer to the forward positions for combat duty. After merely a week in the trenches, her overly romanticized conceptions of warfare were shattered by the brutality of modern combat. She was overcome with fear and suffered from "paralyzing constraint." However, rather than recognizing this as a universal symptom of trench warfare from which men also suffered, Dadeshkeliani was convinced that her poor performance was directly attributable to the fact that she was a woman. Somewhat ironically, considering all of the other distinctively "unwomanly" things in which she had participated, she commented, "a woman is not in her place in the fighting ranks, even when she is disguised, there is an atmosphere of weakness about her." After returning from the trenches, she was assigned to an ambulance company and became the chief medical assistant of the unit. She felt much more comfortable with her duties in this capacity. "I never felt the same feeling of uselessness, of powerlessness, or failing of duty, for in this work there was an abundant scope for my womanly faculties as well as for my energy and my will-power."[82]

The psychological effects of the war were so significant for some sisters of mercy that they found themselves unable to cope with their experiences and chose instead to end their lives. Interestingly, the Red Cross and other organizations providing medical services did not attempt to hide the instances of nurses' suicides. The pages of the various publications of the organizations carrying out medical service during the war report many such cases among wartime nursing personnel.[83] Although sometimes such self-destructive acts were attributed to "personal issues," many others indicate that the pressures of the war, the experiences of frontline service, and the close proximity to death and dying all took a significant toll on the psyches of nurses. A report to the main administration of the Red Cross indicated that Sister Tat'iana Fedorvna Kurysheva, of the Elizavetin community of the Russian Red Cross, killed herself on January 4, 1915. Another revealed that Marina Kuz'menkova, a nurse from the Simbersk community of sisters of mercy working in a reserve field hospital, had also taken her own life that month. Access to medical supplies, particularly drugs, often facilitated such suicides. Evgeniia Borisova, a sister of the Sturdzovskii community, serving in Red Cross infirmary no. 1 in the region of Benderskii, was reported to have died as a result of deliberately poisoning herself with morphine.[84] Male medical workers similarly battled depression, sometimes unsuccessfully. Khristina Semina's husband Ivan, a regimental doctor, became overwhelmed by his experiences in the war, increasingly turning to alcohol and eventually shooting himself in 1916.[85] So heavily did the horrors of war weigh on Furmanov's mind that initially he contemplated suicide to escape them.[86] For some, the war presented too great a psychological burden to bear, and the only way they saw out was to take their own lives. Others managed to cope, but there is little doubt that the experiences of frontline medical service were ineligibly forged in their minds.

CONCLUSIONS

Although Lidiia Zakharova managed to cope with the harrowing psychological impacts of the war, the physical effects proved to be too much for her. In mid-1915 she contracted pleurisy and became too ill to continue her work. She was evacuated to the interior, where she spent several months recuperating in a hospital before she was allowed to return to her home in Moscow. This was the end of her war experience, as far as we know. Her story, however, was considered interesting enough to be published in 1915 by one of the officially sanctioned presses of the war period, while the war was still going on. Perhaps more importantly, it fit with the official prowar narrative that celebrated the brave feats of Russian men in battle, while lauding the self-sacrificing efforts of Russian women in nursing service. For despite the harrowing ordeals that Zakharova endured, despite the tremendous value of the services that she performed for the wounded, in her story the real heroes were the male soldiers, while female nurses such as herself remained secondary players. Indeed, she dedicated the work to the Russian *bogatyr* (epic hero) and spent much of her work lauding his bravery, stoicism, and sacrifice.

This does not, however, reduce the actual value of her service or that of the thousands of other women who carried out medical duties at the front. Nor does it negate the importance of the effects of war on them. Indeed, the experiences of Russia's wartime nurses clearly reveal the war's indiscriminate effects on combatants and medical personnel, men and women alike. As with men who were faced with the inhumane impacts of war, women serving in medical capacities suffered similar psychological traumas. The experiences of Russia's nurses during World War I also belie conventional wisdoms that designate nursing as a naturally feminine endeavor, which assert that the traits associated with normative femininity, such as caring and nurturing, emotional support and comfort, were characteristics particularly well suited to wartime medical service. On closer scrutiny it becomes apparent that wartime nursing moved women well beyond these traditional boundaries into nebulous areas and even into what were considered distinctly male realms. Many of the experiences of Russia's sisters of mercy challenged and demonstrated the limitations and fluidity of traditional conceptions of femininity and conventional notions of female behavior. Ultimately, the further we investigate the phenomenon of modern warfare, the more apparent the intersectionalities of gender become.

6

WOMEN AND MEN AT WAR: RELATIONS AND PERCEPTIONS

N. CHELAKOVA: CAREFREE TEEN TURNED SISTER

Eighteen-year-old N. Chelakova spent the summer of 1914 with her family, as usual, in Finland, relaxing and enjoying herself, oblivious to the impending conflict. In mid-July the family gathered to celebrate Saint Vladimir's Day. "Although dark clouds of international politics were gathering on the horizon," she recalled, "we celebrated happily. We swam in the sea, rode horses along the shore, and in the evening, built a campfire and sang songs around it." When she returned home to Saint Petersburg at the end of the summer, the war was already under way. There she found a letter waiting for her, a request for her services from the nursing community where she had trained as a sister of mercy the previous year. Chelakova expressed a strong patriotic urge to serve her country and showed her father the letter, seeking his permission to enlist. Her father, however, was much less enthusiastic about war as a positive expression of nationalism. He looked at its impact in terms of human costs and was wary of sending his young daughter off to the front. In fact, he only agreed to allow her to go if she could pass a medical exam demonstrating her ability to endure what he knew was to be very difficult service. Worried that her poor health as a child might hinder her chances of being accepted into wartime medical service, Chelakova hid the letter containing her father's demand that she submit to medical scrutiny from the officials of the *obshchina.* With her prior training and the high demand for trained medical personnel at the front, the Red Cross readily admitted her into their ranks of the nursing community without question, and when she requested to be sent to the frontline positions, the authorities immediately complied. The young woman was overjoyed, seeing herself as embarking on a new adventure. Yet, as she excitedly gathered her supplies for the journey, her sister chastised her for taking a camera. Like her father, Chelakova's sister held no romantic illusions about war. "You aren't planning on taking pictures of human suffering, are you?" she chided. Chelakova was perplexed by this response; she was extremely excited to have the opportunity to witness and participate in what she believed were historic events and therefore was convinced of the necessity of recording them for posterity.[1]

After completing her medical training, Chelakova received assignment to a military medical unit on the Russian western front. Prior to her departure for the front, however, she had to receive other "training," in light of deep-seated concerns over the interactions she and other female nurses would have with male personnel. Red Cross officials undertook a number of steps aimed at preventing what they perceived of as inappropriate entanglements. During the ceremony officially consecrating her and her cohorts as sisters of mercy of the Red Cross, the baroness who served as the trustee for the *obshchina* issued a series of stern regulations regarding the nurses' behavior. She spoke at length about the honor of wearing the sister of mercy uniform and the necessity of upholding that honor with proper behavior. Among her prohibitions was the wearing of cosmetics. She then inspected them closely, with the intention of removing from the ranks any women who had contravened her orders. When she came across one sister who was wearing face powder, she sternly reproached her. "You are not respecting the high calling of a sister of mercy," she scolded. "You are excluded from our establishment." The young woman was mortified, but later she was reinstated through the intervention of a well-connected relative who had influence over the baroness. Chelakova was also quick to point out that although the baroness was now highly respected in her advanced age, as a young woman she apparently had a reputation for engaging in "frisky behavior." Nevertheless, the baroness's words resonated long after with Chelakova, and in particular, in her associations with male personnel while in service, she attempted to keep her strong admonitions in mind at all times.[2]

After official induction into the ranks of the Red Cross, Chelakova was sent to the front, initially serving in the hospital located at the fort in Brest-Litovsk. Along the way, she recalled that in their Red Cross sister of mercy uniforms, particularly the long, black head kerchiefs, the nurses were often taken for members of the clergy. Peasants would often come up to them and inquire from which monastery they hailed, referring to them as "little black ones" (the "black" clergy in Russian Orthodoxy composed of monastic monks and nuns who took vows of celibacy).

Soon after her arrival at the front, Chelakova was asked to accompany one of the doctors to a hospital train that had just arrived at the Brest-Litovsk station. As they traveled to the station, they began to get acquainted with one another. The doctor was a bachelor from Vorenezh, where he had a small estate and worked in the local Zemstvo hospital. He had just been called up for military service. Chelakova described him as a very serious man, one who was "a little adverse to having fun." Although he was only thirty-five years old, it seemed to her "that he was almost elderly." In his presence, she commented that she often "felt as if I were a schoolgirl and by old custom often gave reverence when the infirmary doctor came up to me."[3]

After serving for several weeks at Brest-Litovsk, Chelakova's unit was transferred to the military hospital established at the Ivangorod railway station. She recalled the senior doctor of this hospital, Dmitri Ivanovich, in terms similar to the doctor described above. She remarked that he was a man who "always conducted himself with great dignity, smiled rarely, as if his very serious facial expression was an inseparable part of his uniform." She felt great respect for him, as she did for the head of the medication department, Dr. A., whom she described as relating to her like a "kind, patient father."[4] By contrast, she had less regard for the senior surgeon, Dr. B., a younger man, quite inexperienced in performing operations since his area of medical specialization was gynecology. She recalled that he "resembled a big, gentle hound, one that liked to lie on the porch, rarely turning from good-natured growls." Her opinion was even lower of a "scrawny" doctor, who she indicated was of Polish origin, and who, she asserted, "always looked like he was endeavoring to run off somewhere." At the very bottom of the pecking order were the peasant orderlies who worked along with her in the military hospital at the Ivangorod railway station. She described them in largely positive, impersonal, if somewhat humorous and even condescending terms.

> Most of our orderlies were elderly, people unfit for combat service. They were strong, bearded peasants, fully dignified in their gait, which is common for people close to nature, who work on the land and live according to planning by the seasons of the year. They left behind their agricultural work and their large families, but thought

> themselves luckier to work in the hospital. They had names that sounded like bells, names like Ivan Lopata (Hammer), Roman Krasnopera (Redfeather) and Vavila Sinebriukh (Bluebelly).

Chelakova completed this picture by remarking that "all of us, doctors, nurses, and orderlies, gathered from different ends of the country and from different environments (backgrounds), as if to create a colorful pattern of national customs and foundations, beliefs and devotions, that constitute all of the diverse conditions of existence. Soon we became like one big, friendly family." She even included a Jewish doctor in her familial unity, somewhat unusual for the time, and insisted that everyone in the unit was very sympathetic to him.[5]

AMBIGUOUS RELATIONS

Chelakova's reminiscences reveal much about the ways that female nursing personnel and male doctors, officers, and soldiers related to one another, and how sisters of mercy were received. Any study of wartime nursing would seem rather incomplete without an examination of the ways that the women who served as nurses intersected with the men they treated and with whom they worked. The relationships between Russia's wartime nurses and the soldiers for whom they provided medical care and the male medical personnel with whom they worked are highly significant for understanding the phenomenon, and in particular they highlight the gendered meanings of wartime nursing. Her recollections also clearly reveal the anxieties that existed surrounding wartime nursing, especially the interactions between men and women in medical service. Authorities were extremely concerned about intimacy between female nurses and male medical or military personnel. Although sexual interaction was of primary concern to both military and medical authorities, and rumors concerning "immoral" behavior of sisters of mercy spread through Russian society during the war, this was not the primary way that female nurses and male personnel actually interacted. Although there were some women and men who had intimate interactions during the war, interpersonal relations between men and women in wartime service were as varied as the individuals themselves, and they reflect a number of different themes and influences. In many ways, they clearly reflected the familial structure of Russian society, modeled on patriarchal hierarchies of gender, class, and age. Gender, class, religion, nationality, and even politics were important factors in shaping perceptions and relations of female nurses and the numerous men they came into contact with while carrying out wartime medical service. Both men and women, including the nurses themselves, held certain expectations of nurses' behavior, both as sisters of mercy and as women, and when the women did not conform to these idealized notions, both were often critical. By the same token, sisters assumed soldiers and doctors would also act according to conventional notions of masculinity and in keeping with stereotypes, but this was not always the case. The reality of interaction between soldiers and nurses, and their perceptions of one another, are diverse and complex. Studying these relationships as they were portrayed by the women and men involved in them are tremendously useful in helping us understand the phenomenon of war and its reciprocal effects.

Nurses and Male Patients

Official sources that discuss the relations between nurses and male patients and the effect of sisters of mercy on wounded men are rather formulaic. Consistent with contemporary essentialist notions of femininity centered on nurturing and caring, most often they present the wartime nurse as a source of comfort, solace, and even happiness for the recovering soldier and officer. The image is a pure, highly feminized but distinctly desexualized one, which emphasizes the importance of the nurses' efforts on behalf of men. The psychological and emotional impact of their mere presence, rather than their medical work, is presented as the most significant contribution made to the war effort. Relations with nurses were presented as devoid of any sexual overtones or suggestions, with nurses performing roles of motherly care for wounded heroes.

Although they vary significantly based on individual experience, nurses' own accounts often reflected these conventional tropes, revealing the extent to which public discourse shaped their understandings of their service. In particular, many shared a general, romanticized view of the Russian soldier. It was not unusual for representations of soldiers in the writings of Russian sisters of mercy to be consistent with the masculine "myth of war." Soldiers were most commonly depicted as brave, strong, and stoic. A number of the memoirs left by women who served as wartime nurses spend pages extolling the virtues of the "Christ-loving" peasant soldiers, who burn with the desire to serve "for God, for Tsar, and for Motherland." Cossacks, in particular, were frequently extolled for tremendous courage and fortitude, earning them a reputation as the fiercest warriors who would fight to the death rather than allow themselves to be captured.

Indeed, some nurses' stories focused primarily on the soldiers, even to the neglect of their own experiences. Dedicating their writings to the soldiers, they extol their virtues and even recount the heroic deeds that led to their injuries. It was not uncommon for the women who served as wartime nurses to insist that their own experiences were much less significant when compared to the great feats performed by the soldiers. After completing her record of her time spent as a nurse on the front lines, Lidiia Zakharova commented, "Now, when my memoirs lay completed before me, I leaf through them, I review the gallery of fleeting outlines, silhouettes, sketches and my attention stops on one, more significant than all the others: the soldier." For her, all the horrors she had witnessed at the front were seemingly justified by the courageous acts of the soldiers in defense of the homeland. "And in all of my soul in that moment I felt that 'there' [at the front] it was actually good, that there, among the horrors, dangers, and privations, that what was most important, solid, and successful, was man, and that man was . . . our simple, fresh, dear Russian soldier, the true hero of my unpretentious narrative."[6] There were even tinges of guilt that emerged from nurses' writings for having been unable to make the ultimate sacrifice for the nation as defenders. Often this was expressed in gendered terms, indicating that the role of a woman in war could never be as significant as that of a man. Sofia Bocharskaia penned her frustration, as well as that of the other sisters with whom she served, after learning that the brother of one of her fellow nurses had been killed in battle, lamenting that they felt "useless and lamed by being women."[7]

Self-abnegation and placement of the soldier as the central figure of their war stories was not unique to the Russian nursing experience, appearing in many of the writings of wartime nurses in other belligerents. Historian Margaret Darrow has argued that for French nurses of the Great War, this was a uniform model of self-reflection, which she asserts was necessitated by the belief in the central masculinity of the war. As a result, nurses internalized public discourse that insisted only the actions of men in battle, which she argues were being carried out to restore the damaged masculinity of the French nation, were worthy subjects of wartime narratives or even of memoirs written after the conclusion of the hostilities. Accordingly, while French men as soldiers served the nation and the greater cause of the war, French women as nurses could only be seen as secondary players, for they served the men, not the nation.[8] In Russia, I would suggest that while such an explanation is fitting for some of these narratives, for others it is insufficient, as the war for many held meaning beyond the ideal of remasculinization. Moreover, as Karen Petrone has indicated, "the mechanized warfare and mass slaughter of World War I posed a formidable challenge to traditional definitions of the male warrior hero all over Europe."[9] The ways that Russia's female war nurses wrote about their experiences indicate that while they did often see the soldier as the primary figure in the war, they also saw themselves as serving their nation. Moreover, as demonstrated in chapter 4, the female wartime nursing experience shared many features of the male combat experience, rather than, as Darrow has suggested in the case of French nursing, existing to the exclusion of that masculine experience. In France, she asserts, the "policy was to clear the war zone of women and to prohibit women, even nurses, from visiting it; the war was to occur in a zone of pure masculinity. The feminine should cease to exist."[10] True, a number of Russian wartime nurses devoted portions of their writings lauding the soldiers and their actions, especially those written during the war to support prowar efforts (and even a number published after the conflict in émigré presses). Others, however, did not limit themselves to defining their experiences solely vis-à-vis the soldiers. They were distinctly aware of the importance of their actions, particularly on the front lines, where their services were desperately needed. In a letter home, Rimma Ivanova commented on her actions at the front: "I can say without humility that I've accomplished more here over these three days than I did in the hospital over a much longer time." The results of her work had a positive impact on the men, who she claimed "don't look at me as a woman, but as a sister of mercy who deserves enormous respect."[11] Even Zakharova's memoir, written in 1915 and clearly a part of the prowar effort, seems to simultaneously uphold a view of war as the domain of male heroism while also claiming the war experience as her own. As indicated above, she dedicated her work to the Russian *bogatyr,* the warrior hero, and included large sections extolling his virtues. The author recalled feeling ashamed as she sat on the train headed back to Petrograd with wounded soldiers, believing her sacrifice had not been as great as theirs.[12] Nonetheless, she also devoted much of the book to describing her own thoughts, feelings, and actions. She even noted the similarities of her experiences with those of the men, as with the case of the "l'homme qui rit," described in chapter 5. For her, the war was both a transformative experience that allowed her to feel useful and escape the feelings of emptiness that filled her when her husband was called away to the front—an emotional chasm that even her children could not fill. Many nurses even used the device of describing the soldiers that they treated as a means to demonstrate their own worth, by framing their discussion around the thanks and praised heaped on them by the wounded and ill. In this way, they validated their own service against that of the combatant, who, while sacrificing his life for the good of the nation, was being cared for by an equally important member of the national family.

To demonstrate their usefulness, Russian sisters of mercy often included correspondence from soldiers who had been in their care testifying to the benefits of their work. Rimma Ivanova recounted letters from her soldier charges, one of whom was so overwhelmed by gratitude he "could not find the words" to thank her.[13] Tatiana Aleksinskaia included an entire section of letters from soldiers at the end of her book. These refer to "great attention and delicate care" that wounded men received at the hands of nurses in her unit. One former patient wrote, "I am very grateful to you, Sister, for your care and help. If I were to live a hundred years, I should never forget. I am always telling the nurses how kind you are and how much I want to thank you with all my heart." A number of those who had been transferred to rear hospitals for recovery also mentioned the excellent service of sisters of mercy in those facilities. One referred to the nurses in his rear hospital as "cherubim." Another letter from a Russian soldier said, "You cared for us as though we were your children. We thank you. Only Jesus could have cared for us as well as you have done." Patients often asked the nurses for their photographs. Another soldier remarked that his whole family worshipped Aleksinskaia and had put her photograph in a gold frame.[14]

It is certainly not accidental that all those selected for inclusion in her memoir were positive, extolling the virtues of sisters of mercy. As such, they indicated the importance Aleksinskaia ascribed to her work and the positive impact of her actions as much as soldiers' attitudes. Indeed, in one of the first letters Aleksinskaia chose to include, the soldier thanked her "for taking such care of the faithful defenders of our beloved country. May God give you the courage to go on working for the good of Russia." She was not always comfortable with the ways that soldiers wanted to celebrate her contribution, however. One of the wounded wanted to publish an article about her in a right-wing newspaper, to thank her publicly, but she protested. As a socialist, she did not want to be praised in an anti-Semitic right-wing organ. She tried to convince him not to publish the article. But he would not accept modesty as an excuse, instead writing a letter to the Central Committee of the Zemstvos:

> We are very grateful to you for your care of us. And the Sisters of Charity appointed by the Union looked after us with great devotion and kindness. . . . The Sisters on our dear train were never idle for a moment, but renewed our dressings several times a day, did everything possible to allay the sufferings of the wounded, and often stay all through the night by their bedsides, helping them, and talking to them, never sparing their own health, eating nothing for days together, and having never a chance to sleep. There were about four hundred of us in the train, almost all serious cases, and thanks to the Sisters, only two men died in four days. May God keep them all in good health, especially little Sister N. N.![15]

Indeed, in Russia, many argued that wartime nursing was not only the appropriate means for women to carry out national service, but that it was necessary for them to do so in times of crisis that required the full mobilization of society. Moreover, as indicated in chapter 4, many of the writings left by Russia's World War I nurses are explicit about the kinds of sacrifice, the hardships, the depravations, and, particularly, the dangers they faced as part of their service. Rather than diminishing them as less arduous than those of male soldiers, like Zakharova, they often compare them to the experiences of men in the trenches. A number of Russia's sisters of mercy often saw their roles as greater than mere caretakers of the wounded. They believed themselves to be part of a noble effort, one in which their actions were not diminished by the lack of involvement in the fighting. Aleksinskaia, despite her prewar pacifist stance as a socialist, came to view her role as a wartime nurse as assisting the Allies in defeating the evils of German imperialism, which she thought now outweighed the message of internationalism. When talking to a soldier who had suffered fatal injuries, she attempted to shore up his spirits by emphasizing the significance of his sacrifice. "It was death rather than recovery that lay before him. But how could I tell him? You cannot tell the truth to these dangerously wounded men, who are so worn out as well. But I felt I ought to tell them something, and I talked to them, not about themselves, for whom there was little hope left, but of the cause for which they were suffering." Aleksinskaia spoke of the evil of war, but one from which there was no escaping, engulfing the whole world, caused by the Germans and their actions. She related the standard anti-German propaganda about their brutalities among civilians. She recalled that this was her first "prowar" speech but she felt it was necessary to convince the men they were not dying in vain, and soon it became a standard practice for her. Aleksinskaia does not present this as a "secondary" or auxiliary function to the men's "primary" combat role. She was convinced that this was a vitally important role played by nurses, whose words of encouragement had a positive effect, insisting that the men thanked them for "putting heart" into them and giving them the ability to return to the front to finish their work of defending the nation.[16]

Despite the challenge to conventional masculinity centered on defense of the nation presented by the war, it is clear that many sisters held soldiers to these normative standards. More specific to the Russian context, nurses' writings about soldiers also reflected common cultural stereotypes of the fatalistic, long-suffering, but extremely patient, peasant *muzhik*, who never complained about the lot given to him by God. The idea that this stoicism was an integral component of the soldiers' heroism was infused with a conventional wisdom that suffering was a long-accepted part of peasant life. Strongly connected to religious ideals promoted by Russian Orthodoxy, this was sometimes coupled with notions of fatalism, and soldiers were described as uncritically accepting their God-appointed lots. Nurses' writings share this view as well. Lidiia Zakharova watched a regiment of soldiers as they wearily marched along a country road in the burning sun of August in the early days of the war. "Most of them walked slowly and obediently, without lifting their heads, a few of them stopping by the edge of the road to allow our transports to go by and following them with long, indifferent looks."[17]

The peasant soldiers' ability to endure great hardship and pain in particular was a common feature in the writings of Russia's sisters of mercy. Sofia Bocharskaia wrote of her first encounter with wounded soldiers that "they were all excited and paid little attention to their wounds," wanting to be bandaged as quickly as possible so that they could get back to the fighting.[18] Farmborough commented about the soldiers in her care, "They are mostly patient long-suffering men, grateful for what care and attention they receive; seldom if ever, does a grumble pass their lips."[19] A. Ul'ianov, writing in the clearly prowar collection *Liubov sil'nee vrazhdy: rasskazy sestry miloserdiia iz poslednei voiny* (Love Is Stronger Than Enmity: Stories of Sisters of Mercy in the Recent War), included the recollections of a nurse who remarked that the soldiers in her care never uttered a sound while their wounds were being dressed or examined. Even a man with a deep chest wound lay patiently and quietly while the doctor fitted a tube to drain the bullet hole.[20] Tatiana Aleksinskaia pointed to this attribute of soldiers as well. "Never, as I worked all day and night, did I hear a single groan, a single cry; but there were several men who, with their heads pressed hard against the wall, lost consciousness and sank down onto the floor." Later, she recalled that "my experience told me that those who are in the worst condition never cry out: they just lie still and helpless. . . . Where do they get such a power of patience and resignation?"[21] Aleksandra Tolstaia recalled that when she was required to use a strong solution of mercuric chloride to clean the wounds of the man whose buttocks were almost completely blown off by the explosion of a shell, the man emitted no moans or complaints. The only indication she had of the extreme pain he must have been enduring was the faint creaking sound of the grinding of his teeth.[22]

Courage and fearlessness were also essential components of nurses' perceptions of soldiers. While a number of female medical personnel expressed their own fear while carrying out wartime medical service, few did so when describing their patients. For some, this was the result of the view that the soldiers were incapable of understanding the true dangers that confronted them in battle. Zakharova, while remaining faithful to the standard trope of soldier heroes throughout her memoir of war experiences, often refers to the rank-and-file troops as "children." Hers is a somewhat common paternalistic (or in this case, maternalistic) attitude that pervaded much of Russia's educated elite, who tended to view the Russian peasantry as insufficiently mature, especially politically and religiously underdeveloped. Again, this highlights the understanding of Russian society as a large, patriarchal family, wherein the lower classes were conceived of as children needing guidance. Zakharova described the soldiers as "kind, guileless, large children, unconscious of just how much heroism, how much soulful brightness and beauty they possess in their humble ignorance." Yet she also framed her discussion of this childish nature in such a way as to foreground the soldiers' bravery and courage: too immature to know better, he threw himself into battle without caring for his own life, hoping only to serve his motherland.[23]

Wartime nursing seemed to accentuate these perceptions of peasant soldiers as children. An important gendered dimension derived from the close association of nursing with nurturing and thus mothering. Sisters were often transformed into mothers, reflecting their maternal feelings toward their soldier "children" in tender, emotional ways. Bocharskaia commented, "Those we saved we felt had become our children. We were bound to them, even those we liked least held us."[24] Aleksinskaia reflected that "it was strange to have these men, who had gone to the war, who had endured cold and privation in doing their duty, lying there as weak children, patiently awaiting a nurse's care."[25] The idea of mothering allowed Zakharova to derive significant meaning from her war experience and even connect it to her previous life. Indeed, in her narrative, it was her participation in the war that restored her place within the conventional gender order and redeemed her abandonment of her own children when she enlisted in nursing service. While carrying out her duties as a sister of mercy, she experienced something of an epiphany that led her to conclude that the most important things in life were children (whether actual or childlike peasant soldiers), and she suddenly longed to return to her own sons and rededicate her life to them. She recalled thinking:

> This is what never changes! This is what is real, unshakable! Children, relations with them and through all childhood, youth, unspoiled in man. To protect children, to love children, to believe in them! Here is the thread, which connects me with the past, with my previous existence and my new life. And with particular strength, love for my own boys seized my heart, passionate, irrational, reckless thirst to see them right now, without delay, to kiss their cheeks, and hold them to my heart.[26]

This was an aspect of nursing common across nationalities. Nurses in other belligerents often spoke of their patients in similar terms. Allison Belzer has detailed the ways that Italian nurses often "saw themselves as substitute mothers, sisters, or wives, providing love and attention to lonely and injured men."[27]

There were some notable exceptions to the idea of the soldier as blindly courageous, revealing not only that soldiers did in fact experience fear but also that nurses were often acutely aware of this. Often, however, nurses' descriptions of expressions of fear by soldiers fall in line with the divide in views of soldiers based on how badly they were wounded, thereby doing little to disrupt the conventional notions. "True" heroes were conceived of as those who came closest to sacrificing themselves for the motherland and therefore sustained the most serious injuries, while those with lighter wounds not only complained more but also did not perform feats of great bravery that put them at greater risk. Chelakova distinguished the frightened, cowardly soldiers as those with light wounds (especially to the hands, which were suggestive of self-infliction), from the "true" soldiers, brave and stoic, those who were badly wounded and immobilized. Like Aleksinskaia, she insisted that the latter bore their pain without complaint, lying patiently while awaiting medical attention, and did not seem overly concerned even when enemy aircraft flew directly overhead. Reflecting the standard trope of the long-suffering peasant, she mused that perhaps their ability to endure was because they were "already reconciled to the fact that there would be inevitable suffering on their part." She chastised the lightly wounded for making much noise, even crying when their bandages were changed and their wounds cleaned. These were also the soldiers who openly expressed fear, who ran frantically from the hospital seeking cover from enemy bombs. In a further allusion to their cowardice, she suspected that they had come to the hospital "hoping, at least for the time being, to be in a location out of danger."[28] Worst of all were those who came in for treatment of self-inflicted wounds, usually to the hand, suffered in an effort to be sent home. Many nurses were often quick to criticize those they saw as attempting to shirk their patriotic duties. But others were more sympathetic. Florence Farmborough was "aghast" and felt "miserable" as she watched a doctor examining a young soldier's wounded hand, calling him a "coward and fool," and causing the young man to turn his head away and sob.[29]

Some nurses also expressed more critical views of soldiers that do not fit with the heroic tropes of patriotic literature. Aleksandra Tolstaia lamented that Russian soldiers, on entering an abandoned German village, set about destroying the pristine homes and stealing valuable possessions in what she saw as an act of senseless violence. She remembered,

> It was difficult to watch as the soldiers went from house to house, filling bags with various goodies, clothing, wall clocks, linens. The furniture they did not carry out, but simply smashed. Crash! Crash! From the high windows of a clean, comfortable little house flew chairs, tables, commodes, and after them, with piteous groans, the

> striking of hundreds of strings of the bridge of a piano. The soldiers happily bellowed with laughter.[30]

When speaking about the ways that soldiers related to them, nurses were also usually positive, indicating little in the way of animosity or inappropriate behavior on the part of the men toward their female caretakers. Many wrote of the fondness with which soldiers addressed them, calling them "little sister," "little dove," and other terms of endearment. They described tender moments with wounded and dying men who found great comfort in the presence of sisters of mercy while lying in hospital beds. Because nurses performed many basic functions for wounded and ill patients such as feeding, bathing, and clothing them, their relations often acquired a maternal aspect. When nurses performed other tasks, such as writing letters home to soldiers' loved ones and family members, they often found themselves listening to rather intimate details of men's lives. Sisters usually indicated that soldiers were eternally grateful for the care and attention given to them. Without a doubt, much of this gratitude and warm feelings were sincere on the part of soldiers. At the same time, however, it is important to note that nurses recorded such aspects of their interactions with soldiers not only with the intention of demonstrating their good relations with them but also to display their own beneficence and highlight their own importance. It is also safe to assume that some nurses chose to leave out instances of negative interaction with male patients, as they would have disrupted both public and private perceptions of soldiers and called into question the benefit of female medical service.

Class was a significant issue in the relations between soldiers and sisters. As indicated in chapter 3, there was a significant social divide between many of the women who served as wartime nurses and the men who served as soldiers, specifically the rank and file of the Russian armies. While sisters of mercy were supposed to give care and comfort to all patients, regardless of class or rank, the sharp divisions of Russian social structure permeated wartime medical services and sometimes influenced the way medical personnel treated rank-and-file soldiers. Bocharskaia was appalled that the doctor in command of the typhus hospital where she worked early in the war cared very little for his peasant-soldier patients and specifically advised her not to trouble herself much for their sakes. She did not, however, take his recommendation and devoted herself to the care of the ill regardless of their social backgrounds.[31] Vanda Stepanova, similarly from the upper class, noted with displeasure that many of her friends and acquaintances who became nurses during the war expressed a singular desire to serve officers, with little regard for peasant conscripts. She remarked that all of the other nurses in her facility, a dressing station near Riga, spent their time exclusively in the wounded officers' tent, to the neglect of the soldiers. By contrast, Stepanova insisted that she devote herself to caring for the rank and file, believing this work to be more important. She felt compelled to stay at the bedsides of the wounded soldiers who passed through her unit, to whom she had developed a strong emotional attachment. "I didn't want to leave Riga: something strong and incomprehensible made me stay here and wait with patience. I spent all my days with the injured, mainly soldiers, who seemed to me pitiful, helpless, and forgotten by everybody." She spent hours reading to them from books sent from Petrograd published specifically for the lower ranks. She felt so sorry for the conscripted men that she used most of her salary to buy them treats, and she even gave them whatever sweets or other gifts that flirtatious officers bestowed on her in their unsuccessful attempts to secure her affections.[32]

Another distinct separation between many of the women who served as wartime nurses and their soldier patients resulted from the educational requirements for sisters of mercy. This was usually tied closely to class, with middle- and upper-class women being primarily among those able to access education beyond the primary level. While most nurses were literate and usually possessed secondary, and sometimes even higher, education, peasants often were uneducated and even illiterate. Literacy rates, it is true, had been on the rise in Russia for the past half century, particularly among urban populations, and therefore many members of the laboring classes had rudimentary abilities in reading and writing. But many others, from traditional peasant backgrounds, did not possess such skills. Moreover, the ways of speaking differed greatly between the educated elite and the lower classes. Aleksinskaia recalled that when she wrote letters home for wounded soldiers in her care, she was very conscious of this and did her best to write as was dictated to her. In particular, she tried hard not to change anything that his wife would hear as the man's true voice.[33]

Gender also combined with class to act as a barrier between women serving as nurses and their male soldier patients. Again, this resulted particularly from class differences. Sexual difference and gender separation were much more pronounced in the upper segments of Russian society, which had conceptions of female respectability based on sexual purity and fidelity. Thus, exposure to naked male bodies was much more disconcerting to women of these social groups. Aleksandra Tolstaia recalled that she became confused and disoriented the first time she assisted in surgery on a naked male body and that it took some time for her to get used to this sight.[34] As indicated earlier, male officers hailing from the nobility expressed discomfort with and even objected to the prospect of women of their social station being able to view their exposed bodies, and sometimes they even resisted treatment based on this prejudice.

Despite the factors that acted to create divisions between nurses and their patients, a number of sources indicate that these differences were often overcome to allow for the formation of connections across class and gender lines. Some indicate the extent to which soldiers often put great trust and faith in nurses, even more so than in doctors. It was usually sisters whom they called for when in pain, when in some physical need, and, most often, when they felt close to death. As indicated previously, the emotional comfort provided by nurses to wounded and dying men was among the most valued aspects of their service. Doctors were often seen as cold and unfeeling, whereas in keeping with notions of feminine emotionality, sisters were characterized as warmer and more caring. At times, they intervened when doctors prescribed particularly painful treatments, exhorting doctors to find other means or, at the very least, to allow them to provide small comforts to wounded or ill men. Male patients also sometimes confided in sisters of mercy, revealing aspects of their personal lives that they never shared with others. Vasilii Shul'gin, a writer and conservative member of the State Duma, recalled sitting late at night in a hospital ward in Galitsa with the duty nurse, when the latter was called to the bedside of a heavily wounded man. The sister leaned over the soldier and listened closely as he whispered to her for what seemed to Shul'gin to be a very long time. When the nurse finally returned to her desk, she was visibly disturbed. The soldier, believing that he was on death's door after being badly wounded in battle, confessed to the sister that he had killed his wife and his father on discovering them in bed together while on leave from his unit. He had hacked them to pieces with an axe in the middle of the night, and since he had not told them he was coming back to visit, and no one had seen him come or go, he would have never come under suspicion. He did not want to die with a guilty conscience, so he asked the sister to call his regimental commander and to be tried for his crime. The sister was unsure how to proceed and went to church to pray for guidance.[35]

While many soldiers held nurses in high regard, not all held lofty views of nursing personnel. Instances of negative commentary are much less frequently mentioned by nurses, but they did exist. Aleksinskaia recalled a letter from a soldier who apologized for the fact that "there were certain soldiers among us who were lacking in respect, and, instead of giving thanks, used to grumble."[36] Moreover, as will be examined more thoroughly in chapter 8, rumors and speculation about nurses' improper sexual behavior and lack of true devotion to the cause of medical care circulated through the ranks from the very earliest days of the war and seemed to escalate as the war dragged on, war-weariness increased, and Russian politics were radicalized. These undoubtedly influenced relations between soldiers and nurses. Florence Farmborough remembered being on a train bound for Moscow immediately following the Bolshevik Revolution in November 1917. As she moved through the corridors, she recalled that "many disagreeable remarks were heard. The fact that I was in Red Cross uniform seemed to make me a special target for criticism."[37]

Nurses and Officers

Nurses' relations with officers were usually quite different from those with ordinary soldiers, as a result of class distinctions as well as attitudes of both the sisters and the men. The educational requirements for nursing service meant that many women who became sisters of mercy hailed from similar class backgrounds as the men who were commissioned as officers. Many nurses felt more comfortable with and chose to spend their free time with officers, and some even expressed a preference for working with officers. In most medical facilities, officers were separated from rank-and-file soldiers in special wards, where they received distinctly different treatment from the average peasant troops.

For some nurses, however, treating officers presented problems rather than raising feelings of affinity for those of similar social status. A number of nurses were entirely disheartened by the prospect of having to care for men of the officer class. They were often seen as more troublesome, less able to bear pain and suffering, selfish, and difficult to satisfy. Tatiana Varnek expressed significant reluctance treating them when they came into her facility wounded or ill. When assigned to the officers' ward in a hospital in Kiev, she recalled that she "fell into despair" and begged to be assigned to the soldiers' ward. When her request was refused, she "became unbelievably scared," fearing that she would not be able to "manage" them, that she "lacked the authority" to do so. In general, she came to see that her fears were unfounded and that she had good relations with most of the officers, most of whom she claimed came to "love her." However, she did remark that some of them were "capricious, very demanding, and undisciplined."[38] Aleksandra Tolstaia, despite her own aristocratic origins, was similarly hesitant to treat officers. When assigned to the officers' car of her hospital train, she went with great reluctance. She remarked that it was much easier to work with soldiers, because of their simplicity and because they were "more delicate than officers. They turned away, when necessary, in order not to embarrass a sister." By contrast, she lamented that in the officers' car there were often those who lacked such respectfulness, especially the lightly wounded, who, while being bandaged, would tell dirty jokes and make double entendres in front of the nurses. She complained that this often became unbearable, particularly when she was forced to sit in the car with them on the long journeys between stations and listen to the "banal conversations and facetiae of the officers."[39]

In some instances, male medical and military personnel, particularly officers who hailed from the middle and upper classes, were openly hostile to the presence of upper-class women nurses in war service. Some men of the nobility resisted treatment from women of their class because they considered it indecent for them to see their naked bodies. Others believed it was inappropriate for women to be present in military facilities. The senior doctor who ran the infectious diseases hospital to which Sofia Bocharskaia was assigned to bring a typhus patient initially refused to allow her and her companions to enter the facility. Astonished that such "aristocratic" sisters of mercy had been sent to his establishment, he informed them that the hospital, which was in rather poor condition, was not a "suitable environment" for ladies. Turning them away, he asked them to return the next day when the hospital could be "made fit for ladies of their standing."[40]

Sisters of Mercy and Male Medical Personnel

Sources published during the war for public consumption, and even some produced long after the conclusion of the hostilities, usually presented a similarly idealized view of the relations between male and female medical personnel. Doctors were presented as caring father figures to devoted young nurses. Little hint of conflict or intimacy can be seen in most of these sources. In their own writings, the women who served as sisters of mercy in Russia's Great War were often very positive when speaking about the male medical personnel with whom they worked. Doctors were often presented as kind, knowledgeable, paternal figures, as Chelakova depicted the doctors under whose supervision she worked at Brest-Litovsk and Ivangorod in the opening vignette. Lydiia Zakharova's chief doctor, Aleksei Petrovich, was consistently described as honorable, caring, and competent. When he sensed she and the other nurses were having difficulty adjusting to the horrors they witnessed and the rigors they endured, he attempted to cheer and comfort them. When she fell ill with a high fever, he expressed grave concern for her well-being and insisted that she be sent to the rear for treatment.[41] These harmonious relationships are often emphasized in secondary accounts of Russian wartime nursing as well. N. I. Vladimirsteva, in her account of the experiences of sister of mercy F. N. Slepchenko, insists that, when placed in charge of medical service provision in a leper colony, "she worked very harmoniously with the doctor, who she said valued the hard work of the sisters of mercy, and she was very much loved by the patients."[42]

Medics and orderlies were usually solid, strong, helpful peasants. Aleksinskaia had nothing but positive things to say about the reliable group of Mennonites who served as orderlies and stretcher bearers on her hospital train. Excused from combat service as a result of their religious convictions against violence, Mennonites (usually Russo-Germans) were often found in auxiliary military service. Although such relations were often romanticized in the writings of wartime nurses, it is clear that class separation was still a factor in the relationships between members of Russia's elite and the nonprivileged groups of imperial society. Varnek confirmed this concept, despite her insistence on the "excellent relations" she and the other noble sisters had with the orderlies of their hospital, commenting that when the orderlies did seek her opinion on some personal matter, she was often at a loss as to how to help them. "But what could a young, Petersburg lady advise to a married *muzhik*?" She also found it difficult to develop friendships with other nurses when she was transferred to another *obshchina* in mid-1915. The new community was composed of women outside of her social circle, with whom, she remarked, she had little in common aside from their work. Nor did she find it easy to form relationships with the wounded men she treated. Although she found the work very interesting, as the nurse responsible for dressing the wounds of the men when they first arrived at the hospital, she saw the men as little more than the parts of the body she bandaged. "I languished in the bandaging station: I had no relations with lively people. They brought us wounded with gauze on their eyes, so that we almost never saw faces, knowing everyone by last names, not having relations with whole people, rather with legs, arms, stomachs, etc. . . . Although I was always with people, I felt myself to be alone and dreamed of being transferred to the ward."[43]

Other women who wrote about their nursing experiences were decidedly more negative about the men with whom they served. As indicated in chapter 2, Sofia Bocharskaia was less than enamored with the doctors and orderlies she encountered in the infectious diseases hospital to which she was first assigned after completing her training. Both were depicted as corrupt, uncaring, and self-serving. The doctor embezzled funds provided by the Red Cross to finance hospital expenses in order to purchase luxury items for his own benefit, and the orderlies stole food, clothing, and other items from the hospital and its patients. Neither seemed particularly interested in serving the needs of the men whom they were supposed to be treating in their medical facility.[44]

In their relations with sisters of mercy, doctors could be cold, capricious, dishonest, misogynistic, and even sexually predacious. Such negative commentary was found more often in personal writings of nurses than in published sources. Yet even some official publications revealed the tensions that existed between doctors and nurses. The *Red Cross Herald* indicated that there were reports from wounded men concerning the ill treatment of sisters of mercy at the hands of doctors. One report indicated that patients were highly disconcerted by "undeserved rudeness" on the part of doctors, especially senior doctors, toward nurses working under them in military hospitals. Wounded men often thought of nurses as their protectors against doctors, who often ordered painful medical procedures and therapies, which soldiers resisted despite their necessity. One patient, identified only as "B.," protested when the chief doctor of his hospital had ordered that his wounds be redressed each day, a process that caused the man considerable discomfort, and when the nurse asked if this was really necessary, he "yelled and scolded her rudely."[45]

Nurses' own writings are more expressive of these tensions, however. Tat'iana Varnek commented that she, as well as all of the other medical personnel, including the junior doctors, were deathly afraid of the senior doctor in charge of the hospital in Kiev where she worked in 1915. While renowned for being an excellent surgeon dedicated to his work, the doctor, Vladimir Nikolaevich Tomashevskii, had a "despotic character," according to Varnek. He would fly into a rage if things were not done exactly as he wanted them. She recalled how the otherwise silent operating room was often punctuated by his shouting at sisters, even the most experienced surgical nurses, when they failed to anticipate the instrument he desired. He even was reported to have struck an orderly on one occasion.[46] Vanda Stepanova complained about the "depraved talk" she often overheard emanating from doctors and other officers in her medical unit. "I didn't like the all-too-casual treatment of us by the doctors and officers who worked at the station. We were young ladies. There were conversations during dinners that shouldn't have been. They told indecent jokes," she remembered.[47]

Nurses also commented on the female doctors with whom they worked, and they often gendered their commentary based on traditional notions of femininity and masculinity. Aleksinskaia, while praising the abilities of her chief surgeon for treating her subordinates well, also suggested that her success was the result of her possessing "energy . . . equal to that of any man." She further indicated that "her hospitality is that of a great hostess: she makes every guest welcome . . . but she has her little caprices, or rather her peculiarities."[48] Tolstaia was little impressed by the woman doctor who headed her unit, as indicated in chapter 3. Varnek was highly critical of other female professional medical personnel, such as the "nasty" woman pharmacist who worked in her hospital, who rarely troubled herself with care for the wounded but instead sat alone refusing to lend a hand while never missing an opportunity to flirt with the senior doctor.[49]

Nurses were also subjected to unwanted sexual advances from doctors and other male personnel. Vanda Stepanova wrote about continual molestation by the chief doctor of the medical station where she worked as a sister of mercy near Riga, a Jewish surgeon from Saint Petersburg named Lipovetskii. Although Stepanova's resistance to the doctor's amorous attention was at least partially the result of her virulent anti-Semitism (she rarely missed an opportunity in her two-hundred-plus-page handwritten memoir to lambast Jews in some way, usually referring to them using the derogatory expression "yids"), it is clear that this was sexual harassment. From the moment she was assigned to the unit, the doctor had tried to court her. At first, he was merely very courteous and, according to Stepanova, in order to gain her affections, very attentive to the needs of her patients. Over time, however, and especially after finding out that Stepanova often spent her free time with a local military unit where her horse was quartered, his demeanor toward her changed. She claims that he "turned from being polite and correct to being unduly familiar, I would say even with a kind of impudence. He would grab my hand and attempt to hold it for a long time in his hands. I was sickened by this and each time tried to break away." Despite her indication that she had no interest in him romantically, he doggedly continued his pursuit. One evening, Lipovetskii arranged to be on duty alone with Stepanova so that he could ply her with wine and sweets in an effort to obtain her affections. He offered her more wine while he himself drank strong liquor. "His eyes began to burn crazily," Stepanova remembered, "his words became ruder, and then he tried to grab me by the hand in such a way that it scared me so that I ran for the door of the wounded patients' ward." She ran all the way to the commander's quarters, where she immediately fainted on entering. Revived, she recounted the events to the officers present, who acted to have Lipovetskii removed from the unit (after being talked out of dealing with him through more violent means).[50]

Fear of sexual harassment did not only occur between doctors and nurses, but also in other situations where women found themselves alone and vulnerable to male advances. Aleksandra Tolstaia reacted with alarm when she was forced to spend the night alone with her driver as they attempted to cross the mountainous terrain of the Caucasus Mountains. Unable to travel farther in the dark, the two decided to sleep in their car until morning light could aid their movement. When the driver climbed into the back seat where Tolstaia was attempting to rest, she was shocked and frightened. She repeatedly ordered him back into the front seat, but he refused to comply, insisting he could better protect her from the threat of marauding Kurdish bandits from that position. He even asked for her revolver, which she adamantly refused to surrender. Instead, she gripped it tightly throughout what became a sleepless night for her, refusing to let herself doze off and become vulnerable. Although his intentions were not clear, Tolstaia was clearly unnerved by his close proximity and did not trust him.[51]

Moreover, despite the great need for female medical personnel, not all male authorities welcomed women into the sphere of war, even in nursing capacities. Female intrusion into the space of war was met with suspicion by those who believed that the very presence of women was detrimental to military effectiveness. As Joshua Sanborn argues, "the military's bodily and ethical ideals were both explicitly and implicitly masculine. . . . The proper exercise of virtue was conducted in wholly male institutions." Long-standing misogynistic notions of feminine "nature" associated women with untrustworthiness and fears that they would distract men from their military duties, or worse, that the men would be infected with venereal diseases.[52] Even in the setting of the hospital or field infirmary, a female figure was unsettling to some men. Ernst Jünger recalled that he was "always irritated by the presence of women every time that the fate of battle threw me into the bed of a hospital ward. One sank, after the many and purposeful activities of war, into a vague atmosphere of warmth."[53]

Famed revolutionary writer Dmitrii Furmanov revealed the deep-seated resentment some men felt at the intrusion of women into the male sphere of war when he described the sisters of mercy in his unit. He was very critical of these women and lamented that when all was well, everyone would get along fine in the "male half," as long as "there was no answer from the women." Although he admitted being somewhat ashamed to write about these poor relations, he nonetheless believed that he needed to speak about them. In January 1915 Furmanov asserted that relations with the sisters of mercy became untenable for himself and the four other male nurses with whom he served on the Turkish front. He described most of the women in his unit as "extremely unattractive in their pettiness" and complained that "in the dormitory, this turned out to be a major illness. Now and again you would hear their secret sessions and whisperings in the corner: 'I said. He said, that I said, and he said that I . . . ' and so on and so forth, without end. The result was a lot of intrigue—ridiculous, stupid, outrageous." Furmanov complained that all of this was terribly demoralizing and distracted the other members of the unit from their important work. In the evenings he and his fellow male nurses would sit together and smoke in "comradely brotherhood," discussing the disturbing nature of the situation. After they could stand it no more, they decided to act by confronting the command staff with an ultimatum: "Us or them!" They presented their protest to the female senior doctor who refused to accept their demands and instead sent them on to the local administration of the Zemstvo union. A representative of the Seventh Mobile Field Unit named Glebov heard their complaint and promised to help. They waited several days for a response, but Furmanov claimed the situation was unbearable and they despaired that no solution would be found. As a result, the male nurses decided to leave on the first departing train to Sarykamysh, hoping to find work there, citing the "impossibility" of continuing to work with the female personnel.[54]

Even more troubling for some, preserving the masculinity of war was understood as a matter of national security. Many perceived women to be highly susceptible to engaging in gossip and loose talk, which could lead to revealing military secrets and treason.[55] Thus, concerns over the political reliability of sisters of mercy were expressed by both civilian and military authorities. There was a class, as well as a gendered, basis for such anxieties. A number of authorities were particularly anxious that nurses, especially women of the upper classes, coming into contact with ordinary soldiers would become too concerned with the social plight of men of the lower classes. Nurses, as well as other women who volunteered with organizations aimed to aid wounded and ill soldiers, often performed the service of writing letters home for wounded men. Authorities were greatly concerned about the content of such letters, which often included bitter complaints of malnourishment, neglect, and poor treatment.[56] These women were inclined to be sympathetic to their peasant- and worker-soldier patients and listened attentively to their grievances. Some authorities expressed fear that nurses' interactions with "radicalized" wounded and ill soldiers as patients would "politically compromise" the sisters by exposing them to pernicious ideas, including "revolutionary propaganda."[57]

There was considerable concern that revolutionaries had infiltrated the various volunteer civilian groups carrying out medical service during the war. These fears were not altogether unfounded, considering the antitsarist bent of many such organizations. Furthermore, female revolutionaries, recognizing the opportunity presented by wartime medical service to give them direct access to the soldiers, did become nurses during the war. The guise of a sister of mercy was very convenient, often allowing such women to operate in the open without raising suspicion. Bolshevik leader Vladimir Lenin's younger sister, Maria Ul'ianova, served as a sister of mercy on an ambulance train for the duration of the conflict, entering the war effort in order to divert the attentions of the tsarist political police.[58] Sister of mercy Rakhil' Rochko, a member of the Russian Social Democratic Party, was serving on hospital train no. 217 of the Vitebsk community of the Red Cross when, in March 1916, she was discovered "spreading revolutionary propaganda among the troops." The Red Cross authorities recommended that she be expelled from the ranks of the Red Cross and dispossessed of the title of "sister of mercy" for her participation in this "harmful activity."[59] Rochko's Jewish origin likely also played an important part in drawing suspicion to her actions. Despite the recommendation to remove Rochko from nursing service altogether, she was merely purged from the staff of the hospital train at the end of March. In September of that year, Rochko turned up working on another hospital train, no. 198, at which point she was once again discovered and expelled completely from the Red Cross, whose authorities continued to scratch their heads over how she had managed to enter the ranks of another unit undetected.[60]

Perhaps most significantly, while military and governmental authorities expected wartime nurses to follow orders unquestioningly and even adhere to standards of military discipline, they simultaneously continued to apply conventional notions of female respectability with regard to their sexual behavior. As indicated previously, this was a significant requirement for women who served as wartime nurses, accentuated by the fact that nurses served in male spaces of war, in close proximity to male bodies. Both Red Cross and military authorities expressed deep concerns and anxieties over nurses' behavior. Authorities were not simply concerned with preventing female nurses from engaging in sexual activity with male personnel, or even civilians. Any suggestions of sisters of mercy acting in ways that fell outside the very narrowly defined role of nurse, any behavior that suggested that they were anything more than purely angelic devoted caregivers, made male authorities extremely uncomfortable. Echoing the efforts of Chelakova's trustee in controlling female sexuality, Aleksinskaia remarked on the way her female chief doctor attempted to regulate the behavior of nurses. "She keeps a keen eye on the sentimental propensities of the girls working in her train, and intervenes, sometimes very roughly, whenever she suspects a romance in the making. Every now and then she gives them an address, in which she violently attacks what she calls somewhat contemptuously 'the sexual instinct' and revolts against the 'weakness' of women."[61] Even when women engaged in seemingly innocuous activities such as dining in restaurants or going to the cinema, many authorities were highly vexed. As indicated in chapter 2, there were even attempts to put regulations into place that would prohibit sisters of mercy from any public appearances in their uniforms, as their mere presence on the streets or in public venues was tainted with the suggestion of impropriety. The sight of nurses, who were supposed to be devoting all of their time to the well-being of the fighting men, engaging in leisure activities was extremely unsettling to many. Police interceptions of letters sent from the front indicate this unease. For example, one P. Kukol', writing in January 1915 from Odessa to Countess E. A. Uvarova in Moscow, complained that "sisters play tennis, dine and supper in restaurants and they are almost never without flowers, and in general they are extraordinarily elegant and joyous. Throughout all of Galicia among the medical personnel there is a tone of a happy picnic and vulgar ostentation."[62]

Although the Red Cross had significant religious associations and imposed the strong moral proscriptions of Orthodoxy on its female volunteers, the vast majority of women who became wartime nurses were not members of the clergy (indeed, not even all were Orthodox) and could not, therefore, be expected to behave as such. Despite the unrealistic nature of such expectations, they formed an essential part of the nurses' code of conduct, and the women would be judged by these standards regardless of the context in which they operated. When nurses did not conform to these codes of conduct, they risked removal from the ranks of medical service personnel. Sisters Shevetera, Bratukhina, Zhukova, and Shetakova, of the Tobolsk *obshchina,* were stripped of their titles of sister of mercy for "depraved behavior."[63] The implication of the language used in the expulsion order is clear: the women were engaging in what was considered sexually improper activity. Sisters Valentina Grishenko, Ruslana Pirumova, and Adele Iankovskaia were similarly expelled from the Tiflis Nadhezhinskii *obshchina* for their immoral conduct, deemed "intolerable for sisters of mercy."[64] What frustrated command personnel of military medical units to which Red Cross nurses were assigned was that, while they could request that women be removed from their units, only the trustees of the communities had the authority to expel nurses from the ranks of the Red Cross and deprive them of the title of "sister of mercy."[65]

Despite efforts to desexualize sisters of mercy and prevent sexual interaction between female nurses and male personnel (military and medical), numerous instances of this occurred. A number of nurses even wrote about their relationships with doctors. Mary Britnieva fell in love with and eventually married a doctor in her unit, as did Sofia Bocharskaia. While ultimately such relationships were legitimized by their culmination in state- and church-sanctioned legal unions, other, more casual, sexual interactions also occurred between nurses and male military and medical personnel. These encounters caused the most consternation among authorities and usually led to punishment of the women. The Viatka *obshchina* reported the expulsion of nurses Marianna Koriakina and Vera Viatkina from its ranks in mid-March 1917. The two women had been caught visiting the quarters of male medical personnel (feldshers), with one of the sisters in the throes of "intimate relations" with one of the feldshers.[66] Ultimately, it would be impossible for either the military or medical authorities to stop men and women from engaging in sexual relationships, but both continued to insist on the impermissibility of these interactions. Efforts to curtail them, however, rested almost exclusively on attempts to control female behavior, and it was the women, not the men, who would be held responsible and punished for any transgressions of these rules of conduct.

Sisters of mercy who engaged in sexual and romantic interaction with male personnel (either military and medical) faced significant criticism from their fellow nurses as well as from authorities. Such activities were seen as damaging to the reputation of wartime sisters of mercy. Tat'iana Varnek expressed irritation with her close friend Ksenia Ispolatova, who was "very excitable and easily carried away with love." Varnek complained that her friend was "constantly falling in love, losing her head, and imagining that she was going to be proposed to." When Varnek tried to dissuade her from these amorous inclinations and focus her attention on their work, Ispolatova would grow angry and accuse her friend of jealousy.[67] Vanda Stepanova insisted that she and the two other nurses that shared her quarters attempted to maintain strictly professional relationships with doctors and other male personnel, and they even distanced themselves somewhat from the other sisters in their unit, whose deportment they openly criticized. Stepanova expressed her significant disapproval that these other women often went out in the evenings with officers and sometimes returned to the nurses' quarters very late and visibly intoxicated. This led to tension between the nurses themselves, especially when the command personnel of the unit reprimanded the nurses who "cavorted" with doctors and officers and used Stepanova and her cohorts as examples of good behavior. The problem apparently became so bad that the chief doctor, Saksen, removed a number of nurses from the ranks of the unit and imposed very strict discipline governing the behavior of the nurses. The result was that the unit was nicknamed "the convent."[68] Despite her irritation with the behavior of other sisters in her unit, Stepanova herself developed a personal relationship with an officer from a nearby military unit named Basmanov, whom she eventually married.

Sexual behavior on the part of female nurses was certainly seen in an extremely negative light, but, as in the case of the Crimean War, perhaps even more troubling for male personnel was female authority. Conflicts with male personnel were particularly pronounced when sisters of mercy were given positions as head or senior nurses, which often placed them at odds with the men in their facilities serving as medical and military commanders. In theory, the head nurse's line of authority extended only over other female medical personnel. Yet, although all sisters of mercy, even head and senior nurses, were supposed to be subordinate to male doctors and officers, some women found themselves giving orders to such men. Male military medical personnel complained bitterly about certain head nurses and senior sisters who meddled in affairs of the hospital considered outside of their purview and who tried to command male doctors, despite their lack of military or medical rank or knowledge. Solov'ev urged both the military and Red Cross authorities to rein in the wives of high-placed officials and other well-connected women who believed it was acceptable to tell doctors how to run their facilities and to more clearly delineate the chain of command in medical establishments. He bemoaned that although Red Cross regulations dictated that senior nurses be appointed exclusively from staff sisters (i.e., those who had been part of the Red Cross societies prior to the outbreak of war), aristocratic women without staff designation used their "social positions and their connections in society" to secure senior nurse status.[69] The doctor who complained about the lack of martial discipline of nurses Sirenova and Osipova (described in chapter 2) was further irked by their tendency to "constantly take liberties to 'teach' doctors and openly, in the presence of the ill and wounded lower ranks, speak with extreme disdain about their medical knowledge." For him, however, gender was not the only issue. Indeed, he insisted that "at war, there are no men or women, only soldiers."[70]

Nurses sometimes went against doctors' orders in attempts to provide comfort and solace to patients, even when their efforts may have had detrimental effects. In many cases, despite strict doctors' orders against giving water to men with stomach wounds, sisters of mercy found themselves unable to resist their agonized pleas. Knowing that it was only a matter of time before the soldiers eventually succumbed to their injuries, sisters would sometimes give dying soldiers a last drink. This often hastened the inevitable, but it allowed the men some relief at the end of their lives. Doctors were infuriated by this gross insubordination, but they could do little to stop the practice. Once, when Farmborough gave water to a man she was certain was near death, her head doctor fumed at her, accusing her of deliberately killing the man. Yet she, and many of her fellow nurses, continued to disobey orders and did what they believed was best for men who would otherwise die in a state of tortuous thirst. Nurses such as Farmborough did not take this lightly, and it weighed heavily on their consciences. They believed that, as part of their comforting mission, it was more important to provide a little respite to a dying man than to adhere to military orders.[71]

Even when female medical personnel had proven medical training and knowledge, and when their advice was scientifically sound, men did not welcome their input or respect them as authorities in their field. Sister of mercy Tat'iana Aleksinskaia related several occasions in which she attempted to act in contradiction to what she considered to be her male supervisor's medically unsound orders, to the great consternation of the former. Although she was a doctor herself (though serving as a nurse in the war), the male doctor in charge of her hospital train would not accept her medical opinion as valuable. Nor did the female doctor who headed her unit have power over male doctors who were her subordinates in the organizational hierarchy. Aleksinskaia related several episodes wherein her medical expertise was dismissed and the advice she offered to doctors not only rejected but angrily resented. In one instance she recalled seeing a soldier on his hands and knees on the floor of her hospital train, with his face "in the dust," and thought this was a sign of the man's distress. She begged the doctor to examine the man, but he insisted that he could wait. By the time the doctor attended to him, the soldier was already dead. Reflecting common racial prejudices, Aleksinskaia attributed the doctor's obstinacy to his Caucasian ethnicity, rather than to the fact that the advice had come from a woman. Another instance of conflict with the same doctor came when she asked if two very serious cases could be left at a station where they could be transferred to local hospitals, fearing they would not survive the journey to the town that was their terminus. The doctor refused, stating, "I know better than you who ought to be left." She argued, "But you haven't even examined them. They need careful examination." The doctor, however, "would not budge." Overnight, one of the men developed a high fever and his bandages soaked through with blood. His wounded leg "turned bluer and bluer." Aleksinskaia worried he would not make it if he were not immediately sent to a hospital for surgery. Fearing for the men's lives, when they arrived at the next station, she appealed directly to the chief medical officer there, without waiting for the approval of her doctor. The officer agreed to take the men. When the surgeon of the local hospital examined them, he insisted that they remain there; both soldiers needed their legs amputated to ensure survival. Aleksinskaia knew she was disobeying chain of command, but she acted anyway to save the men's lives. "My doctor will not be pleased with me, in all probability," she mused. "I had acted without authority in contravention of 'orders.' If subordination is a good thing, so is human life."[72]

Furmanov did not hide his contempt for female authority figures in his diary recounting his experiences as a male nurse (brother of mercy) during the Great War. He remarked,

> One of the biggest mistakes of all of the medical organizations turned out to be the appointment of women in the capacity of senior doctors. Where it was necessary for bravery, hard, and direct words, there was weakness and even a few ridiculous methods of the female psyche. Many problems remained unresolved: you can't go to women with them, and if you do, you risk being only half understood. It is not enough for a soul to be warm and loving, there is a deficit of firmness and certainty that is covered to a certain extent by affection and comfort.

He described the woman who served as the senior doctor of the hospital train unit with which he served on the Turkish front as a "distracted person" and "desperate coward" whose words they took no notice of. He surmised that perhaps she would have made a "good, quiet wife or a peaceful office worker, but only that."[73] For him, leadership was clearly a masculine trait, one that was necessitated by the exigencies of war.

Furmanov's remarks further the reveal the paradox of wartime nursing, wherein certain essentialist components of femininity were valued while other assumptions about conventional womanhood were seen as completely inappropriate, even detrimental in the context of the war zone. This resistance to women exercising, or attempting to exercise, authority should not be surprising considering the history of the development of wartime nursing in Russia. As indicated in the first chapter, male military and medical officials, by and large, were fundamentally opposed to this kind of activity on the part of women. Even the most well-intentioned efforts by women to contribute to better management or facilitate improved conditions in medical units and establishments were met with hostility on the part of most men, who could not tolerate female authority. This continued to be a serious obstacle throughout the war period. Nor is the kind of mistrust and attribution of weakness to women by those such as Furmanov unusual, considering the deeply engrained cultural assumptions about women and negative associations of "female nature." Like many others, Furmanov attributed indecisiveness and lack of strength to women. Although only one of the two doctors in his unit was a woman, he described them both as "typical, slobbering, cooing *baby* (broads)." "It did not matter that the second doctor was a man," Furmanov complained. "He, indeed, could be even worse . . . than any woman." He attributed "unbelievable spinelessness" and superficiality in thought to him. For Furmanov, the fact that the male doctor was "soft and gentle" was a distinct disability in military medical service.[74]

Although they complained about women in positions of authority, in reality male military medical personnel, especially chief and senior doctors, had considerable power over the nurses assigned to their units. Often they were in complete control over the fate of the nurses that came into their facilities, regardless of whether the nurses' actual behaviors were positive or negative. They could often punish women, even when charges of misconduct leveled against them were false. While in many cases male doctors acted in ways they believed to be in the best interests of their units, they could use their positions arbitrarily and take action against sisters for strictly personal reasons. They could fairly easily have sisters removed based on their individual prerogative, in cases where mere personality clashes or failure to respond to sexual advances led male personnel to want to rid themselves of unwanted sisters of mercy. In many cases women, even those in authority, were powerless to stop male action against nurses. Not all doctors treated their nursing staffs well, and senior sisters or other nursing authorities had little ability to remedy this situation. The baroness who served as trustee of the Riga community of sisters complained to the main administration of the Red Cross that nurses were "completely dependent" on the goodwill of doctors. She claimed that many were prone to mistreatment of women assigned to their commands. As a result, sisters of mercy often came to her in tears asking to be transferred to different medical units, to be "rescued from persecution by doctors." While the baroness made such requests on behalf of the sisters of her *obshchina,* the ultimate decision for reassignment usually rested with the chief doctors of the units.[75] Similarly, there was little recourse for nurses who were targeted for dismissal by male medical authorities, even when the evidence was in their favor. Despite her record of capable service, a report from one individual doctor indicating that sister Glikeria Ponamera was not competent not only resulted in her removal from the ranks of his unit but also prevented her from reassignment, even to the reserves. Ponamera had worked in the Eighth Evacuation Hospital for more than two years and had proved herself an able and knowledgeable nurse. She was removed from its staff because the chief doctor, Dr. Likydi, expressed his discomfort with having her remain at the hospital as a result of her "increased inclination toward errors." The doctor did not provide any evidence of his accusations; nonetheless, his word was taken as the ultimate authority, and Ponamera had no means to appeal the decision.[76]

Red Cross officials often favored doctors over nurses when it came to settling conflicts, and they often mistrusted the intentions of sisters of mercy. When Tat'iana Varnek and her fellow sisters began to suspect that the senior doctor in charge of their field hospital was sympathetic to the enemy, they attempted to draw attention to his actions. According to Varnek, Dr. Kiummel, who hailed from a Baltic German family and had a poor command of the Russian language, seemed to favor the Austrian patients that came into the field hospital he ran on the southwestern front. She reported that he would spend long hours conversing with Austrian officers in German while redressing their wounds, but he paid almost no attention to the Russian soldiers being treating in the hospital. On one occasion, the sisters walked in on the doctor engaged in a conversation with a group of Austrian officers and pointing out locations on a military map. This incident was very disconcerting to Varnek and her fellow nurses. But they were completely outraged by his behavior shortly thereafter, when they learned that a train full of wounded had come into the nearby railway station and had been left completely unattended, their wounds undressed, without having been fed for days. When the nurses informed Dr. Kiummel of this situation, they expected him to dispatch them to the station to care for the soldiers. Instead, he categorically forbade them from doing anything for the wounded. The sisters and orderlies defied his orders and went to the station regardless.

Immediately following this event, the nurses decided to bring his actions to the attention of the Red Cross authorities. After writing individual letters "in all directions" and obtaining no results, the women appealed collectively to the Red Cross administration to intervene, or at least investigate the doctor. This act did pique the interest of the organizational authorities, but not in reaction to the doctor's suspected traitorous behavior, but rather because of what was perceived to be a "nurses' revolt." Sisters of mercy were expressly forbidden from undertaking such actions, and even in this case, when the nurses in question were members of Russia's elite (including the niece of the chairman of the Red Cross), it was their activities that raised eyebrows rather than those of the male doctor and head of the medical unit. The Red Cross immediately sent a plenipotentiary to the field hospital, who reprimanded the women. Three of the nurses were transferred out of the hospital to other units, in order to separate the troublemakers and prevent any further rebellious activity. The doctor was not "touched," and Varnek and her fellow sisters were "in despair" as a result of their inability to do anything about the situation.[77]

CONCLUSIONS

Chelakova's experiences as a nurse during the Great War tell us much about the ways that women and men intersected through medical service. Despite the image of the happy patriarchal family as structuring the relations between male and female personnel at the front, Chelakova's memoirs also reveal the deep-seated concerns about sexual interaction between them. She recalled that while traveling to the front, she and her fellow sisters were waiting to transfer trains at a station when they were approached by a group of officers, who asked to sit with them. The nurses agreed, but only on the condition that the men did not converse with them, suggesting that the mere act of speaking with unknown men might have deleterious effects on their moral value and damage the reputation of sisters of mercy. Their answer, Chelakova was certain, would have made the baroness proud. On a train ride back to the hospital, Chelakova and a doctor traveled in a car with a number of officers, all of whom were very attentive to the single woman in their midst. She stated that they treated her with "chivalrous attention" because she "now shared their service." Yet her description of their actions, as well as her own reaction, indicates that they may have been interested in her for other reasons, or that this was her perception. "They tried to engage me in conversation, offered me candy," she related. "But according to the instructions of Baroness I., our great service and the honor of our uniform sounded louder in my ears and I maintained an impregnable serenity." The doctor with whom she was traveling was somewhat perplexed by her aloofness. "'Why don't you want to talk with them? They seem like nice young men,'" he asked. "'I am a sister of mercy,' I said with sincerity. "'I came here to work and not to chit-chat,'" she replied, again, indicating that even engaging in conversation with strange men might cast aspersions on her reputation. Her actions surprised the doctor somewhat. "His eyes reflected disbelief and sincere admiration," she wrote. Indicating the prevalence of negative associations of sexual promiscuity with nurses, she remarked, "through his practice as a Zemtsvo doctor he had had dealings with another sort of sister, one who loved and sought out male attention."[78]

The multiple ways that men and women interacted through medical service indicate the complexity of gender relations, further complicated by the circumstances of war. The conflict often drew men and women together in ways that would have been unlikely in peacetime conditions. In many ways, conventional stereotypes and expectations regarding female behavior significantly colored the ways that men viewed and related to women. Power structures and social designations that held sway in prewar society were expected to be maintained despite the tremendous upheaval caused by the war, and the rearrangement of traditional hierarchies was expected to accommodate the necessities of wartime medical service. Class and social status similarly influenced gender relations, and similarly, relations between the classes affected by the ways the war brought those of divergent origins together in common situations. The incongruities of a nation at war presented significant challenges to what were perceived as "normal relations" between men and women.

Despite the changes wrought by war, many of the old structures and attitudes of imperial Russian society remained firmly in place. Even when faced with direct challenges to conventional notions, many men and women clung tenaciously to ideas that were forged long before the conflict but failed to hold up when their boundaries were pushed by total war. Ultimately, few questioned the cultural assumptions about women's essentialist nature as caring nurturers. Men often refused to accept female power or authority as something desirable or beneficial—even in some cases, possible—despite its necessity under the circumstances and despite empirical evidence of its feasibility. For their part, women continued to view masculinity in terms of bravery, stoicism, and courage. Many men and women accepted the notion that sexual interaction in a military context was unacceptable, while men continued to hold women accountable for transgressions of such taboos, in spite of their own actions. This attitude was closely linked to misogyny and suspicion of women, which was heightened by their presence in the perceived masculine space of military endeavors.

7

IMAGINING SISTERS: REPRESENTATIONS OF WARTIME NURSES IN RUSSIAN POPULAR CULTURE

LIUDMILA AND ELIZAVETA BYCHKOVA: MOTHER AND DAUGHTER TURNED SISTERS

Following the enlistment of both of her brothers into the army, Elizaveta Bychkova, a young noblewoman from Moscow, desperately wanted to join the war effort as a sister of mercy. Her young age of twenty, however, dictated that she could not do so without parental permission. Her widowed mother, Liudmila, was extremely reluctant to allow Elizaveta to go. Faced with the fear that she would lose all of her beloved children to the war, Liudmila implored her daughter to reconsider, pointing out the danger of such a venture and appealing to her not to leave her alone. Elizaveta was sympathetic to her mother's concerns but continued to press the issue. Liudmila finally relented and gave her daughter permission to enlist in Red Cross nursing training courses, but she insisted that the young woman take a letter to the medical unit, entreating the Red Cross authorities to protect her only daughter from danger. The next morning, Elizaveta set off to present herself to the nursing unit called "Young Aid" (*Iunaia Pomoshch'*). She returned shortly thereafter, informing her mother that she had been instructed to reappear at 5:00 p.m. that day. She was to be ready to depart for Petrograd that very evening, where she and the other enlistees would train (for a brief week) prior to being sent to the front.[1]

The story of Elizaveta and Liudmila Bychkova was detailed in a pamphlet clearly produced as part of the prowar effort. While the first half of the text describes Elizaveta's efforts to secure permission to enlist as a sister of mercy, the second half moves far from the comfortable domestic space of the Bychkovas' Moscow home to a scene graphically describing the horrific conditions on the battlefields during an enemy attack:

"Bullets buzzed, grenades exploded, cannons thundered, shrapnel flew, the earth trembled, and smoke burned their eyes, as the Russian heroes (*chudo-bogtyry*), with great dignity, repelled the combined Austro-Germanic forces, 4–5 times greater than ours. . . . The noise, bloodcurdling, hair-raising, heart-pounding, was a hellish pandemonium."[2] The male combatants were not the only heroic figures present, however. The story continues, bringing our attention back to the subjects of the tale:

> Amid this turmoil, amid bursting bullets, amid dead bodies lying in graves dug out by shells, walk two sisters of mercy. One is forty-five years of age, the other, not more than twenty, they move through and pick out the wounded; they are mother and daughter, the Bychkovas. And here now, amid the noise, amid the flying bullets, the constant risk to their lives, she and her daughter gather the bodies of the wounded, carry them to a safe place, and dress their wounds.[3]

It seems that her daughter's patriotic exhortations were so strong (combined with what is presented as the mother's maternal impulse to protect her youngest child) that, despite her age, Liudmila also decided to become a nurse and accompany her daughter to the front. The two women, we are told, left behind a life of luxury in an "exceptional mansion," equipped with servants, "a happy life, a future that promised much" in order to dedicate their lives to serving soldiers wounded in battle. It is not known whether the mother/daughter nursing duo were real historical figures, or whether they were invented for propaganda purposes, to highlight the selfless, hard work of nurses in the war effort. Regardless of their questionable existence, it is notable that the pamphlet did not merely describe women as passive, caregiving figures on the sidelines of the main action of the war but emphasized the great danger they faced as well as their active participation at the front. The author asks the reader, "Is this indeed not an act of bravery? Is this indeed not deserving of attention?" The answer, of course, was yes. "This great feat will not go unnoticed, their valiant name will be recorded in the pages of history in gilded letters!"[4]

PATRIOTIC CULTURE AND THE SISTER OF MERCY

During the course of the war, the Russian patriotic press produced numerous tracts such as the one described above, detailing the efforts of many citizens in the war effort. These were published as part of the attempt to shore up public support for the war. Although they may have been sensationalized and even exaggerated the activities of their subjects, they are nonetheless important to official efforts to shape public opinion, and they indicate what kinds of activities were deemed acceptable, in fact, laudable. For women, no wartime activity was accorded higher esteem than nursing. The outbreak of war in 1914 had dramatic effects on popular culture in Russia. In particular, the media and entertainment industry immediately shifted its focus to the war, which is reflected in the cultural productions of the period. Contemporary periodicals not only reported on the factual events and circumstances of the conflict but also published texts and images that revealed public opinion and popular imagination concerning various aspects of the war. Plays, films, and other performance arts created new works that placed the war at center stage. Visual representations of those participating in the war effort were widely disseminated through cheaply produced media such as posters, postcards, and other popular prints such as *lubki* (illustrated broadsides). They featured depictions of the war both realistic and fantastic.

Although most cultural productions of the war period focused mainly on male action in combat, women were also featured in a number of such sources. The most common form of female representation was that of the wartime nurse. As with those of men, images of women were employed in textual and visual forms to represent both actual nurses participating in the war effort and symbolic figures meant to signify abstract values or ideas. The sister of mercy was an important cultural figure during the First World War in Russia. In many ways she became a national symbol, an important exemplar of appropriate women's roles in the war. Nurses were featured in the periodical press, in posters, postcards, *lubki*, and other popular artistic productions, and in wartime films, plays, and other forms of performance art. Contemporary commentators on the war also made reference to wartime nurses, usually expressing distinct opinions about these women.

Representations of wartime nurses were particularly prevalent in the Russian press. During the last decades of tsarist rule, periodical publications proliferated throughout the empire. Literacy rates in Russia had increased significantly in the prewar period, making newspapers and journals increasingly accessible to the population. By 1914 dozens of popular titles were circulating around the empire. Some of the most widely distributed were illustrated journals and magazines, which had large readerships.[5] Contemporary periodicals not only reported on the factual events and circumstances of the conflict but also published texts and images that reflected public opinion and popular imagination concerning various aspects of the war. The wartime press was highly interested in the activities of women as nurses, featuring stories, photographs, and artistic representations of sisters of mercy in their pages.

Sisters of mercy were also highlighted in numerous printed images, particularly posters and postcards, which had broader reach across the Russian public as they did not require literacy. Encouraged by the state, dozens of new publishing houses were established during this period to print thousands of copies of posters featuring war scenes. Illustrations were created by some of Russia's leading artists during the war period, representing the diverse genres prevalent at the time: realism, impressionism, and the developing avant-garde. These were some of the most important cultural productions of the war period: extremely popular and readily available, cheap to produce, easy to distribute, and able to depict the war in pictures, thus accessible to even the uneducated peasant.

The *lubok* in particular is an extremely important component of Russian culture: its ubiquitous presence came from a long tradition of production in Russia, reflecting popular views since the seventeenth century. *Lubki* were significant enough that peasant homes often featured them in their icon corners, hanging next to images of saints.[6] For some families, these images were their only connections to their sons serving in the Russian military. Posters were also highly visible and accessible; as historian of Russian wartime culture Hubertus Jahn has demonstrated, they "bloomed on the walls of buildings in Russian cities on an unprecedented scale."[7] The images used in posters and *lubki* were even more widely disseminated because they were often reprinted in contemporary periodicals, particularly in the numerous illustrated journals that circulated during the war period. Moreover, these prints were commercially produced and therefore driven at least partially by what printers believed people wanted to see and buy. When reproduced in contemporary periodicals, they reflected not only popular cultural views but also the desires of their publishers who were motivated to move copy. As such, the viewers helped shape the images and the attitudes about them.

All of these images were important representations of official and popular public opinion, which worked both actively and passively to shape the way Russians understood and expressed their perceptions of the war.

Simultaneously, cultural productions were influenced by the ways they were perceived in popular imagination, created in what scholars such as Jahn have called a situation of "mutual conditioning." Thus, they express both the values and the worldview of the society in which they are produced and are shaped and modified by those that produce and view them. As a whole, popular culture represents the views that collectively go into the creation of, or the attempt to create, national identity.[8] As Ernest Gellner has argued, it constitutes a "system of ideas and signs and associations and ways of behaving and communicating" that comprise a nation.[9] The images of wartime nurses are thus further significant because they reflect the attitudes of not only those who produced them but also those who consumed them. One of the major obstacles, however, to analyzing cultural productions in this formula of "mutual conditioning" is that, as historian Stephen Norris has pointed out in his study of wartime *lubki*, "people who view posters, art works, and other visual sources rarely write down their reactions." This presents one of the most significant challenges in attempting to contextualize cultural productions in order to understand their impact on their "eyewitnesses" and the ways such images were shaped by the attitudes of the times. To further complicate matters, all Russian wartime publications had to undergo heavy censorship, which dictated appropriate and inappropriate subject matter. It is also important to consider the sources of such images, which ranged from conservative ultramonarchist periodicals to official government publications to liberal and satirical journals highly critical of the regime and its prosecution of the war. Nonetheless, as Norris demonstrates, these images are extremely useful, as "the evidence available suggests that while we can never know every way in which a consumer understood these patriotic images, we do know at a basic, more general level that most Russians who came into contact with *lubki* found them to be inspiring. At the same time, some Russians who encountered the wartime prints believed that they promoted false ideas about Russia and Russian national identity."[10]

Images of sisters of mercy produced in patriotic prints and in the wartime periodical press are representative of the effort to construct national identity in gendered terms. They convey cultural attitudes about wartime nurses and their place in the war effort while simultaneously revealing anxieties and concerns that broke with patriotic tropes and thus demonstrate a range of ideas about these women. Much of the existing scholarship on the image of Russia's Great War–era nurses tends to portray them in oversimplified generalizations.[11] This usually means a highly positive representation of the selfless, asexual, passive, devoted provider of emotional care and support frequently employed in patriotic rhetoric, which Jahn contends promoted nurses as "caring mothers, hand-holding lovers, and untouchable beauties."[12] Echoing this view, historians such as Barbara Engel argue that these women were portrayed as passive, "gendered symbols of patriotic virtue, the feminine counterpart of the masculine soldier," thereby serving the propaganda needs of the state.[13] These conceptualizations fit with the overt efforts to preserve the masculinity of warfare, so often seen in visual and textual images celebrating the Russian soldier.

Although such images were prevalent, they were not the only ones used to portray sisters of mercy. In fact, the Russian nurse of World War I was imagined in much more richly diverse ways. Visual as well as textual depictions of Russia's sisters of mercy vary significantly, even within similar types of sources, and move well beyond one-dimensional views. Through a careful examination of a variety of sources representative of Russian patriotic culture during the war, a number of significantly different tropes in the representations of Russia's sisters of mercy emerge. Although the passive, self-sacrificing woman is one of the most common tropes employed in images of the nurse, figuring prominently in many wartime productions, even this archetype is more nuanced than has been suggested. In addition to the sisterly connotation (as well as denotation) of nurses, women in medical service also appear as motherly figures. A number of representations have strong religious overtones, whereby nurses take on the characteristics of the Mother of God. Others are represented as somewhat ethereal, as "angels of mercy." Nurses could also be featured as allegorical figures or abstractions, representative of the nation (Mother Russia), the people, or womanhood in general. Nor are all of these passive representations; many placed women in much more active roles. Even when nurses appear as motherly figures, they are often portrayed as considerably stronger than the men whom they serve. Perhaps most strikingly, the distinct trope that depicted wartime nurses as forceful, daring, and heroic participants in dangerous events contrasts significantly with the standard passive images. Other sources emphasized the weakness of women, particularly within the context of the war zone, which highlighted the vulnerability of wartime nurse, based on her gender and sexuality, while simultaneously emphasizing the brutality and inhumanity of the enemy.

All of the preceding tropes could be and were manipulated for patriotic purposes. The passive nurse who provided comfort and solace was used to motivate women to enlist in medical services, while simultaneously reassuring men that should they be wounded in battle, they would be well cared for. Those with religious themes affirmed the righteousness of Russia's participation in the war, with a Christ-loving army protected by angelic nurses in their sacred mission. Sororal and maternal representations confirmed the idea of the nation as family, wherein brothers served with brothers under the command of fathers and were aided and comforted by sisters and mothers. Sources that portrayed or hinted at women's sexual violation based on women's perceived weakness as a means to motivate men into military service by playing on traditional conceptions of male chivalry and their roles as protectors and defenders of women, especially of their "honor."

Moreover, some representations of sisters of mercy that appeared in Russian cultural productions were decidedly less positive in their attitudes about the war. These kinds of sources should not be seen as less patriotic, as patriotism is itself multifaceted and can take on various forms, including social and political criticism. This is especially poignant in Russia during the First World War, when many members of society questioned the actions undertaken by the tsarist government during the conflict. A number of the representations that emerged during the war demonstrate deep ambiguities of the Russian population. While strongly supporting the efforts to repel German aggression, they also revealed the horrors of violent conflict, exposed the difficulties associated with conducting a total war, and sharply rebuked those that were seen as shirking responsibility during a time of national crisis. In this vein, images of nurses could be used critically, to highlight problems with the prosecution of the war. In particular, they were often utilized to disparage those (both male and female) seen as not doing their part for the war effort. And even when women did enlist in wartime medical services, sometimes their intentions and activities were questioned, especially when they failed to conform to normative expectations of female behavior. They exposed deep-seated angst surrounding female participation in the male zone of war.[14]

The result of evaluating the image of Russia's wartime nurses is a series of challenges to simple dichotomies of representation that feature women as passively supportive to the active, male heroic figure. They offer the opportunity to consider the multiple ways that women's wartime activity reflected the values and anxieties of a transforming society. The complex and often contradictory images of Russia's nurses of World War I indicate that ambiguities about women and war continued to resonate in Russian public opinion. As such, they are indicative of the ways in which the war both supported and challenged prevailing notions of gender and separate spheres, and thus of national identity. Public opinion largely embraced the role of women in the war, despite the disruption of traditional conventions, and incorporated the wartime nurse into the pantheon of national servitors (although in a secondary role). However, such acceptance was not without some significant reservations and concerns about gender identities.

The Nurse as Patriotic Symbol

Nurses appeared frequently in both the periodical press and the patriotic prints circulated throughout the empire during the war. In keeping with long-standing popular cultural traditions, women appeared more often in religious and folk art, as well as commercial, charitable, and educational productions, than they did in official wartime sources, which heavily favored depictions of male combatants.[15] Publishing houses produced books and pamphlets describing the activities of sisters of mercy in the war, such as the story of the Bychkovas detailed above. Articles about nurses were featured in contemporary periodicals, but even more often, their pages were filled with photographs and artistic renderings. They were not just featured in illustrated journals but also in numerous other printed sources produced during the war, such as posters, postcards, and *lubki.* Indeed, there was a concerted effort to include the service of nurses in publications dedicated to patriotic culture, indicating their importance to the successful prosecution of the war.

A highly positive, but passive and secondary, image of the nurse featured prominently in the pages of the Russian press and in the prints produced during the war depicting scenes from the conflict. However, it is also important to note that images of soldiers and male participants in the war greatly outnumbered those of sisters of mercy in these types of sources. Of the approximately 650 different Russian war posters contained in the collections of the Hoover Institution on War, Peace, and Revolution at Stanford University, only roughly a dozen feature nurses, while hundreds feature male soldiers and officers. This is not surprising, considering the masculinist conception of war and the infrequency with which women were represented in tsarist political propaganda.[16] Moreover, the ways in which women were often depicted reveal a perception of their actions and presence as secondary to men. Nurses appeared in most of the widely circulated periodicals of the war, but frequently only as isolated photographs or illustrations, often without captions to identify them, or with no connection to the text that surrounded the image. For the most part, only noted personalities (such as celebrities or members of the royal or aristocratic families) serving as sisters of mercy were given individual attention. More often, nurses were pictured in groups, and in many cases, with men, either male patients or male medical or military personnel, who were the true focal points of the images. While their presence in the sources attests to the consciousness of their participation as significant to the war effort, the lack of exposition about their activities and their identities indicates that many considered them less important players. Stories about the exploits of soldiers and officers, commanders, and officials, all men, dominated the text. Women appear in pictures, but they do not seem to be the main focus of the images. This can be seen in the example of the page from the popular illustrated weekly journal *Iskry,* featuring photographs of nurses and wounded men (figure 7.1), as compared to the exploits of fallen heroes detailed on the following page (figure 7.2). While each male figure is given a detailed caption indicating his identity, rank, and specific circumstances of his service, the sisters are rarely identified by name, and little information is provided regarding their activities in the war. Instead, they appear somewhat akin to accessories to the male figures.

By contrast, the women's journals of the war period, especially progressive publications, took a particular interest in women's wartime nursing and often portrayed sisters of mercy in much more prominent ways than the mainstream press did. Their primary aim was the representation of female medical personnel as patriotic counterparts to male combatants. Seeking to "present themselves as responsible citizens who recognized their obligations as well as their rights," women's organizations such as the Mutual Philanthropic Society and the League for Women's Equality were quick to express their support for the war, including women's enlistment in wartime medical service.[17] Progressives viewed nursing as an appropriate form of female behavior, consistent with traditional notions of femininity centered on caring and nurturing, and a means by which women could positively affect the war. The editors of the journal *Zhenskoe Delo* indicated that "women's calling is to be compassionate, helping and healing; hence when men become soldiers, women should become nurses."[18] Even those who had

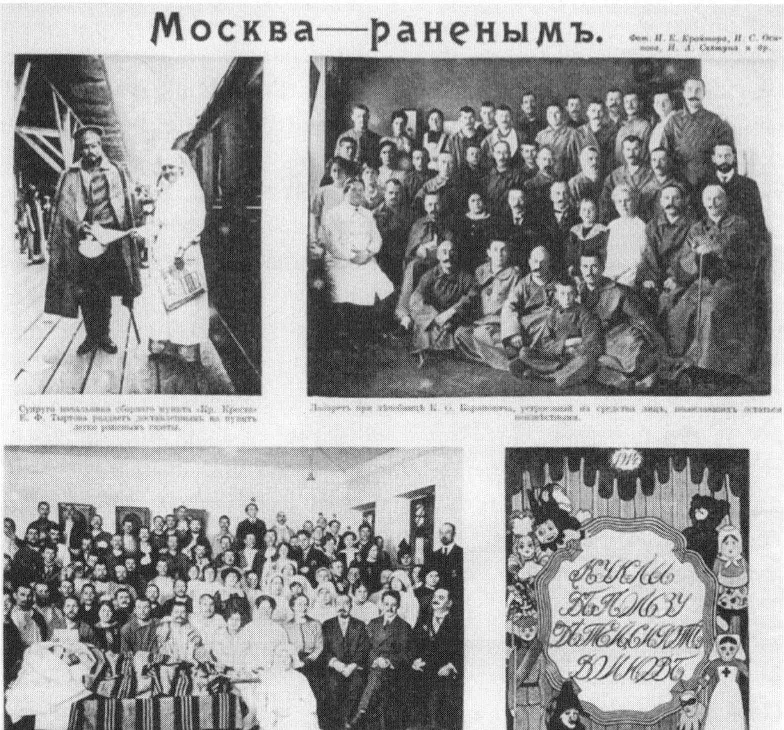

Figure 7.1. Female figures were usually featured alongside men but rarely individually and rarely identified (unless members of the elite). "Moskva-ranenym" [Moscow wounded], *Iskry*, November 30, 1914, 374.

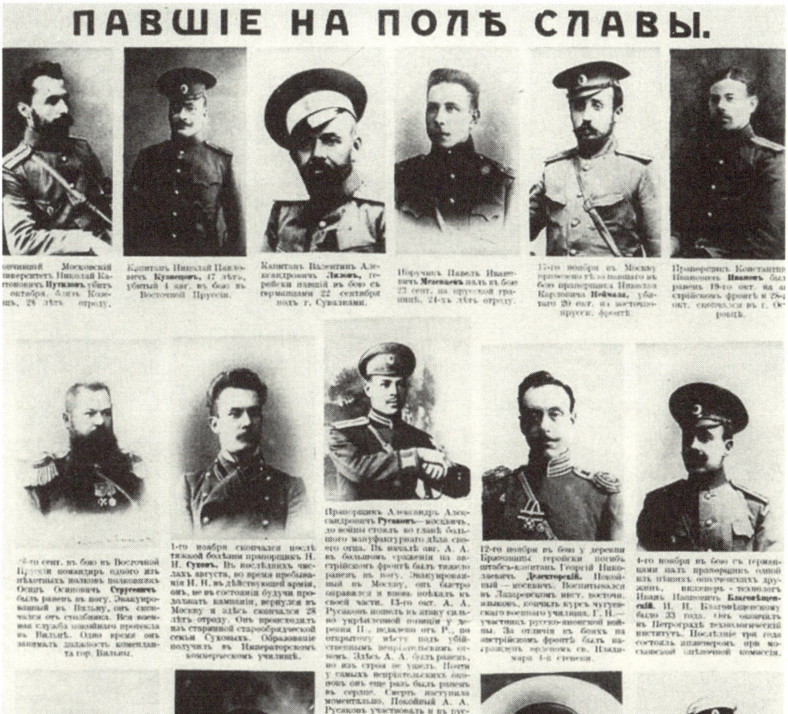
ПАВШІЕ НА ПОЛѢ СЛАВЫ.

Figure 7.2. Publications most frequently featured images of individual male soldiers, identified by name. "Pavshie na pole slavy" [Fallen on the field of glory], *Iskry*, November 30, 1914, 375.

previously expressed staunchly pacifist attitudes could embrace nursing for its life-giving rather than violent and destructive aims. A number of the journals' covers were dedicated to images of wartime nurses at work caring for soldiers, such as the October 15, 1914, issue. The painting by E. A. Klodt, titled "At the frontline position," featured on the cover of this issue depicts several nurses attentively bandaging the wounds of soldiers at a field dressing station while the smoke of a battle raging in the distance billows up behind them.[19]

In the prowar literature produced by officially sanctioned sources, soldiers' views of nurses also reflected stereotypes and standard tropes. The most common of these was the nurse as caring, comforting figure that brought wounded and ill men solace in their suffering. In official sources, the views portrayed of nurses on the part of their wounded charges were sanitized, idealized constructs that emphasized the qualities identified as feminine, as well as the self-sacrificing aspects of nursing service. In the official organ of the Russian Society of the Red Cross (*Vestnik Krasnago Kresta*), this type of portrait of the wartime nurse was quite common. One article, titled "One among many," details the inspiring example of a sister of mercy named Nadezhda Nikolaevna (surname not given), according to the reports given by the wounded men in her charge:

> What joyfulness she brings each time she appears in the infirmary. The wounded who are able to stand up, on hearing her gentle voice, get out of their beds and go to greet her. Nadezhda Nikolaevna goes up to the bed of each of the wounded in turn and inquires at length about his health. What mercy, what care is felt in this questioning. . . . She carries out her work with such attention, with such gentleness, that the soldiers say: "We have never seen a sister of mercy like Nadezhda Nikolaevna." With her own money, she often purchases items for the wounded, shirts, scarves, shoes, etc. For one wounded man she bought an entire suit, which cost around fifty rubles. Of course, N. N. turns out to be one among many numerous such self-sacrificing Russian sisters of mercy.[20]

Celebrity Nurses

Many of the images and stories produced in the patriotic press and in propagandistic sources focused on the activities of well-known women of the Russian elite. Pamphlets, brochures, and posters frequently featured stories about the activities of such women in nursing service. Reports in the periodical press, often accompanied by photographs, emphasized the heroic and patriotic activity of these women, who gave their time and energy to the cause of the war. These kinds of publications continued through the war, focusing on both visual and textual representations. This was especially true with regard to women of the imperial family. Photographs of the Empress Alexandra and her two eldest daughters Ol'ga and Tat'iana wearing nursing uniforms, attending to wounded men, bandaging their wounds, or assisting in surgeries were extremely common in prowar sources. Other well-known women were also depicted quite frequently carrying out medical service. They were intended to demonstrate the devotion of the tsarist family to the war effort, especially that of the Empress Alexandra, whose loyalty to the nation had been questioned as a result of her German origins and her seemingly cold and aloof personality. They were also clearly meant to serve as examples for other women, who, it was hoped, would follow the imperial example and enlist in wartime medical services. As such, they presented powerful symbols of appropriate national roles for women. Such images appeared in a number of periodicals published during the war period, from the very outbreak of hostilities in the summer of 1914. The official periodical of the war, published by the tsarist government and titled *Letopis' Voiny* (Chronicle of the War), while focusing mostly on the prominent male figures involved in the war, particularly the commanders of the Russian military forces, also featured women of the imperial family serving as sisters of mercy. A number of images of the empress and her daughters as nurses, such as that seen in figure 7.3, were first printed in this publication but later reproduced in a number of other periodicals. Most of these images, however, were highly constructed, staged specifically for propaganda purposes, portraying the women in unrealistic settings and unnatural poses. Figures 7.3 and 7.4 demonstrate the kind of images taken by official photographers during the war to promote the appearance of the royal women as dedicated nurses.

Other efforts to demonstrate the devotion of the imperial women to the war effort were made in the form of textual representations. In 1916 the Petrograd publishing house Rus' put out a brochure titled "Our Tsarina and the Tsarevnas in the Second Fatherland War: A short description of the activities of Her Imperial Highness the Empress Alexandra Fedorovna and Her Most August Daughters the Grand Duchesses Ol'ga

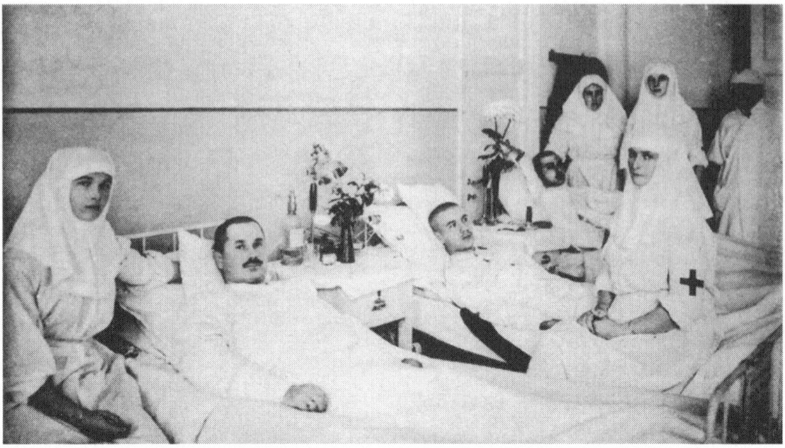

Figure 7.3. Empress Alexandra and Grand Duchesses Ol'ga and Tat'iana with wounded men in a rear hospital. *Letopis' Voiny*, May 28, 1916, 1484.

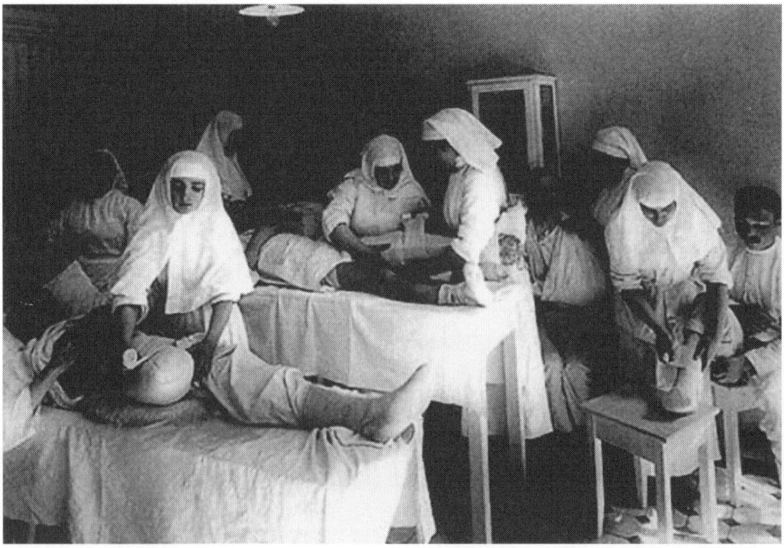

Figure 7.4. The Grand Duchesses Ol'ga and Tat'iana bandaging the wounds of men recently operated on. Photographed by K. Bulla, 1914.

Nikolaevna and Tat'iana Nikolaevna in the Second Fatherland War in the care of our warriors and their families." In the same year, a poster was produced similarly depicting the empress and her eldest daughters at work in medical service.[21]

The extent to which these efforts were successful in rehabilitating the tsarina and endearing her to the Russian population is somewhat ambiguous. Negative rumors and offensive gossip about the imperial family, particularly the empress, did not abate despite the pristine and self-sacrificing image produced in wartime propaganda. According to Boris Kolonitskii, the actions of Alexandra in the war effort did little to improve her popularity, particularly because she preferred to spend her time in the small, private hospital established at the tsar's summer home at Tsarskoe Selo, rather than involve herself in efforts being undertaken in the capital.[22] As a result, she remained aloof and seemingly inaccessible. She and her daughters certainly did not work on the front lines in positions that would have put their lives in danger. However, there is little doubt that many of Russia's elite women looked to the female members of the tsarist family as role models, and that this inspired a number of other women to become wartime nurses. Indeed, as discussed previously, being a sister of mercy was considered "fashionable," which drove a number of women to don the nurse's uniform and attend to the wounded in local hospitals. Moreover, some members of the royal family did serve in the forward positions, such as Grand Duchess Ol'ga Aleksandrovna and Grand Duchess Maria Pavlovna.

Ol'ga Aleksandrovna, in fact, was a favorite subject of visual images of nurses in Russian patriotic culture. Her portraits, in a variety of poses, wearing the uniform of a sister of mercy and engaging in a number of different activities associated with providing medical assistance to wounded soldiers, were featured in several different media. Ol'ga was particularly popular as a result of her reputation for eschewing the benefits and trappings of her privileged position and living like a "common nurse." A photograph published in *Letopis' Voiny* in November 1914 featured the grand duchess in a staged pose next to a wounded man covered in bandages (figure 7.5), which also included a lengthy caption praising her efforts and emphasizing her devotion:

> Her Imperial Highness the Grand Duchess Ol'ga Aleksandrovna, from the very start of the war, has given herself fully to the care of the wounded. In the city of Rovno, Her Imperial Highness works at

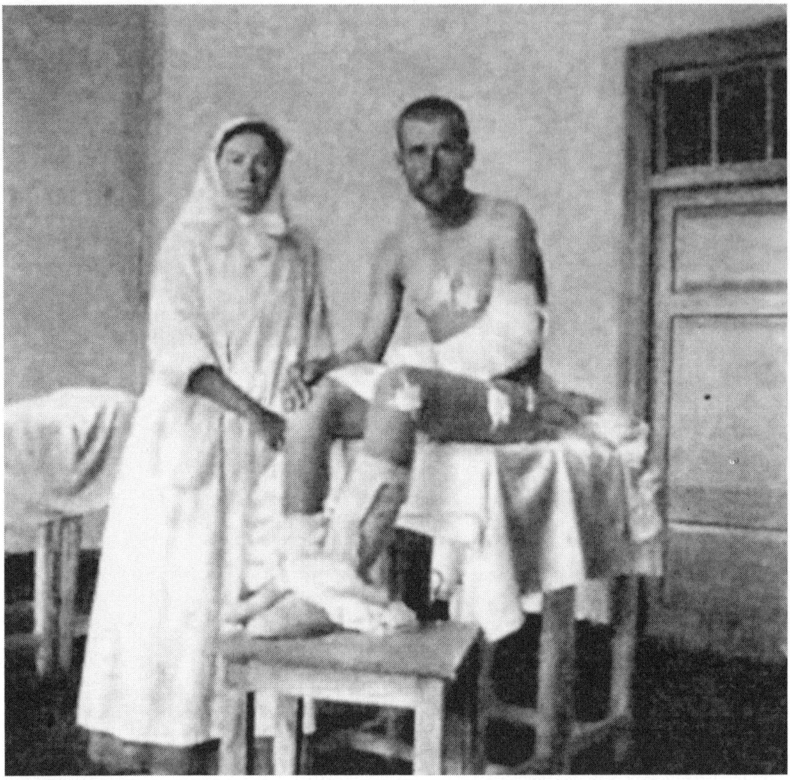

Figure 7.5. Her Imperial Highness Grand Duchess Ol'ga Aleksandrovna at the front. *Letopis' Voiny*, November 15, 1914, 205.

> the same level as a sister of mercy, from 7:00 in the morning until very late in the evening. During especially difficult days, when the hospital at Rovna named for Her Highness receives hundreds of wounded, the Grand Duchess sleeps very little over the course of several days. Very often, the Grand Duchess personally bandages and washes the wounded soldiers. Without any exaggeration it is possible to say that Grand Duchess Ol'ga Aleksandrovna exemplifies the heart of a sister of mercy.[23]

The royal women were not the only famous figures represented in the patriotic press and other cultural productions during the war. Actresses, singers, ballerinas, noted aristocratic women, and other well-known individuals were similarly featured in such publications. Even those known only through their connections to other celebrated Russians were photographed and written about. The illustrated magazine *Stolitsa i usadba* (The Capital and the Estate)[24] dedicated a number of pages in its issues throughout the war to photographs of prominent women, posing in their nursing uniforms, such as the example featured in figure 7.6. Other popular periodicals with wide readerships, such as *Niva, Ogonek, Solntse Rossii,* and *Iskry*, also gave such women significant attention in their publications.

The notion that entering nursing service was a noble endeavor was widespread in contemporary writings. Indeed, so ennobling was becoming a sister of mercy that it was sometimes accompanied by the idea that it could bring honor and purpose to those whose lives before the war were seemingly purposeless. A poem by O. Liatkovaskaia titled "Sestra" ("Sister"), published in the popular illustrated literary magazine *Ogonek*, expressed this well:

Yesterday I was so tired
Completely unnecessary, sad . . .
I had long since ceased to create life
I was cursed with a hateful fate . . .
But today I am light and sweet!
On my arm a band of white
And there, into death, light and happy
I go, humble and courageous
Bullets whistling by us crazily
Countless ranks of fighters fall
And the crosses of sisters, crimson-red
Flashed tenderly, welcoming . . .
I, as mother, bend over the dying
Giving him constant tenderness
And light the burning fire myself,
Completely unnecessary, forgotten.
If death comes, I will die calmly.
After all, I blossomed with fraternal love,
And now, perhaps, I am worthy
To lie in the common grave of a soldier . . . [25]

Further indicating the extent to which the role of wartime nurse had come to be seen as not only acceptable but even desirable were images

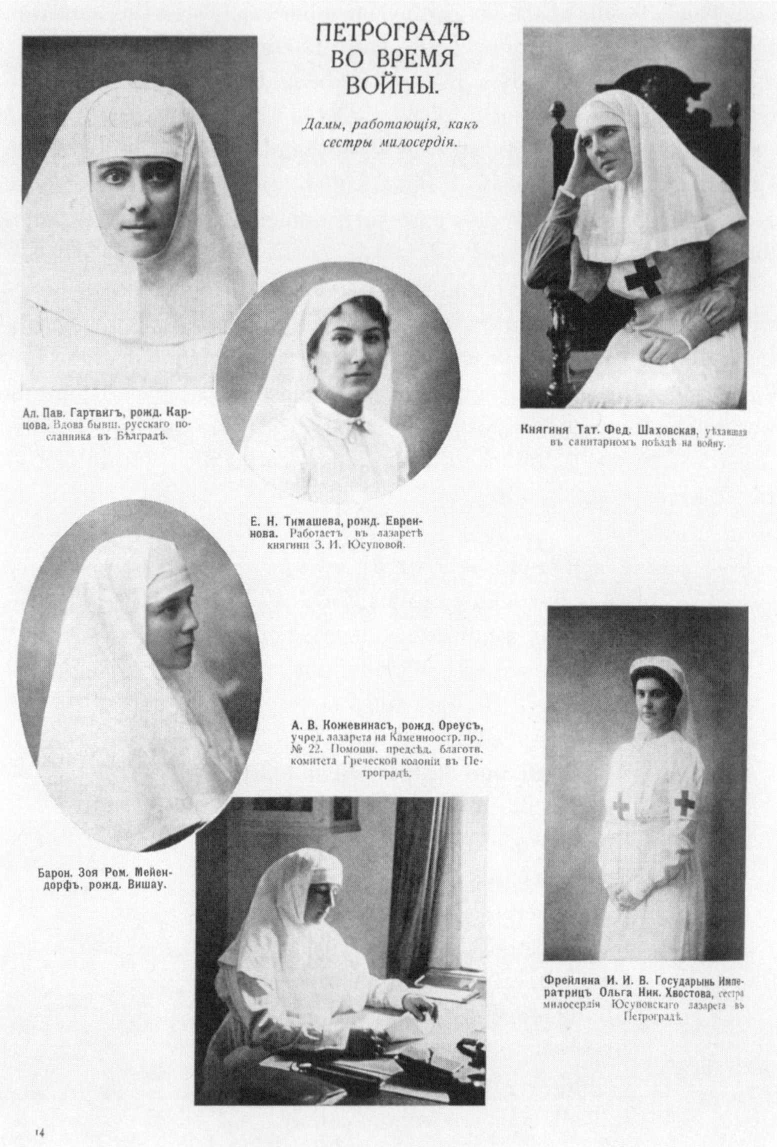

ПЕТРОГРАДЪ
ВО ВРЕМЯ
ВОЙНЫ.

Дамы, работающія, какъ сестры милосердія.

Ал. Пав. Гартвигъ, рожд. Карцова. Вдова бывш. русскаго посланника въ Бѣлградѣ.

Е. Н. Тимашева, рожд. Евреинова. Работаетъ въ лазаретѣ княгини З. И. Юсуповой.

Княгиня Тат. Фед. Шаховская, уѣхавшая въ санитарномъ поѣздѣ на войну.

А. В. Кожевинасъ, рожд. Ореусъ, учред. лазарета на Каменноостр. пр., № 22. Помощн. предсѣд. благотв. комитета Греческой колоніи въ Петроградѣ.

Барон. Зоя Ром. Мейендорфъ, рожд. Вишау.

Фрейлина И. И. В. Государынь Императрицъ Ольга Ник. Хвостова, сестра милосердія Юсуповскаго лазарета въ Петроградѣ.

14

Figure 7.6. Photographs of elite women who volunteered for wartime medical service. *Stolitsa i usadba*, February 1, 1915, 14.

that featured children dressed as sisters of mercy. As such, they were presented as appropriate role models for young girls. A number of depictions of children dressed as nurses appeared as posters and in photographs in the patriotic press. One charity poster illustrated by artist L. M. Brailovskii, featuring a doll in the uniform of a Red Cross nurse, appealed to members of Russian society to purchase toys for orphans of the war.[26] The poster was distributed widely and even printed in *Iskry* to increase public exposure (as seen in figure 7.1).[27] Such images often featured children of various ethnicities, seemingly in an effort to emphasize the cooperation among the various nationalities of the empire as well as to indicate gender-appropriate notions of national service. Early in the war, *Iskry* published a picture of a young girl named Zina Kotliarova dressed as a sister of mercy and a young boy identified as Volodia Shenfein sporting a soldier's uniform, holding a collection bucket (figure 7.7).[28] Another picture presenting two very young girls from Mariupol' in nursing uniforms appeared in *Iskry* the next month, urging Russians to donate to the fund for victims of the war (figure 7.8).[29] Perhaps even more interestingly, in December 1914 the journal ran a short article with a photograph of two Muslim girls, Fatima and Mariam Ishukova, dressed as sisters of the Red Crescent, who were collecting money on behalf of the Simbirsk Muslim community. The event, organized by a man identified as Mr. Ishukov (perhaps the father of the children pictured), was held to collect gifts to send to the troops at the front for Christmas, including tobacco, sugar, and biscuits.[30]

"Caring Mothers, Hand-holding Lovers, and Untouchable Beauties"

As one might expect, the images of nurses in prowar Russian wartime sources often emphasized characteristics that were consistent with traditional femininity in early twentieth-century Russia. Time and again one encounters similar descriptors: "selfless," "self-sacrificing," and "devoted." Such representations placed the wartime sister on a pedestal, romanticizing nursing service and making the depictions of her less than realistic. The books and pamphlets published during the war aimed at presenting the nurse assisting the male soldier, and in so doing featured the tasks she performed in devoted service to the wounded and ill men in her care. While the publications did often highlight how difficult the work was, particularly the long hours associated with wartime nursing,

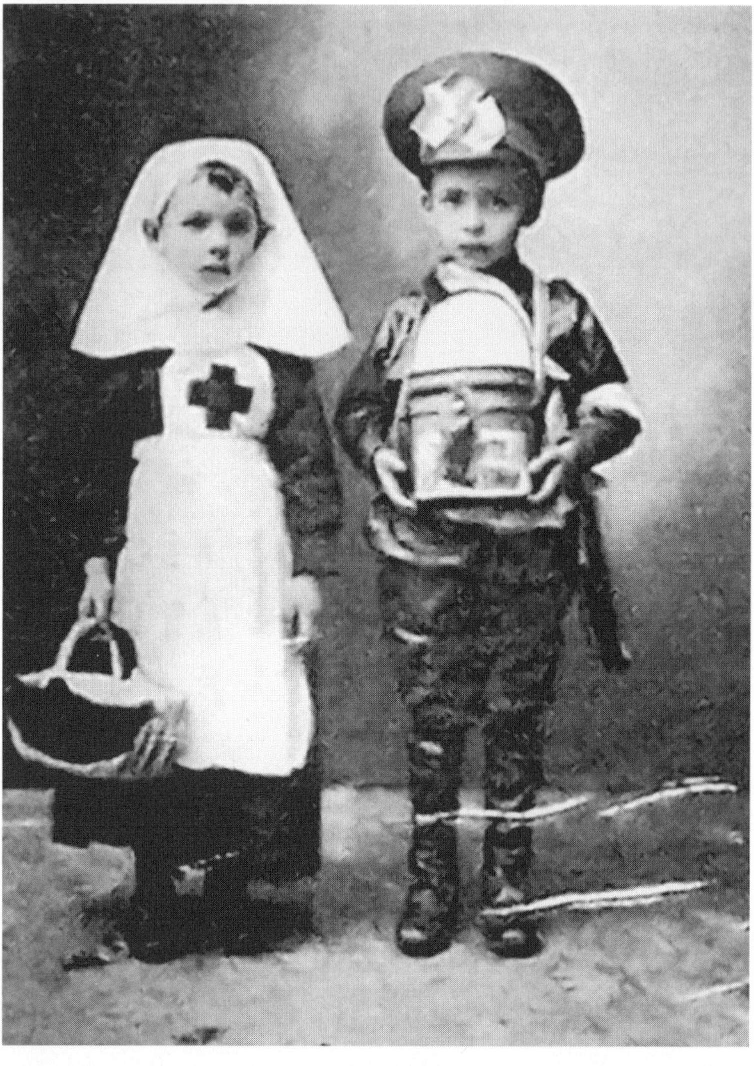

Figure 7.7. A young girl dressed as a nurse and a young boy in soldier's garb, used to elicit patriotic support for the war, but also indicative of appropriately gendered roles. "Zina Kotliarova. Volodia Shenfein," *Iskry*, August 31, 1914, 271. Digitized image courtesy of Boris Kolonitskii.

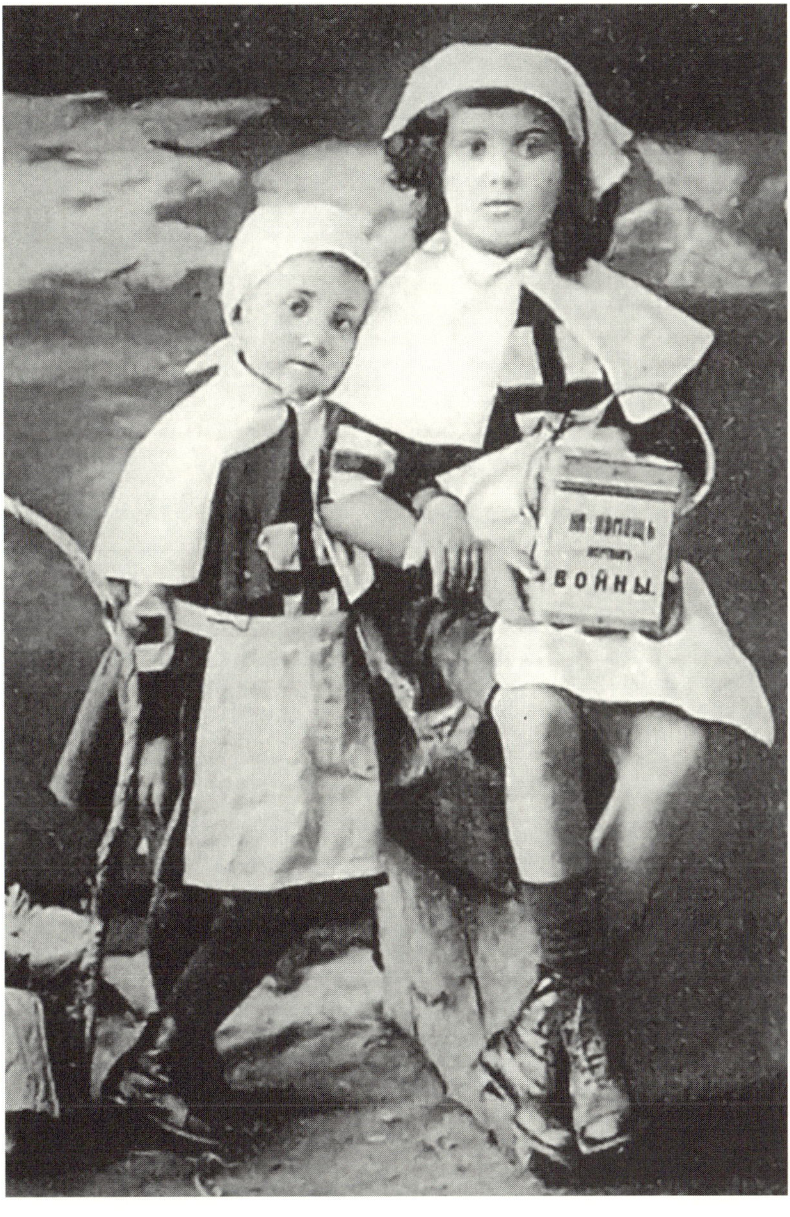

Figure 7.8. Young girls dressed as nurses, used to raise money for war victims. "Pomogite zhertvam voiny. Mariupol'. Malenkiia prodavshchitsi v den' flazhkov 31-go avgusta" [Help the victims of the war. Mariupol'. Little salespeople on Flag Day, August 31], *Iskry*, September 21, 1914, 295. Digitized image courtesy of Boris Kolonitskii.

the main focus was more often the male combatants and their relationships with the nurses. Without much variation, Russian soldiers were nearly always presented as stoic and patient, grateful for everything done for them by their gentle, compassionate caregivers.

Indeed, most of the women who appeared in these stories share the features of compassion and self-sacrifice. Visual representations commonly depicted sisters of mercy as devoted, compassionate, and altruistic. Nurses were usually featured in soft, passive tones, in nurturing poses, displaying compassionate expressions toward their patients. The sister of mercy standing over the bed of a wounded soldier, tending to his needs while he looks up at her with gratitude, was repeated in various iterations in prowar illustrations and photographs and disseminated through a number of different sources: posters, postcards, *lubki,* and the periodical press. The settings for such images were the sanitized, bloodless, and safe "domestic" spaces of rear hospitals, completely removed from the front lines. One such archetypical representation of this trope was featured on the cover of the March 12, 1916, issue of the literary journal *Lukomor'e* (figure 7.9). The idealized depiction by artist G. Georgiev fit well with the publication's strong emphasis on the aesthetic as well as its conservative political bent. The color illustration, titled "Sister," shows a matronly nurse bringing tea to an officer with a bandaged arm lying in bed and looking up gratefully at his caretaker. The sister does not perform any medical treatment but rather provides the wounded hero with comfort, in a clean, safe environment appropriate for women. Another, produced by the wartime publisher Tamarkin, features an extremely saccharine image of a nurse gazing tenderly at a wounded man in bed, set against a completely blank, white background that seems to suggest that the two figures are floating in a heavenly cloud. The only hints of the hospital setting are the iron bed frame and the side table next to the bed. Yet another (figure 7.10), also set against an equally nebulous background, depicts a nurse sitting by a man's hospital bed and reading to him from the popular newspaper *Russkoe Slovo.* This image was produced by the Nikolskii Community of the Red Cross and distributed as postcards, sold to raise funds to manufacture respirators for victims of gas attacks. Photographs were similarly constructed to feature nurses in this manner, showing sisters attending to men in ways that strongly suggested their nurturing and concern. Figure 7.11 depicts a nearly identical photographic image as that of the artistic rendering in figure 7.10.

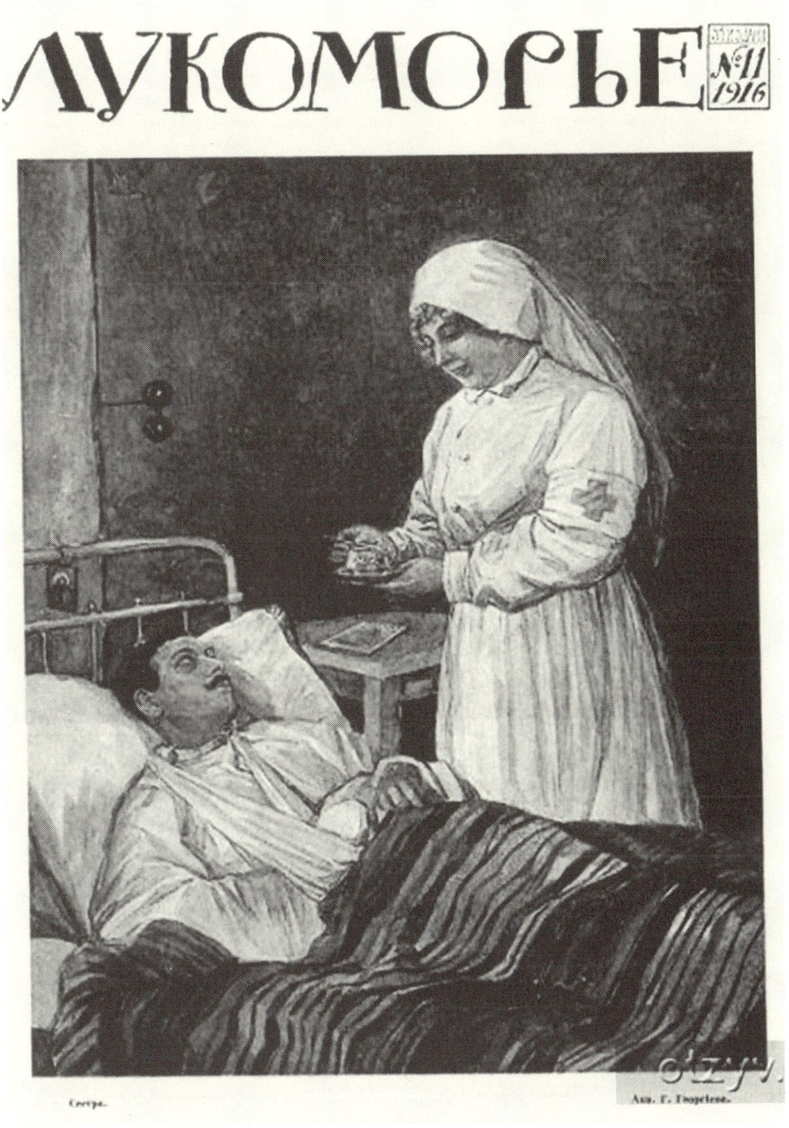

Figure 7.9. A cover of the literary journal *Lukomor'e* depicting a nurse in the conventional, passive role. G. Georgiev, "Sestra" [Sister], *Lukomor'e*, March 1916, cover. Digitized image courtesy of Boris Kolonitskii.

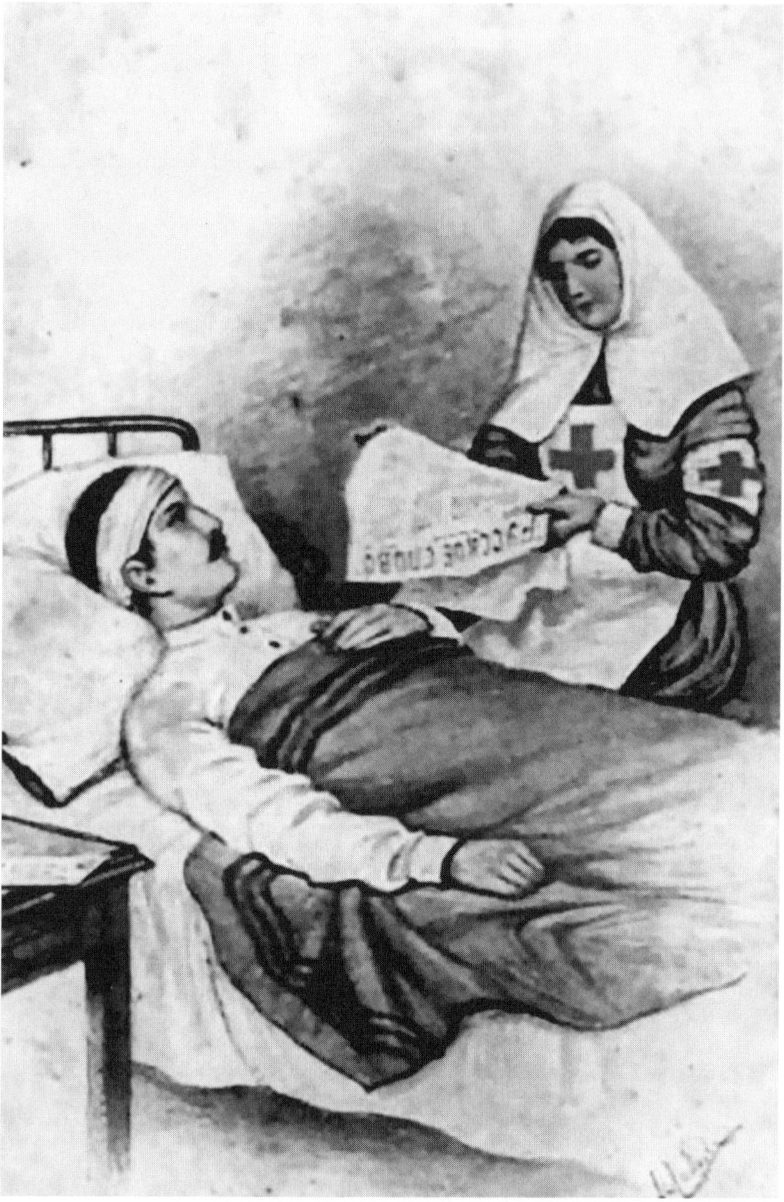

Figure 7.10. Illustrated image of a nurse reading a newspaper to a wounded soldier. Publishing House of the Nikolskii Community of the Russian Society of the Red Cross.

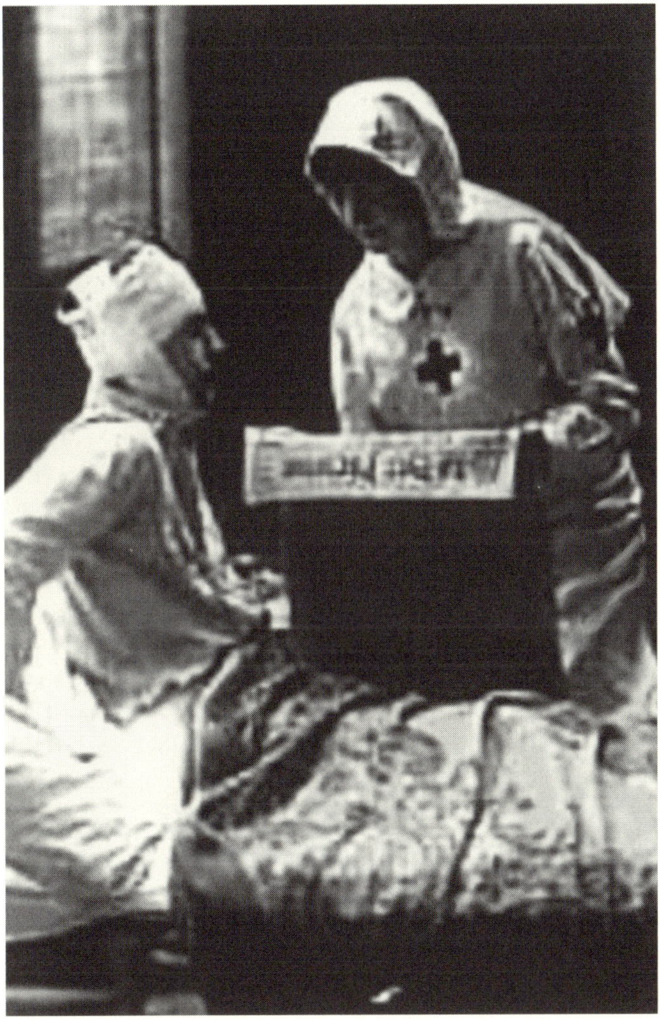

Figure 7.11. Photograph of a nurse reading a newspaper to a wounded soldier. Note the nearly identical composition of this image as compared to the previous image. Unknown title and source.

Not surprisingly, many of these images do not focus on sisters of mercy providing any kind of medical treatment. As indicated previously, Russian nurses were highly valued for the emotional support they offered to wounded and dying men, and comforting the troops psychologically was considered by many as one of the most important aspects of the sister's work, perhaps even more significant than the medical services they provided. The Russian press often described nurses as providing wounded and dying men with "cheer" and "easing their souls." The women's journal *Zhenskaia Zhizn'* (Woman's Life), dedicated to issues concerning women and their relationship to the war, referred to nurses as "sister-comforters" in its very first issue, published in October 1914.[31] Some visual representations such as posters and *lubki,* Jahn contends, "transformed these dedicated women into Red Cross beauties who piously held the hands of wounded soldiers or read newspapers to them in the garden of a clean and homey hospital."[32] Nurses were often portrayed as developing strong emotional attachments to their patients in a familial context—as sisters to brothers. Numerous images, such as the one featured on the *Lukomor'e* cover above, also depict this emotional aspect of nursing. There was nothing particularly threatening about these images, no eminent danger for either sister or soldier, no blood, no dirt, and certainly no hint of sexuality. But this did not mean that such representations were devoid of any notion of how difficult wartime nursing could be. Indeed, they did not shy away from demonstrating how this emotional component could take a heavy toll on nurses. A poem by S. Mikheev titled "The Sister of Mercy," published in September 1914 in the journal *Novyi Satirykon,* emphasizes the impact of nursing on the women who engaged in this wartime activity:

She has a brown dress,
A white apron with the symbol of Christ on it,
Her faith is happily simple:
All around are her brothers . . .
In her heart is pain, but this kind of pain is a response
To long-faded love . . .
Accustomed to everything . . . the walls of the hospital
And the bandages, and even the blood . . .
Before her are new losses
And she meets them with jest,
Only occasionally, she leaves the room,
Suddenly crying bitterly, like a child! . . . [33]

Religious Connotations and Imagery

The religious aspect of Russian nursing, as previously indicated, is extremely important in understanding the Russian nursing phenomenon, even during the war when medical service was largely secularized. The nursing communities of the Russian Red Cross retained their loose affiliations with the Russian Orthodox Church, and the quasi-religious nature of nursing was reflected in a number of representations of nurses. Not only was quasi-religious veneration for nurses not uncommon among soldier-patients toward their caretakers, but this was also reflected in depictions of nurses in wartime patriotic culture.[34] One journalist referred to nurses as "saintly humanitarian ascetics."[35] Nor was the resemblance of the sister of mercy's uniform to the habit of a nun accidental, and nurses were often taken for nuns. One historian has argued that the effect was dramatic, so as to even suggest the Virgin Mary.[36]

In writings about nurses produced during the war, references to religious ideas were not uncommon. Texts emphasized the spiritual devotion of sisters of mercy, which was portrayed as a strong motivating factor for enlistment in medical services. Visual representations of wartime nurses also often evoked this kind of religious imagery. One wartime poster (figure 7.12) shows a nurse standing behind the bedside of a wounded officer. Her pose can be compared to that of representations of the Madonna in a number of Orthodox icons. Her head is tilted slightly to the left, her expression is one of spiritual devotion: her arms crossed over her breast, her saintly gaze turned upward toward the heavens, in seeming reverence.[37] In another artistic rendering (figure 7.13), featured on the cover of the illustrated journal *Solntse Rossii,* a sister of mercy sits on a bedside gazing up with reverence at an icon hanging on the wall. Interestingly, there is only a suggestion of a wounded man lying in the bed next to her. The focus is clearly on the devotional image of the female nurse. A number of others also closely mimicked iconography in style and construction. A portrait of a nurse holding a wounded soldier in her arms (figure 7.14) can be compared to the icon of the Don Mother of God by fourteenth-century Russian iconographer Theophanes the Greek (figure 7.15).

Another common religious trope portrayed the wartime nurse as an "angel of mercy," a term often used in textual descriptions as well. Sometimes this figure literally descended from the heavens to provide care and comfort to the wounded soldier. This often occurred on the battlefield, with

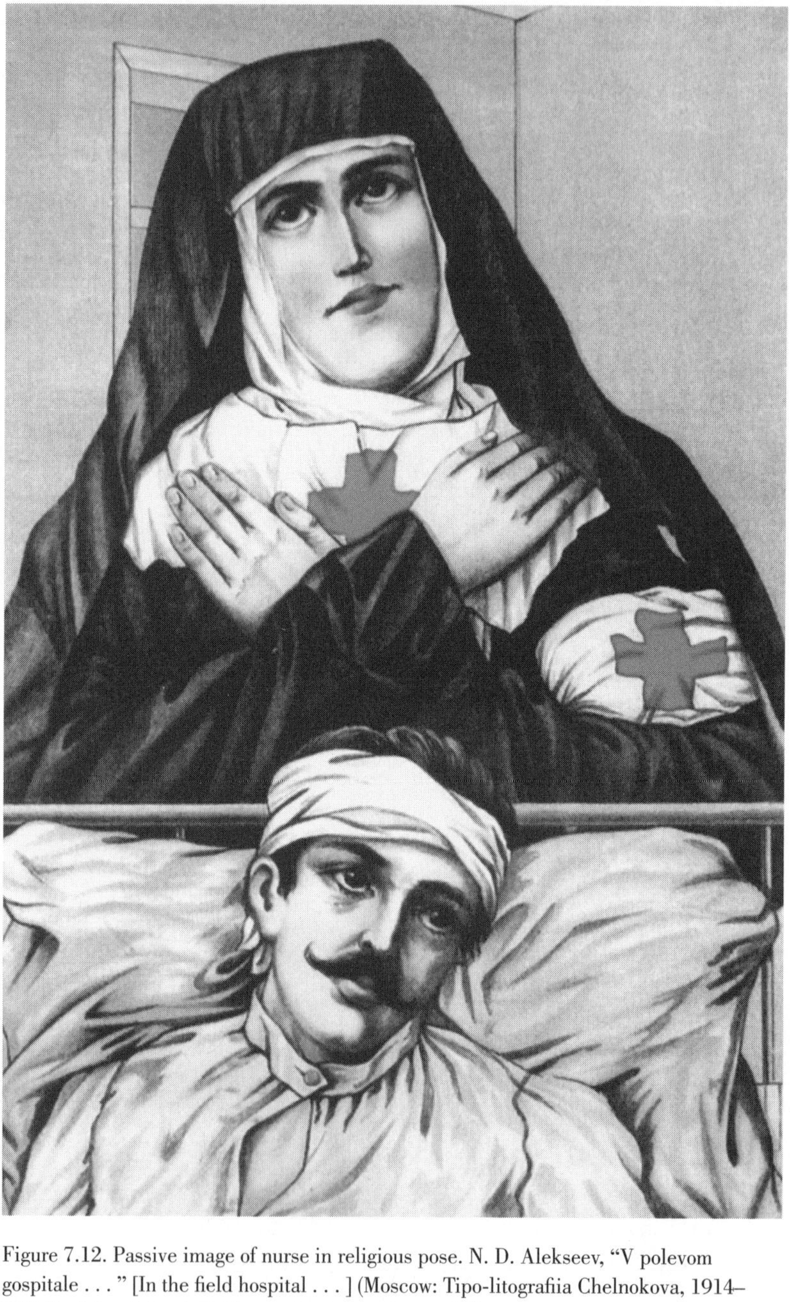

Figure 7.12. Passive image of nurse in religious pose. N. D. Alekseev, “V polevom gospitale . . . ” [In the field hospital . . .] (Moscow: Tipo-litografiia Chelnokova, 1914–1916?). Color. 22" x 16". Hoover Institution Poster Collection, RU/SU-32.

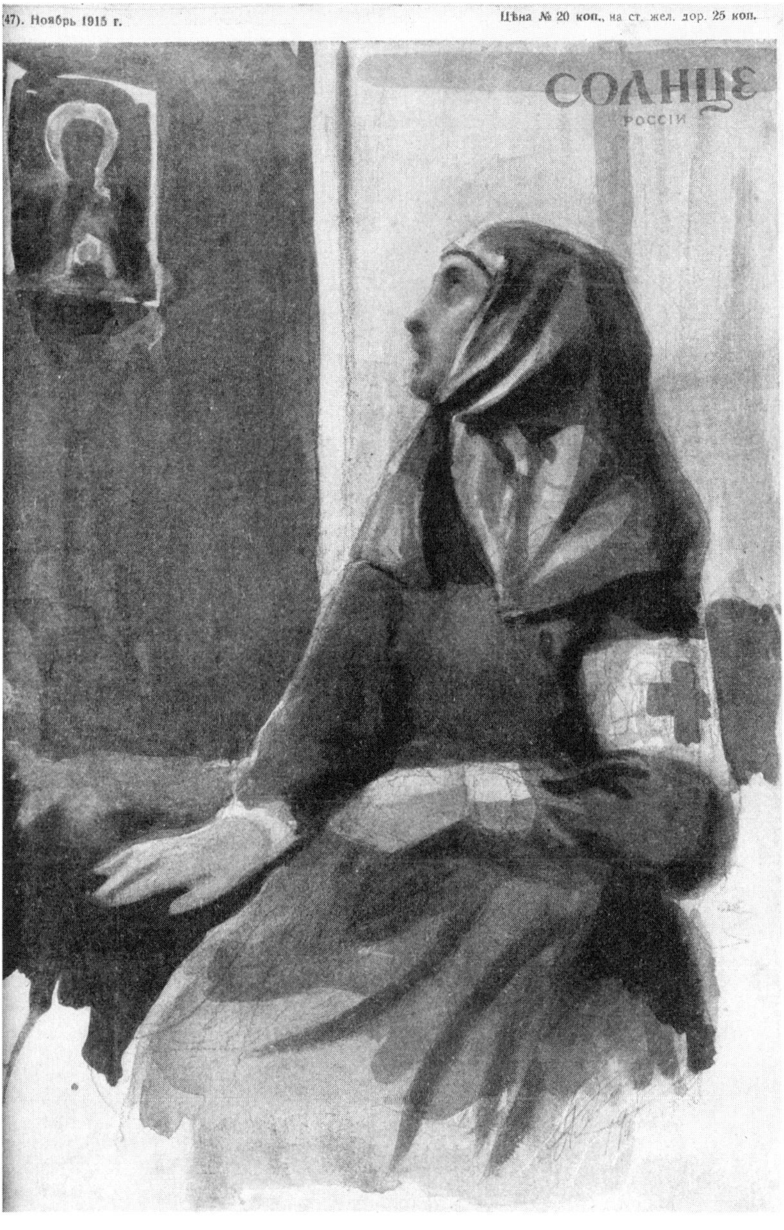

Figure 7.13. Idealized image of sister of mercy with heavy religious association. *Solntse Rossii* 47, no. 302 (1915): cover.

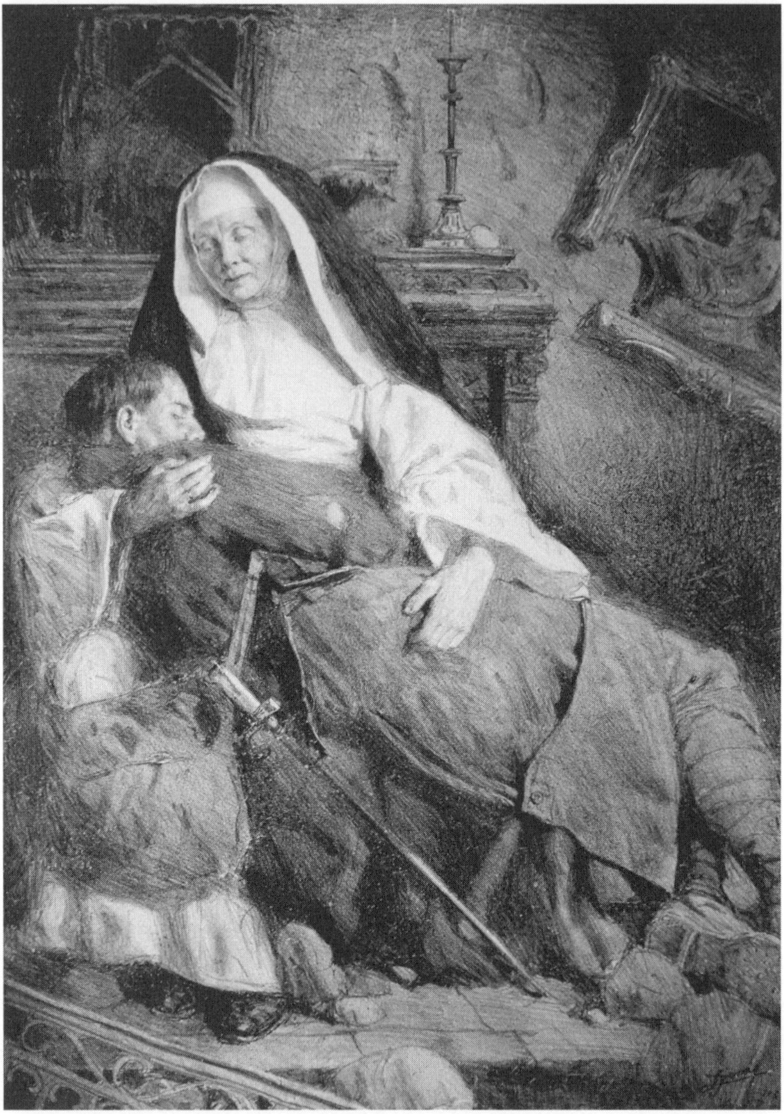

Figure 7.14. Image of nurse with soldier in religious pose, resembling iconography. "Miloserdiia" [Mercy], *Letopis' Voiny*, August 20, 1916, 1687.

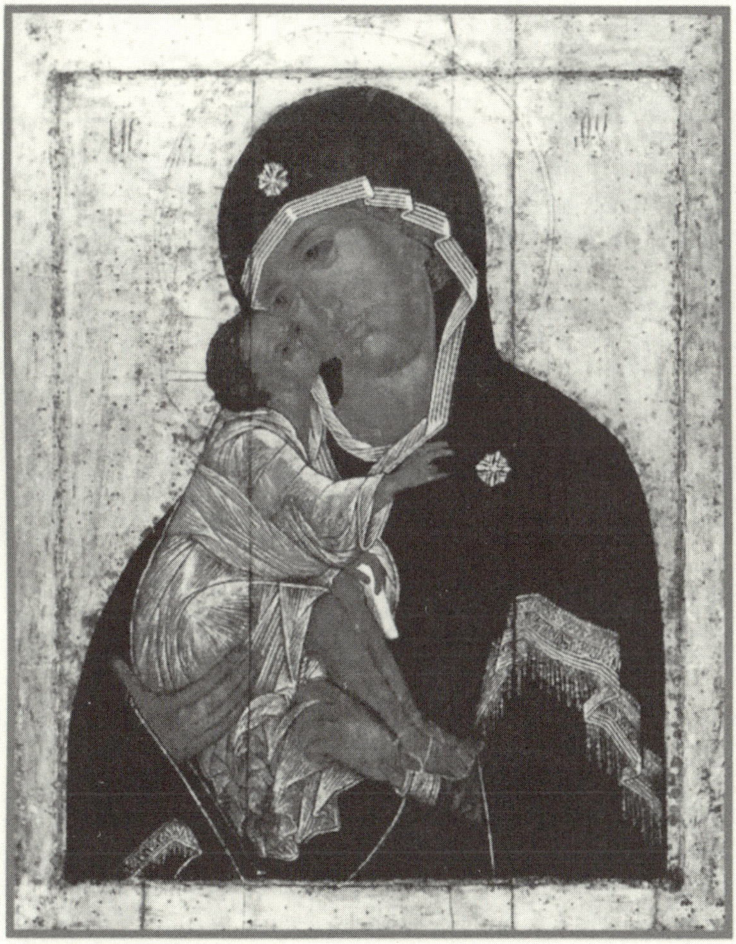

Figure 7.15. Icon with nearly identical composition as figure 7.14. *The Don Mother of God*, Theophanes the Greek, fourteenth century.

nurses appearing among the casualties either as angels themselves or accompanied by the winged figures of seraphim hovering close by or even assisting in providing medical care. The idea that Russian nurses possessed the ability to provide heavenly protection fit well with the Christ-loving Russian soldier, those that fought not only for tsar and country but also for God. The image titled simply "Voina" (War, figure 7.16), which was featured in the satirical illustrated journal *Novyi Satirykon*, is a stylized

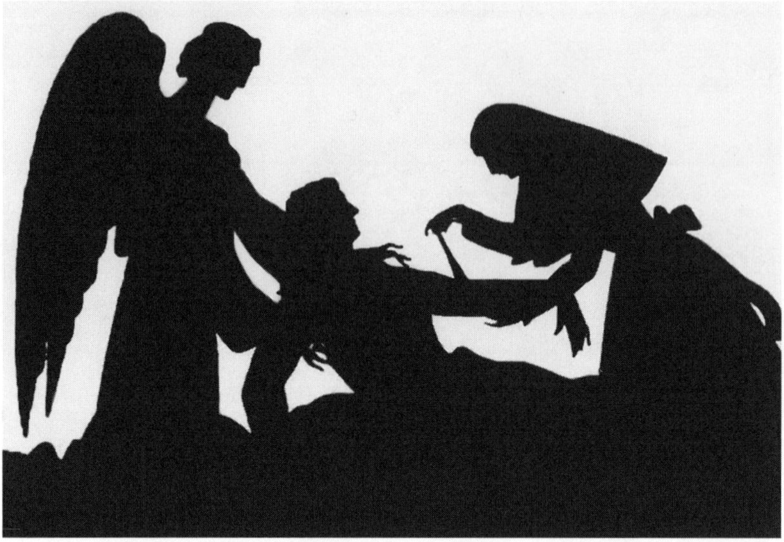

Figure 7.16. Nurse as "angel of mercy" alongside actual angel. "Voina" [War], *Novyi Satirykon*, March 1915, 3.

silhouette showing a nurse bandaging the arm of a soldier while an angel provides support for the wounded man. Although *Novyi Satirykon* was published by and for the Russian intelligentsia and tended to be critical of the tsarist government and the prosecution of the war, it clearly represents a highly positive, idealized representation of the sister of mercy. This image contrasts sharply with many of the other images published in the journal, which tended to be cartoons and illustrations that lampooned the enemy as well as those who shirked their patriotic duties.

The image of the angel of mercy was also used in representations of wartime nursing indicating that when there was little hope for a soldier's survival, the nurse brought the dying man comfort and solace in his last moments. Some illustrations even seem to suggest that the sister of mercy acted as a conduit to the eternal. In a war with a tremendously high casualty rate, the importance of providing such spiritual succor was highly valued. This representation is seen in the painting published in *Letopis' Voiny* titled "Last vision on Christmas Eve" (figure 7.17).

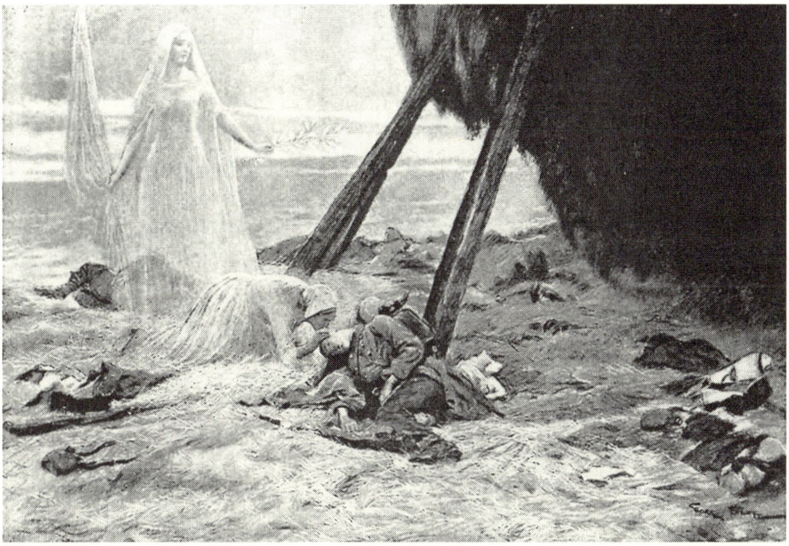

Figure 7.17. Nurse appearing with an angel descending from the heavens. "Poslednee videnie v Podzhestvenskuiu noch'" [Last vision on Christmas Eve], *Letopis' Voiny*, December 26, 1914, 1137.

Sisters as Mothers and Mothers as Sisters

The conception of the wartime nurse as a life-giving and preserving force often manifested itself in images of nurses as mother, or at least mothering. One of the main assets many believed women had that made them effective nurses was their "natural" inclination to motherhood. Fitting into conceptions of the imperial family, nurses were akin to "sister-mothers," acting as surrogate for female caregivers left behind by men sent to the battlefields. Not only were nurses portrayed in maternal ways, but actual mothers figured prominently in a number of wartime productions. Several of the short prowar booklets featured mothers as the protagonists in idealized stories about nurses' selfless service. They were often presented initially as the mothers of young women who wish to enlist in wartime nursing service, as in the story of Liudmila and Elizaveta Bychkova. Although they fear for the safety of their daughters, they ultimately agree to allow them to enlist out of patriotic duty and the ideal of self-sacrifice for the good of the nation, just as they had done with their sons called to duty in the active army. Some are so moved by the selfless motives of their children that they, too, decide to enlist in medical service. A similar story was fleshed out in "The Love of a Sister of Mercy, or Mother under Bullets and Bombs," written by Kristofor Shukhman in 1915. The text described how Maria Petrovna, the "tall and stately" mother of four sons who had enlisted at the outbreak of war, was swayed by the desire to be useful during the national crisis, but also by the possibility of being closer to her sons. After receiving word that one of her sons, Petr, had been killed in action, Maria Petrovna and Petr's young widow, Olenka, cried bitterly. To overcome her sorrow, the latter immediately decided to enter nursing training courses with the intention of going to the front. Explaining her motivations to her mother-in-law, Olenka stated, "I will never again love, never again be able to marry. . . . I want to be useful to those who suffer so much and lay down their lives for us." Inspired by this example, Maria Petrovna decided to enlist in medical services as well. "'I will go with you,' she said resolutely. 'I don't want to cry any more. I want to die where my sons are dying or have died.'"[38]

These were not simply passive figures, playing secondary background roles against the primary actions of soldiers, strong and brave. Mothering, too, contained a significant element of strength and power. This was demonstrated in visual as well as textual images. A poster clearly intended for purposes of recruiting women into wartime medical service featured a matronly looking woman standing above a young officer seated on the ground at her feet (figure 7.18). While the text of the print reads, "When men are at the front—this is your place, women!" suggesting a decidedly secondary role for women, the image presents a somewhat contradictory message. Indeed, the gendered associations of strength with masculinity and weakness with femininity are reversed. The female figure of the nurse appears very strong and physically capable, standing above the man with one hand on his back and the other offered to him as if to help him get up. The male figure, by contrast, looks thin, weak, and vulnerable, perhaps even lame, with one arm hanging limply by his side.[39] This poster suggests that nurses' roles could be strong and active, rather than subordinate and passive, and again was intended to inspire women to enlist in medical services rather than sit at home and wait for their men to return from the battlefields.

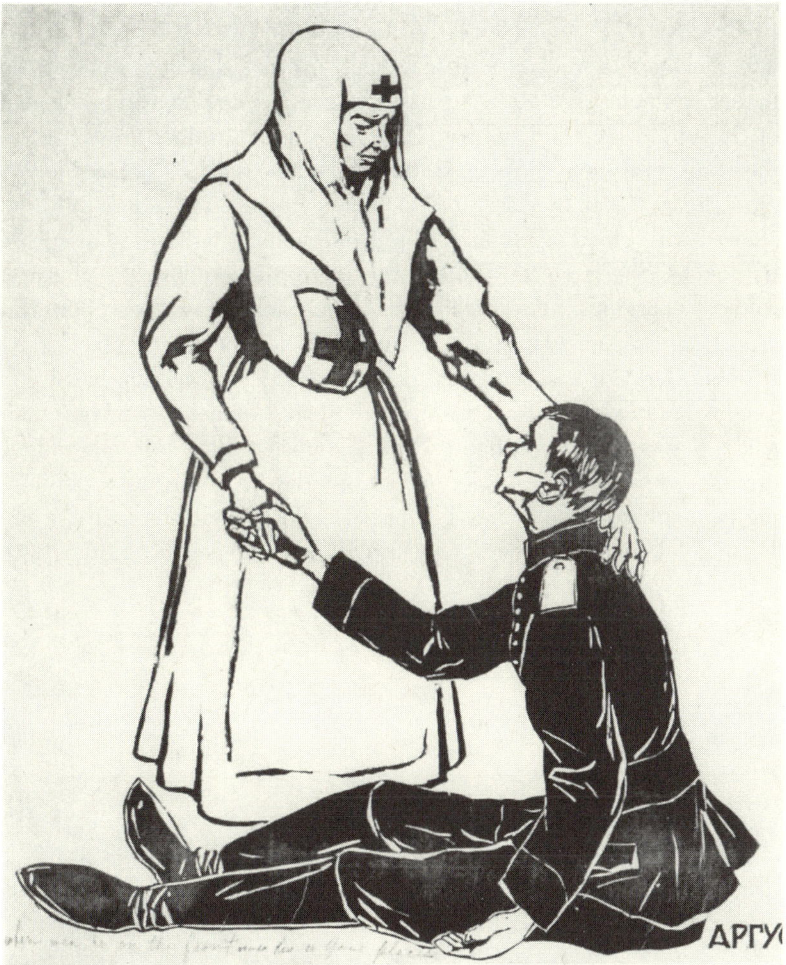

Figure 7.18. Recruitment poster for nursing service. Argus, "Kogda muzhchiny na fronte, vot gde vashe mesto, zhenshchiny!" [When men are at the front, this is your place, women!] (Russkoe Obshchestvo Pechatnogo Dela, n.d.). Black and white. 25" x 36". Hoover Institution Poster Collection, RU/SU 1107.

Mother Russia

Other images used nurses to represent abstract concepts such as the nation, particularly "Mother Russia." In a work strongly reminiscent of Delacroix's depiction of *Marianne* (*la France*) leading the charge in the 1830 revolution, the print titled "The heroic feat of a sister of mercy . . . " (figure 7.19), by Ivan Simov, features a nurse, dressed all in white, stained with blood of the man (the people) she is helping limp off the battlefield. She is clearly the central figure, rising above the melee of soldiers charging in the foreground.[40] Such images were also powerful as prowar propaganda, aimed at appealing to women to enlist in the Russian Red Cross or other medical services as wartime nurses.

Other examples portrayed wartime nurses as national symbols, such as the poster depicted in figure 7.20. The image, titled "Moscow during the days of sacred war," was produced by the A. A. Levenson publishing company to raise money for the war effort. Here, the figure of the nurse is labeled as "Moscow" and is collecting money and valuables to

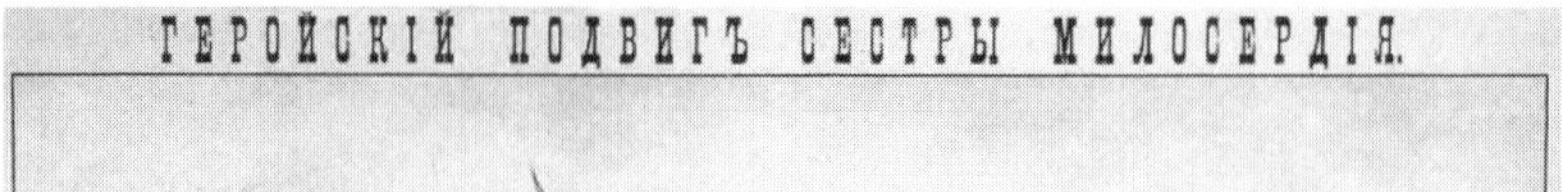

Figure 7.19. Active portrayal of nurse rescuing wounded men from the battlefield. I. Simov, "Geroiskii podvig sestry miloserdia" [The heroic feat of a sister of mercy.] (Moscow: T-vo Tipo-litografiia I. M. Mashitova, 1914–1917). Color. 17" x 23". Hoover Institution Poster Collection, RU/SU 353.

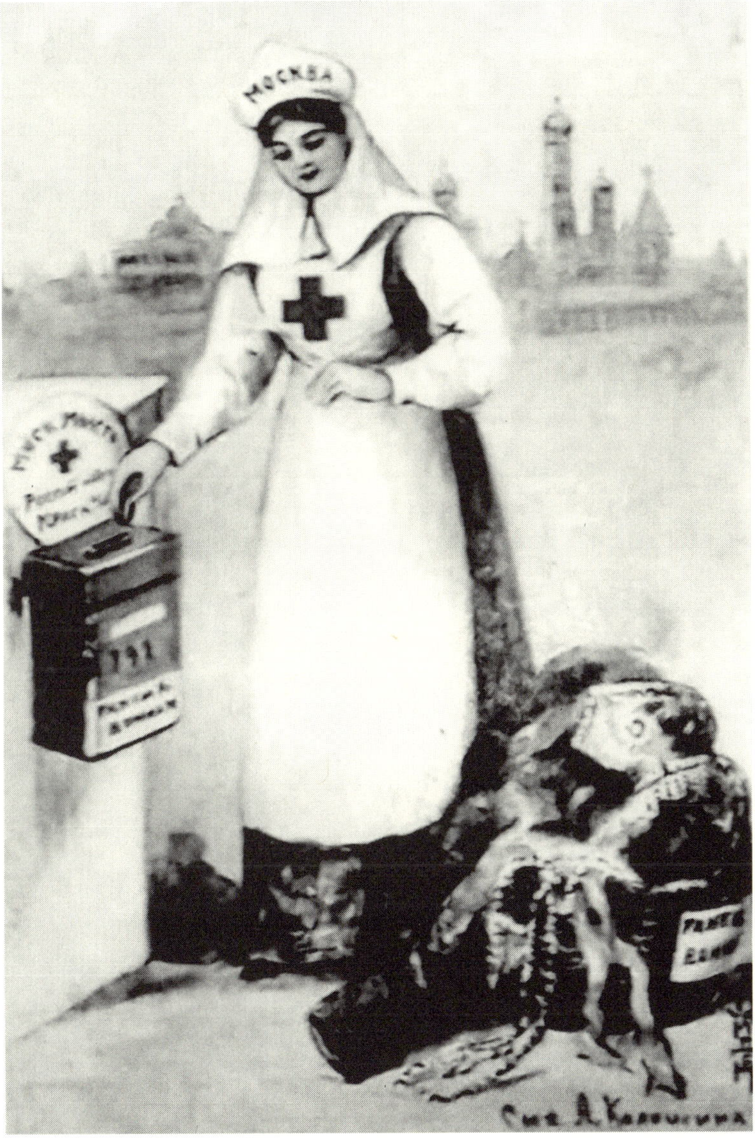

Figure 7.20. Nurse depicted as national symbol. "Moskva v dni sviashchenoi voiny" [Moscow during the days of sacred war] (Moscow: T-vo Skoropechatni A. A. Levenson, 1914). Digitized image courtesy of Boris Kolonitskii.

assist those who had been wounded at the front. She is not performing any medical duty but clearly indicating her secondary, supportive role in the war. This image contrasts significantly with those like the Simov poster above. The chaos, smoke, and blood of the battlefield in the first image is completely absent; instead, the Levenson poster is set against the outline of the center of Moscow, with the towers of the Kremlin visible in the soft background light. The figure of the nurse is pristine with no hint of the violence of the war at all. Under her Red Cross smock, the sister of mercy is dressed in traditional Slavic garb, further indicating her symbolism as a representative of the nation.

The Active, Heroic Nurse (Heroine or Virago)

A number of other representations also place wartime nurses squarely in the center of the action and highlight their strength against the weakness, vulnerability, and passivity of male figures depicted with them. The Russian press and other cultural productions emphasized the immense value of services provided by these women and their undertaking of acts of great courage and bravery to treat the wounded. In fact, the story of the "heroic" nurse who "endured enemy fire without regard to her own life" in order to attend to the needs of the soldiers was a standard trope. This was especially true with regard to depictions of nurses serving at the front, as opposed to those serving in the rear. Women who served as nurses on the front were often portrayed in more positive and masculine terms, as active, heroic, strong, composed figures.[41]

Many such sources emphasized the willingness of wartime nurses to sacrifice their own lives for the benefit of the soldiers they served, demonstrating that their work placed them in positions of great danger. While the safe, sterilized image of the nurse in a pristine hospital setting may have been strongly prevalent in Russian popular imagination, the war led to the creation of an entirely different image. These were considerably edgier images, depicting nurses amid blood, dirt, and violence—a pronounced difference from the images of sisters in rear medical facilities, which placed women in spaces that were discordant with conventional notions of femininity that centered on the protected, safe sphere of the domestic. These images, while still highly idealized for propagandistic purposes, more accurately reflect the reality of service for nurses working on the front lines.

A number of textual representations of wartime nurses reflected this trope. In his book titled *War, Women and Children,* writer V. V. Brusianin extolled the self-sacrificing and difficult work of nurses, detailing the hardships they endured. "There have already been sisters of mercy who have been killed, those who have been wounded, and those who have had to be relieved of duty as a result of the strain on their health, health that had undergone such excessive testing at the frontline positions or near them."[42] The periodical press similarly celebrated the actions of nurses on the battlefields, often emphasizing characteristics of strength, courage, and fortitude. The rather dry and heavily statistical official journal of the Russian Society of the Red Cross, *Vestnik Krasnago Kresta* (Red Cross Herald), is filled with reports on the activities of Russian women performing medical services in both rear and frontline hospitals.[43] Popular publications also featured the heroic exploits of nurses at the front. A favorite subject for both photographic and textual representation were the nurses who had been awarded medals for their bravery and self-sacrifice, especially the coveted Saint George's medals and crosses. The widely circulated journal *Niva* published a short article titled "Sister of Mercy—Hero" that described the actions of a nurse named Ksenia Bondarenko. Bondarenko was serving with a field hospital on the front lines in the Carpathians, near the village of Moshchenitsa. She was awarded a Saint George's Cross, fourth class, for her care of wounded men on the battlefields. The text highlighted one particularly heroic feat, whereby she ran to the aid of a wounded commander and carried him on her shoulders for about two kilometers under heavy enemy fire until they reached safety.[44] Numerous portraits of nurses who had put themselves in harm's way, often resulting in death or injury, were featured on the pages of Russian wartime periodicals, with those having famous names more likely to appear. The journal *Letopis' Voiny,* although primarily dedicated to the great feats of soldiers and officers on the battlefields, often ran stories or photographs with explanatory captions lauding nurses for acts of courage, as figures 7.21 through 7.23 demonstrate. The first image describes sister of mercy M. F. Kokh, who was attached to the Second Flying Hospital Train. She was awarded the Saint George's medal for her bravery in attending to the wounded while her train was stopped on a bridge and was being bombed by an enemy zeppelin.[45] The second tells of the courageous, self-sacrificing feat of sister Iulia Puchkovskaia, who was the first to run to the aid of wounded men on the front lines, despite being under heavy shelling and bullet fire. She too received a Saint George's medal.[46] The third image

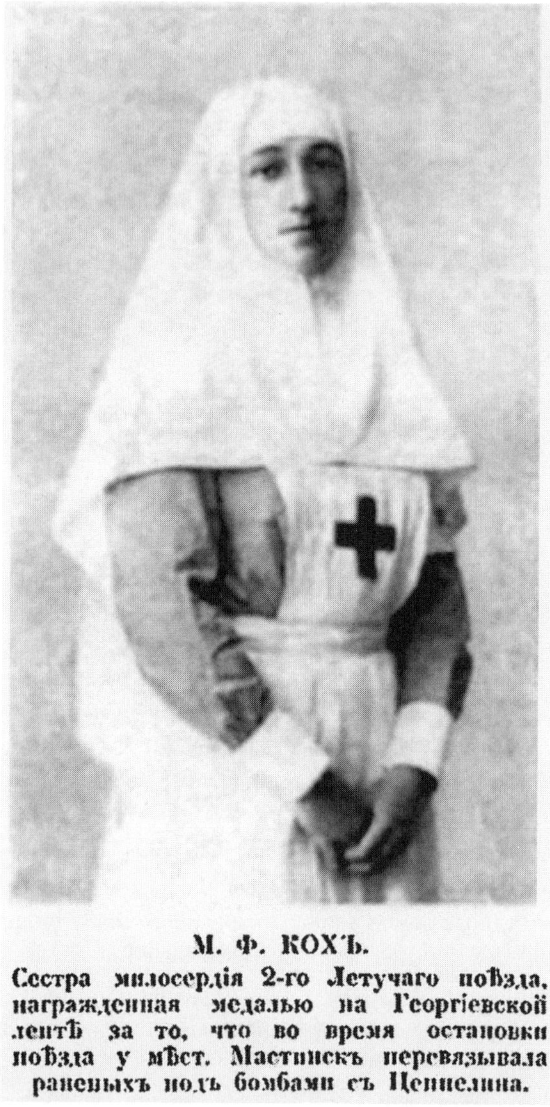

Figure 7.21. Sister of mercy M. F. Kokh, awarded military honors for courage and self-sacrifice. "M. F. Kokh," *Letopis' Voiny*, November 29, 1914, 248.

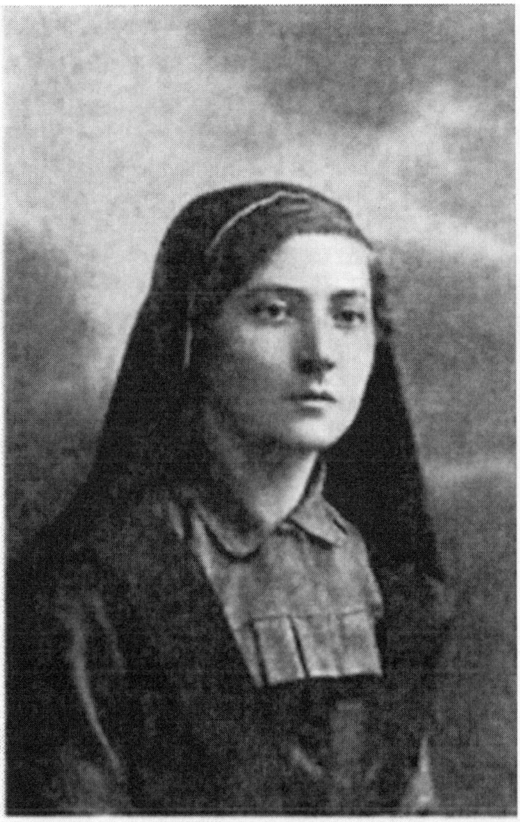

Сестра милосердія Юлія Пучковская,
нагр. Георгіевскою медалью 3-й ст.
за самоотверженную храбрость и по-
двиги, выразившіеся въ томъ, что на-
ходясь подъ дѣйствительнымъ огнемъ
непріятельскихъ снарядовъ и будучи
оглушена сама, оказывала первую
помощь раненымъ съ явною опас-
ностью для собственной жизни.

Figure 7.22. Sister of mercy Iulia Puchkovskaia, awarded the Saint George's Medal, Third Class, for self-sacrificing bravery. *Letopis' Voiny*, November 21, 1915, 1062.

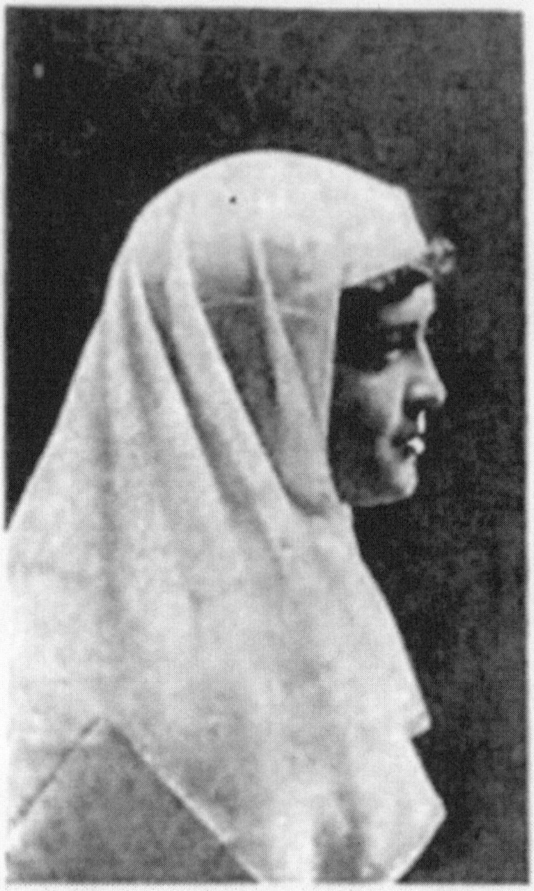

Сестра милосердія Ольга Плахова, слѣдуя въ военно-санитарномъ поѣздѣ, съ полнымъ самоотверженіемъ и опасностью для жизни дважды подобрала раненыхъ въ поѣздъ и сдѣлала имъ перевязки. Награждена Георгіевской медалью.

Figure 7.23. Sister of mercy Ol'ga Plakhova, awarded the Saint George's Medal for courageous work on a hospital train. *Letopis' Voiny*, April 23, 1916, 1414.

features sister of mercy Ol'ga Plakhova, similarly a recipient of a medal for her bravery and self-sacrifice in bringing the wounded to her hospital train, despite the risk to her own life.[47]

Visual images published during the war also portrayed nurses as active, courageous, and willing to put themselves in grave danger. A number of contemporary prints showed nurses in the midst of combat, images that contrast sharply with scenes depicting sisters of mercy in rear medical establishments. Images printed in the form of *lubki* and posters, and even distributed as postcards circulated during the war, depict female nurses on the battlefields, tending to wounded men while under direct threat of enemy fire. Numerous artistic renderings of nurses featured in contemporary illustrated journals showed sisters of mercy caring for wounded men on the front lines and even on the battlefields. Often bombs exploded in the background, menacing-looking airplanes flew overhead, and bullets and shells flew past them as they bandaged soldiers. One image (figure 7.24), created by the artist A. Lavrov for the Nikol'skaia *obshchina*, was distributed on postcards used for fund-raising, specifically to raise money to produce gas masks for soldiers at the front. The image depicts a nurse kneeling on the ground next to a wounded soldier, whose unconscious body she supports. As she bandages his chest, she looks up with grave concern while a shell explodes in the air above them. The barbed wire in front of the trenches is visible just behind her.[48] Here the nurse is portrayed as delivering lifesaving medical care to the wounded soldier with an injury to his chest who is seemingly completely dependent on her in his unconscious state (although the wound is presented as bloodless, and both the soldier and the nurse are portrayed as very clean). They are both in a position of considerable vulnerability, but the sister continues the work despite the grave danger to their lives.

The *lubok* titled "The Feat of Sister E. P. Korkina" (figure 7.25), produced in 1915 by the wartime publisher Ivan Sytin, shows a nurse, standing serenely in the foreground of a scene depicting a German attack on Red Cross transports, with the bodies of wounded and dead Russian and German officers lying around her. One hand rests on the head of a wounded officer seated at her feet, and the other is outstretched to the right, indicating a scene on the road where a Red Cross transport cart is in the process of being blown to bits. Behind her, Russian Red Cross stretcher bearers (male) load wounded men into another transport cart. The nurse is clearly the centerpiece of the image, and she is the only woman in the picture, despite the presence of a number of other medical personnel. The extensive

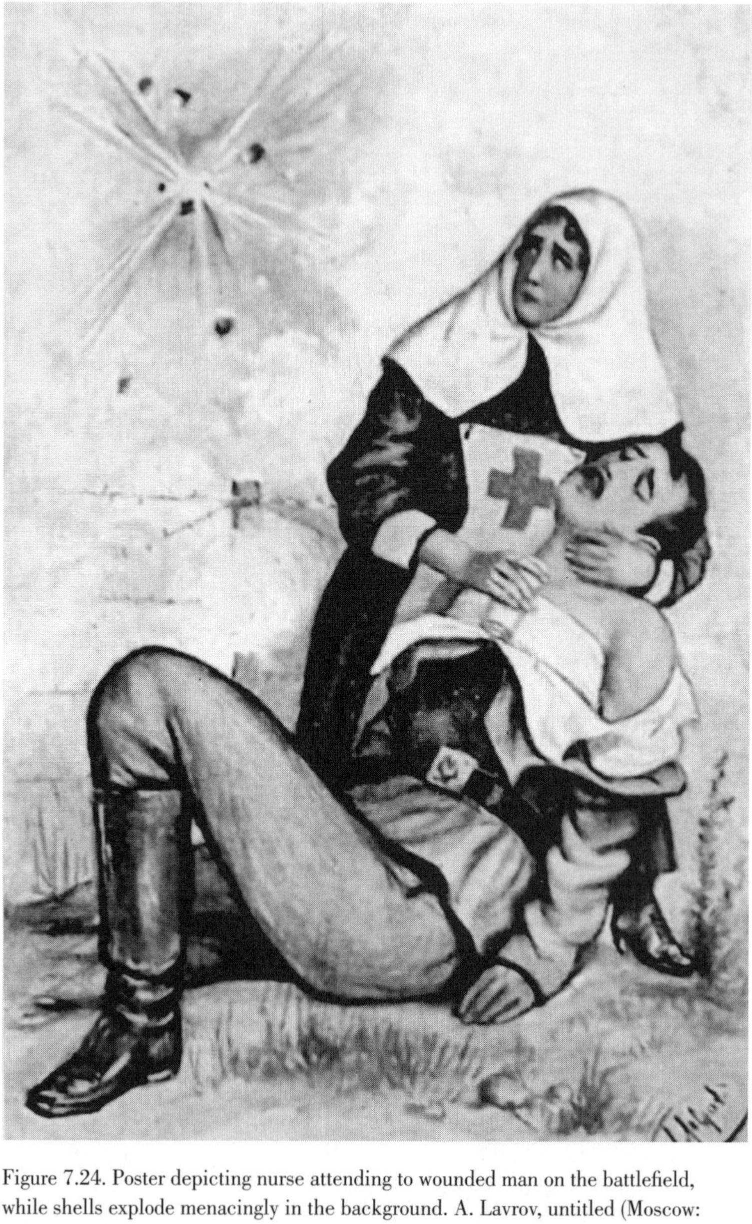

Figure 7.24. Poster depicting nurse attending to wounded man on the battlefield, while shells explode menacingly in the background. A. Lavrov, untitled (Moscow: Nikol'skaia Obshchina R. O. Krasnago Kresta, n.d.). Digitized image courtesy of Boris Kolonitskii.

text below tells the tale of the scene, wherein Korkina is described as a valiant hero who worked calmly under deadly enemy fire to rescue nine wounded officers after the Red Cross transport they had been traveling in was shelled by the Germans. Both the picture and the caption emphasize Korkina's strong, composed action and identify her clearly as the central heroic figure on whom the men, wounded and thus passive (perhaps even emasculated), must rely.[49]

Figures of nurses were also featured in artistic productions such as sculptures, celebrating their heroism and devotion to the war effort. One particularly striking work titled "The saving of the flag" (figure 7.26) by the artist Maria Dillon depicts a nurse holding both a wounded man and the flag he was apparently carrying for his unit, indicating her commitment not only to the welfare of the male combatant but also to the patriotic cause of the war as symbolized by the flag. The sculpture appeared as part of a "patriotic exhibit of artwork in Petrograd," and photographs of the work were run in various periodical publications, including *Letopis' Voiny* and *Niva.*[50]

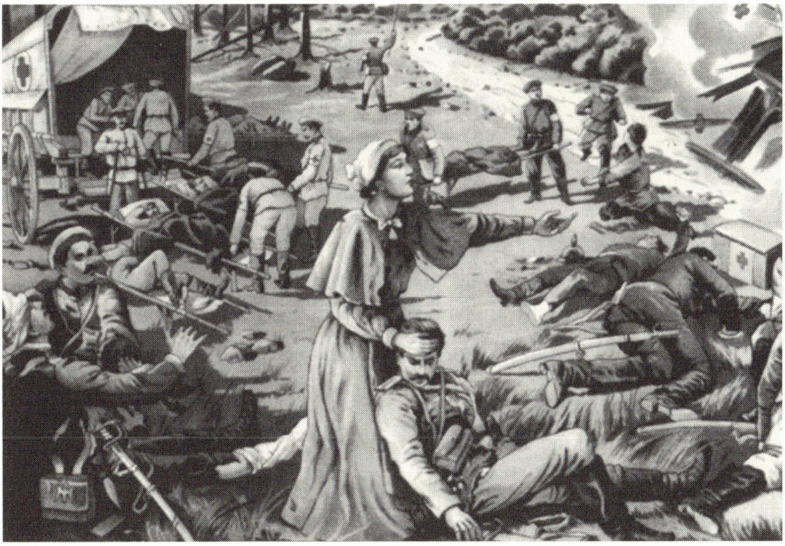

Figure 7.25. Heroic actions of a sister of mercy when her medical transport was attacked by the enemy. P. Petrov, "Podvig Sestry E. P. Korkinoi" [The Feat of Sister E. P. Korkina] (Moscow: Litografiia T-va. I. D. Sytina, 1915). Color. Various sizes. Hoover Institution Poster Collection, RU/SU 322.

A number of these images seem to suggest that although women were often perceived as weak and passive, participation in the war as a nurse could transform them into strong and active, even fearless, figures. This idea was expressed visually in an illustration titled "Metamorphosis: At Home and at the Front," published in *Sinii Zhurnal* (Blue Journal). The first frame of the drawing depicts a woman standing on a night table like a fixture near her bed, looking fearful and trepidatious (afraid of what appears to be an insect on the bed—perhaps a cockroach in a Kafka allusion). In the next, she appears physically transformed, wearing the uniform of the sister of mercy, looking confident, even happy, seemingly oblivious to the danger as shells burst all around her.[51]

Some images even celebrated women who stepped outside the boundaries of the roles as medical workers to engage in combat activities. The participation of nurses in violent activity was not seen as unacceptable by some Russian sources.[52] The media response to the actions of Rimma Ivanova, a nurse who led her unit into battle after all of the male commanders had been killed in battle, is a salient example.[53] The Russian press reported Ivanova's deeds as feats of great heroism and bravery, comparing her to Joan of Arc. Stories about her personal history filled the pages of local and national periodicals. Ivanova's picture was featured in multiple publications, including the front page of *Iskry* in October 1915. A depiction of her actions in battle even made it into the British press, displayed on the cover of *The War Illustrated* (figure 7.27).

This is not to say that there was no ambiguity regarding the implications of her deeds. The Germans in particular expressed their objections that she was a woman, and especially a member of medical services who was clearly prohibited from participation in combat by the Geneva Convention. For some Russians, Ivanova's gender was similarly paramount to their misgivings. These sentiments have been echoed in secondary sources. Iu. N. Khristinin believes that the award was not granted to Ivanova until January 1916, and that the long space between the time of her deed and her award should be seen as an attempt by the Russian military authorities to hide the event. Joshua Sanborn argues that the army was embarrassed that a woman had carried out such actions, as they did not fit with the masculine military ethic.[54] To many Russians, however, Ivanova was a hero, whose actions on the battlefield were laudable regardless of the fact that she was a woman and a nurse. The military authorities posthumously awarded her a Saint George's Cross, which was a specific combat medal. The soldiers and officers

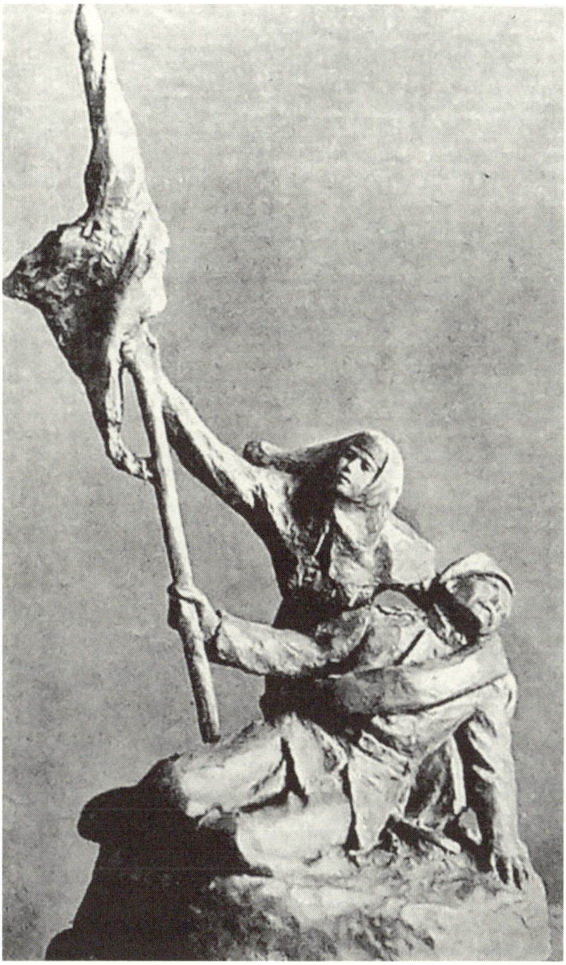

Figure 7.26. Sculpture depicting nurse saving both wounded man and Russian flag while under attack. "Spasenie znameni. Gruppa M. Dillon (Patrioticheskaia vystavka kartin v Petrograd)" [The saving of the flag. M. Dillon Group (Patriotic exhibit of pictures in Petrograd)], *Niva*, June 6, 1915, 442.

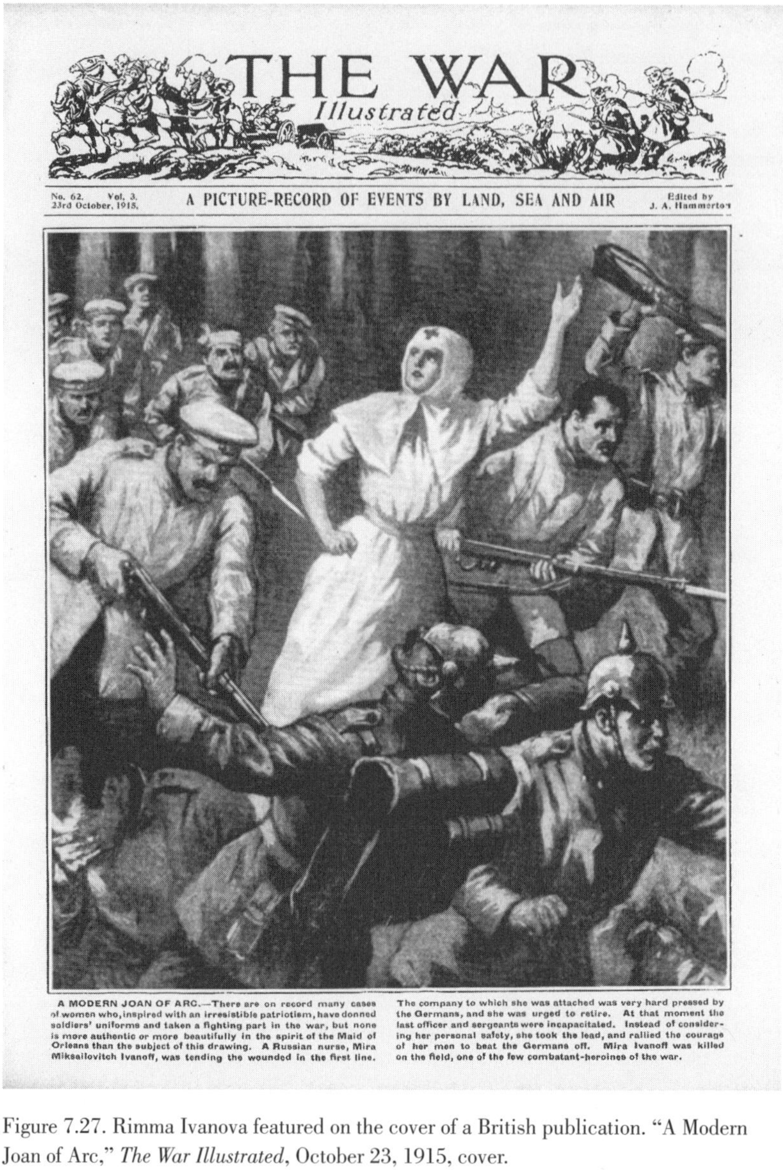

THE WAR Illustrated

No. 62. Vol. 3. 23rd October, 1915.

A PICTURE-RECORD OF EVENTS BY LAND, SEA AND AIR

Edited by J. A. Hammerton

A MODERN JOAN OF ARC.—There are on record many cases of women who, inspired with an irresistible patriotism, have donned soldiers' uniforms and taken a fighting part in the war, but none is more authentic or more beautifully in the spirit of the Maid of Orleans than the subject of this drawing. A Russian nurse, Mira Miksailovitch Ivanoff, was tending the wounded in the first line. The company to which she was attached was very hard pressed by the Germans, and she was urged to retire. At that moment the last officer and sergeants were incapacitated. Instead of considering her personal safety, she took the lead, and rallied the courage of her men to beat the Germans off. Mira Ivanoff was killed on the field, one of the few combatant-heroines of the war.

Figure 7.27. Rimma Ivanova featured on the cover of a British publication. "A Modern Joan of Arc," *The War Illustrated*, October 23, 1915, cover.

of her unit seemed to have no misgivings about her, calling her a heroine, requesting a special railway car to take her body back to her native Stavropol' and soliciting the tsar to bestow a combat medal on her following her death. The procession of her body and her funeral, held in one of the city's most important cathedrals, attracted large crowds of spectators. The archpriest Simeon Nikol'skii, who presided over the service, suggested that Ivanova be canonized by the Russian Orthodox Church, and the Grand Duke Nikolai Nikolaevich, commander in chief of the Russian armed forces at the time, sent a silver wreath wrapped in the Saint George's ribbon to adorn her grave. In November 1915 the military authorities actually commissioned a film titled *The Heroic Feats of Sister of Mercy Rimma Mikhailovna Ivanova.* The first screening of the film caused a tremendous scandal—not because a woman was being portrayed carrying out combat feats, but because the actress playing the nurse appeared on the battlefield waving her sword while wearing high-heeled shoes and trying not to dishevel her fashionable coiffure. The officers who had served with Ivanova were so outraged by this misrepresentation that they threatened to "capture the entrepreneur [filmmaker] and make him eat the film."[55] These actions indicate that Ivanova was perceived by many as an example of courage and bravery, with little equivocation regarding her gender. Indeed, the clear response of the veterans to the film, which attempted to make light of her in gendered terms, was rejection.

The aggressive, violent nurse was also featured in a wartime film by famed director Evgenii Bauer. In "Glory to Us—Death to the Enemy," the female protagonist becomes a Red Cross sister at the front to avenge her husband's death. As historian Denise Youngblood indicates, this was not an unusual role for women in the war period in Russia: "the idea of a nurse as a murderous avenging angel might strike those familiar with the conventions of Western, especially American, cinema of this period as strange, but the strong, independent, even murderous heroine was a recurring motif in prerevolutionary Russian film melodramas."[56]

The Victim

Seemingly at the opposite end of the spectrum were portrayals of female nurses as victims of violence perpetrated by the enemy. Although they reflect real anxieties about what might happen when "weak" women were exposed to the aggression of war, such concerns could also be used as powerful prowar propaganda to incentivize men to fight. Women, especially nurses, were often used in visual images that highlighted enemy violence perpetrated against innocent civilians completely undeserving of such attacks, thereby dramatizing the inhumanity of the enemy. These depictions are entirely consistent with efforts to construct strong patriotic support for the war and, as Stephen Norris has argued, represent a successful attempt at building national consciousness.[57] The use of nurses in these efforts was intended both to demonstrate the active participation of women in the war effort, as members of the national community, and to emphasize the need for male defenders of that national community. A *lubok* by the artist B. V. Kudinov titled "German Cruelty. Cruelty that . . . " (figure 7.28) contains such a scene that reflects the latter, wherein German soldiers destroy a village, burn homes to the ground, and kill innocent women and children. In the right front corner of the poster, a Red Cross nurse is featured on her knees, arms outstretched as if seeking aid from the heavens, as she is being shot in the back by a German soldier. The text below the image implicates the Germans in acts of brutality "surpassed in no other war, by no other earthly people, not even African savages."[58] Another *lubok* features two panels, "Cruelty at Kalisz" on the left and "Events at Kalisz" on the right. The latter shows a group of Red Cross nurses and medics being fired on by a group of German soldiers in the town of Kalisz, Poland. The brutality of the Germans is punctuated by the fact that the nurses and medics were traveling in a medical transport flying the Red Cross flag. One of the nurses who has not already been shot dead is on her knees with her hands in the air, indicating surrender and perhaps an appeal for mercy. The caption under this panel indicates that thirteen sisters of mercy were killed in this attack.[59] The use of nurses in these posters was an effective means to convey the message of a vicious enemy that resorted to the killing of women, even nurses who were supposed to be protected by the international symbol of the Red Cross.

Of particular concern was the sexual violation of Russian women by enemy troops. Numerous examples in both visual and textual sources depict nurses as victims of sexual violence perpetrated by the enemy. Posters produced as official propaganda often reflected this fear in striking visual as well as textual ways. The left panel of the image described above, "Cruelty at Kalisz," depicts a group of Germans in the process of executing a father and his two sons by sword. In the foreground lies the lifeless body of his daughter, whose torn upper bodice and exposed breasts, as well as her

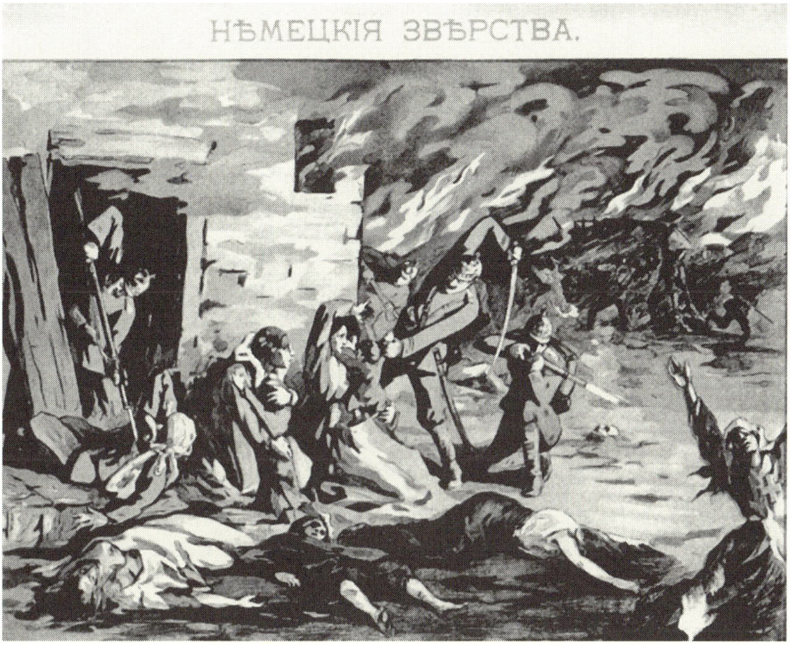

Figure 7.28. *Lubok* featuring cruel acts of Germans. B. V. Kudinov, "Nemetskiia zverstva. Zverstva kotoryia . . . " [German cruelty. Cruelty that . . .] (Moscow: Tipo-lit. T. D. Br. Evdokimy, 1914–1917?). Color. 17" x 24". Hoover Institution Poster Collection, RU/SU 355.

bloodied skirt, clearly indicate that she had been raped. The text below the images reveals that the violence had been perpetrated against her in front of her father and brothers. Another *lubok* by N. D. Alekseev, titled "The cruelty of Germans" (figure 7.29), features a heroic Cossack soldier riding to the rescue of a Russian nurse, who is being dragged along the road tied to the tail of a German officer's horse. The nurse is disheveled, her veil missing, her uniform torn open in the front, with bloodstains on her abdominal area, similarly indicating that she had been raped. Her expression, and even the positioning of her body as she is being dragged by the horse, is stoic, saintly, as she passively endures her torture. The text, however, points to the psychological impact of the ordeal on the young woman, describing her as "hysterical and suffering from nervous shock."[60] An image titled "Innocent victim in the hands of cultured butchers" (figure 7.30) depicts a small room with three Germans, one of whom sits at a table calmly drinking beer and chatting with a fellow soldier, while the lifeless body of a bloodied, disheveled nurse lies dead on the floor.

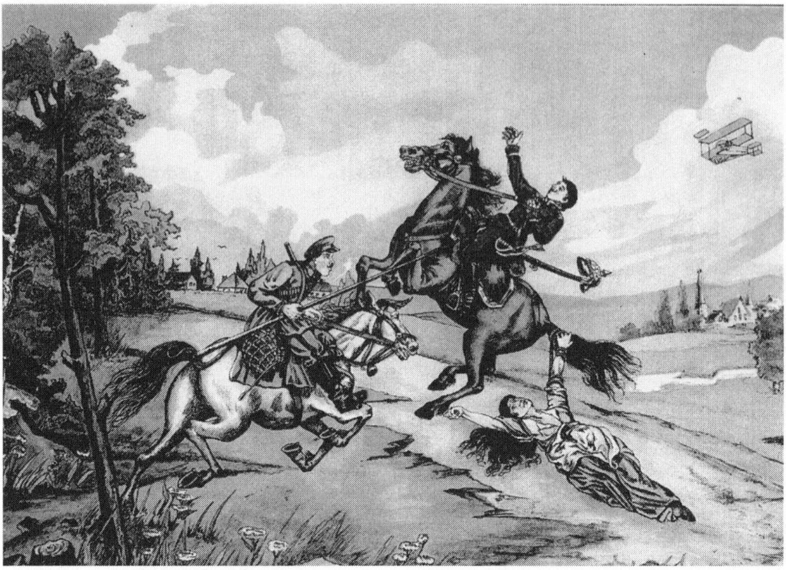

Figure 7.29. *Lubok* depicting rescue of a Russian sister of mercy being dragged behind a horse by a German. N. D. Alekseev, "Zverstvo nemstev" [The cruelty of Germans] (publisher unknown, 1914–1917?). Color. 16" x 22". Hoover Institution Poster Collection, RU/SU 445.

The text below the image describes how a "drunken horde" of Germans descended on the nurses, who were carrying out their "lofty Christian work in healing the suffering wounded," and began mocking and harassing them. The innocent nurses could not endure such abuse, which left one of them dead. The text insists that the shedding of her blood would elicit cries from the entire civilized world.[61]

Thus, in these posters female vulnerability was also used as a means to expose the inhumanity of Russia's enemies. Such images were intended as sources of propaganda to inspire men to enlist in combat. In a *lubok* titled "Education of a barbarian" (figure 7.31), another Sytin image, a young nurse is depicted lying seemingly unconscious in the arms of an officer. By his side lays the bloodied corpse of an enemy soldier. The Russian officer looks behind him with grave concern as his comrade pursues another German on horseback and engages him in a sword fight. The sister of mercy in this image has an angelic, though decidedly vulnerable, look about her. The male officer is clearly the strong, active figure, propping up the limp, unconscious body of the female nurse, the

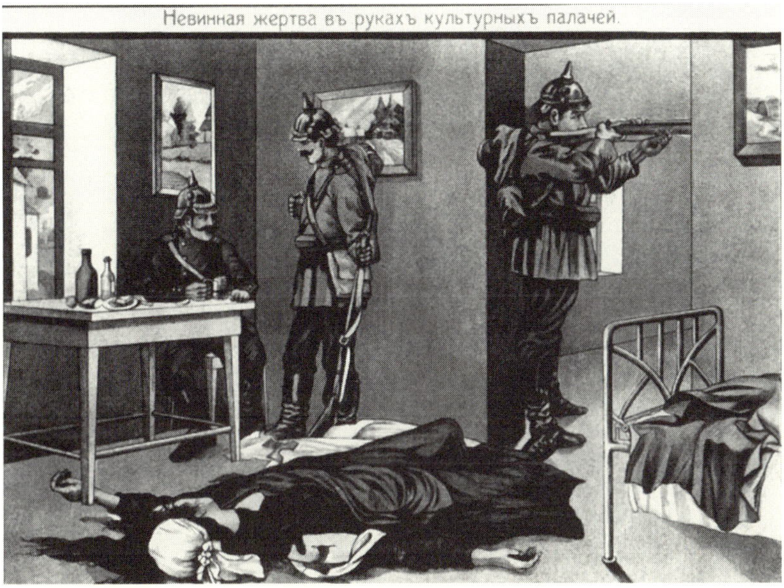

Figure 7.30. *Lubok* featuring a nurse raped and killed by Germans. "Nevinnaia zhertva v rukakh kul'turnykh palachei" [Innocent victim in the hands of cultured butchers] (Moscow: Tipo-lit. E. F. Chelnokova, 1914–1918?). Color. 15" x 20". Hoover Institution Poster Collection, RU/SU 334.

weak victim in need of male protection. The caption tells us that the young woman has just been saved from a "fate worse than death" by a Russian dragoon, who killed her German attacker in the nick of time, making the "barbarian pay for his villainy."[62] These types of images fit with a more general trend of presenting the enemy in the worst possible light, as barbaric invaders who violated the principles of honor and the conventions of war. Other artistic media reflect these tropes as well. The climax of the film *The Horrors of Reims*, directed by Grigorii Libken, is a dramatic scene in which a German's attempts to rape a nurse on the altar of a cathedral are thwarted by a priest. Such an act, as Hubertus Jahn has argued, "violates religious, moral, and patriotic values all at the same time."[63]

Such images were predicated on notions of the vulnerability of women in the war zone while simultaneously appealing to traditional ideas about masculinity and men's obligations to the national family in times of crisis. The trope of women's sexual vulnerability was thus used as a means of promoting male enlistment in military service by playing on

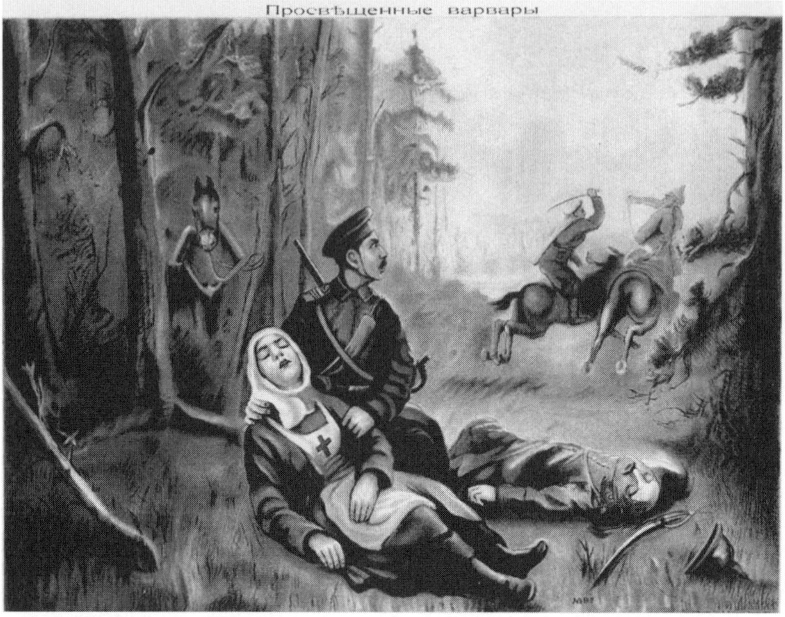

Figure 7.31. *Lubok* depicting rescue of a Russian sister of mercy from the hands of Germans. "Prosvieshchennye varvary . . . " [Education of a barbarian . . .] (Moscow: Litografiia t-va I. D. Sytina, 1915), copy #97. Color. 17" x 22". Hoover Institution Poster Collection, RU/SU 382.

fears of enemy aggression against innocent civilians and notions of male chivalry. One might assume that such images might be counterproductive to the recruitment of women into wartime nursing, but clearly women were not the intended audience for these posters. However, they simultaneously functioned, if not explicitly but subconsciously, as conveyors of deep-seated anxieties about the vulnerability of nurses to violence at the front and the suitability of women in the zone of war. While the nation was dependent on women to carry out medical services in order to prosecute the war effectively, there was, nonetheless, concern that such activity put women at risk, specifically to sexual violence, which, for many, was "a fate worse than death."

Images of Nurses as Instruments of Social Critique

Depictions of wartime nurses could also be used by the Russian illustrated press to express criticisms about the war and the participation of women in the conflict. A number of observers worried about the effects of the gruesome realities of the masculine war zone on women. Would they lose their femininity and what many considered women's most valuable assets, their life-giving, life-affirming, life-preserving natures, when faced with the violence and destruction of combat? The idea of women going to the front to "mother" soldiers similarly proved problematic for those who worried that if women were attending to the wounds and illnesses of soldiers in the public sphere they might neglect what was regarded as woman's primary function in the domestic realm. "First and foremost," wrote Valentina Kostyleva, a journalist in the popular women's journal *Zhenskaia Zhizn'*, "women are obligated to maintain the value and sanctity of the family hearth, to maintain a healthy, cheerful atmosphere, in which the younger generation can grow up freely and without sadness." Without the mother's presence in the home children would not receive an emotionally supportive upbringing, Kostyleva argued. Without the wife at the hearth, she maintained, men would wonder for what they were fighting and to whom they would come home.[64] Although the Red Cross preferred to accept unmarried and childless women, there were thousands of nurses that left families behind in order to serve in the war. While acting as surrogate mother to wounded soldiers was largely commendable, abandoning one's own family was extremely disconcerting.

Despite fears of abandoning children in the rear, one of the most common complaints was the notion that some members of Russian society were not "doing their part" for the war effort. These, too, can be seen in the vein of patriotic culture, as expressed by those who believed that some of Russia's citizens were shirking responsibility to the nation in its time of crisis. Men who used connections or bribes to obtain exemptions from military service were often targets of social condemnation, but so too were women who were believed to be capable of participating in the war effort but chose to focus on their private lives instead. Nursing was thus depicted as the means to transform women from useless socialites into contributing members of society, as indicated by the image titled "Metamorphosis." Those who did not undergo such a change were compared negatively to those who did. The illustration from the popular journal *Ogonek* from June 1916 (figure 7.32) depicts this in gendered terms, suggesting that in civilian life not only had women become selfish and decadent, but also the gender order had been disrupted, even unnaturally inverted. The first pair of images illustrates this well, wherein

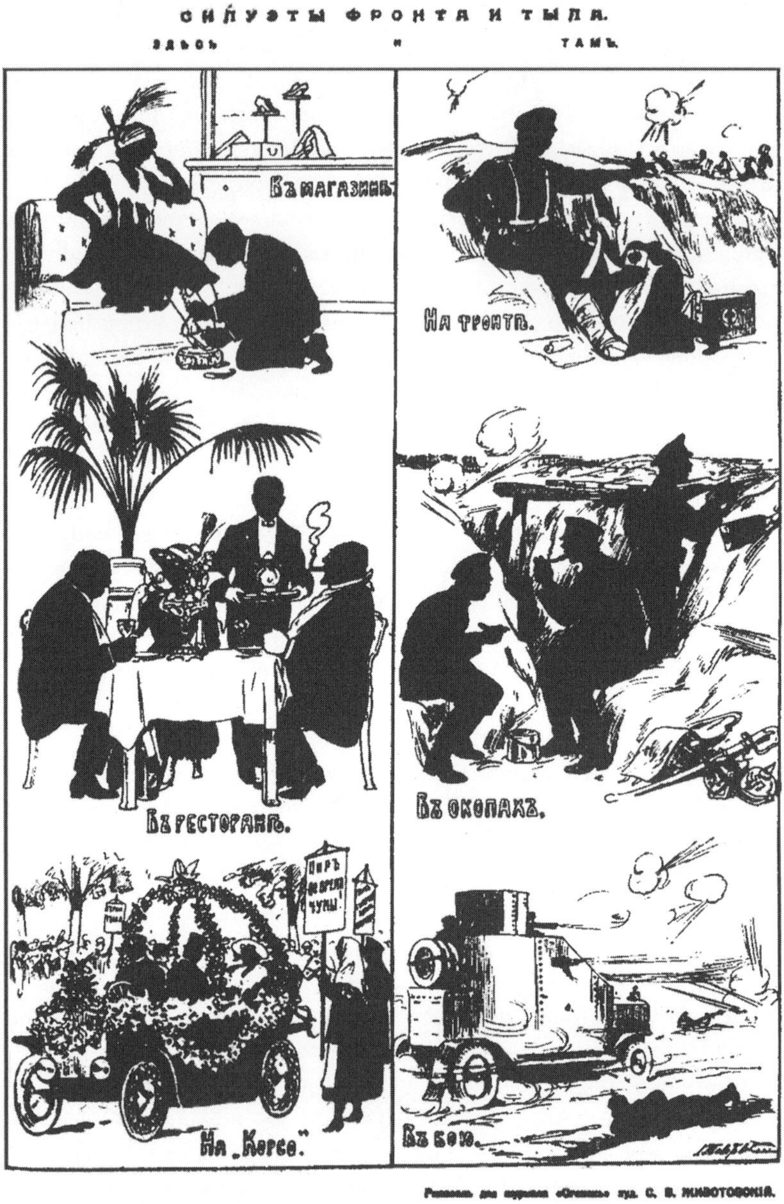

Figure 7.32. Contrasting images of front and rear. "Siluety fronta i tyla" [Silhouettes of the front and rear], *Ogonek*, June 16, 1916, 5.

the "rear" image shows a man at the feet of a woman, while its "front" companion portrays a reversal of male and female physical positions to reflect what was considered the appropriate arrangement.

CONCLUSIONS

An examination of use of images of wartime nurses in Russian patriotic culture during World War I reveals both the extent to which women's activities in the public sphere were accepted and the ambiguities inherent in wartime nursing. The plethora of positive nursing images indicate the degree to which this entrée into public service was successful, presenting new ways of imagining women: dynamic, active, and strong. At the same time, many such perceptions remained bound by convention, portraying women in ways consistent with traditional notions of femininity: passive, caring, nurturing, and supportive. They reflect the fact that by the time of the outbreak of World War I, the use of women in medical capacities was seen as highly desirable, specifically because of the characteristics thought to be natural to women.

The war, however, revealed that such conventional conceptualizations were problematic, even paradoxical. As indicated previously, retaining passive and emotive aspects of femininity was difficult and impractical for wartime nurses. Moreover, the very change of space in which women's activities were performed was potentially very troubling. In peacetime society, the caring and nurturing activities of women were conducted in the private realm, the feminine arena of the home. Women had begun to move outside these boundaries by serving in public health capacities beginning in the late nineteenth century. These activities were still carried out in the sphere of domestic society, in the rear or "home front." The rear was traditionally perceived of as a "feminized" zone, and thus women's activities within it would not have been challenging to such conceptions. The front, by contrast, was considered to be a kind of hypermasculine realm, one from which women had traditionally been excluded. The realities of war in Russia dictated the tremendous need for nurses' participation at the front, not just in the rear. One might assume, therefore, that taking women's service out of the domestic realm and into the war zone would have been the most disconcerting aspect of wartime nursing. So, while nursing was seen as appropriate for their gender, wartime nursing presented a challenge because it required women's presence in a sphere that had been deemed largely inappropriate for them, indeed one that many men had worked to preserve as purely masculine. However, the images of women as passive sources of comfort in military medical establishments demonstrate the extent to which many did not see a problem with taking the caring and nurturing out of the home.

Thus, the indication of such a shift to public activity during the war is even more salient in the images of nurses serving at the front. In many of these representations, women were not only commended for their participation in the war zone, they also had the intention of inspiring other women to enlist in wartime medical services. As such, they acknowledged the important contributions made by nurses in the war effort and sought to expand the participation of women in these endeavors, drawing them out of the private sphere into public activity, even into the distinctly male zone of the war front. Moreover, frontline nurses were portrayed with traits generally considered to be masculine in early twentieth-century Russian society: active, strong, heroic, cool, and composed. This corresponds to gendered associations of the front as a masculine sphere: women gained gender-appropriate attributes through their participation in this arena. Celebrating, even encouraging, women's active heroism in the face of danger can be seen consistent with the traditional "strong woman motif" present in Russian culture.[65] But what is unique about the war experience is that the nurse is clearly operating in a nontraditional sphere of activity for women. The Russian cultural trope of the strong woman was usually seen as positive only when anchored within the context of the family. However, the active, frontline nurse who worked heroically in the face of great danger, subsuming her own needs into those of the male soldier, and who retained a standard of sexual purity, was not usually targeted for criticism. Removing her from the domestic context did not damage her image. As long as her efforts were being undertaken in the service of others, she was lauded. Within the context of the patriarchal nature of Russian society that portrayed the nation as an extended family, with the tsar as the father figure to millions of subject children, nurses were the mothers and sisters coming to the aid of their sons and brothers. Their actions were acceptable even in this sphere because they worked for the good of the family of the nation.[66]

Not all public imagination was positive concerning nurses. Representations emphasizing their vulnerability, especially sexual, revealed ambiguities about wartime nursing, even when used to inspire men to join the fighting or promote the war effort. In these depictions, women were seen as innocent victims, suggesting some misgivings over the wisdom of placing them in harm's way. Much more negatively imagined, however, were women engaged in wartime nursing who were perceived as acting for personal benefit—when they were placed in safe, secure, rear assignments, when they were given authority over men or intervened in an attempt to gain personal power, when they responded to romantic overtures from men, or worse, when they initiated such interaction themselves, and worse still, when they sought to gain from such relationships. Thus, it was when she seemed to focus her attentions on her own needs or desires that public opinion often turned against the sister of mercy. It is these disparaging images and sordid reputation of Russia's wartime nurses that are explored in the next chapter.

8

"SISTERS OF COMFORT" AND "SISTERS WITHOUT MERCY"

VANDA STEPANOVA: REFUGEE TURNED SISTER

At the start of the summer of 1914, Vanda Kazimirovna Stepanova, a young woman from a Baltic Russian family, had just completed the seventh class in secondary school. She returned home to her family estate near the town of Shavli (present-day Šiauliai, in northern Lithuania) to help her mother look after her younger brothers. On the declaration of war in July, many of Stepanova's friends hurried to enlist in nursing courses. Many of them went to serve in Riga, where "the hospitals were overflowing with wounded." Vanda desperately wanted to go join them, longing to "be useful" in the war effort. But her mother would not hear of it, believing it to be much too dangerous of an endeavor. And while Stepanova expressed her motivations in patriotic terms framed around a sense of duty, she was quick to criticize other young women of the elite who she believed had less honorable, more personal motivations. "I didn't like that most of the young ladies going off to the front were not really interested in nursing, but only wanted freedom and independence," particularly from strict parental control, Stepanova lamented. She chastised those who were attracted to the salaries paid to wartime nurses as well, as an unseemly expression of selfishness. The financial independence they could achieve by earning their own money could not only liberate them from familial dependence but also allow them to spend money on things they personally coveted. "You will be able to dress well," her friends and acquaintances argued. Moreover, free from constant adult chaperoning, these young women would have the opportunity to engage in other activities that previously had been off-limits to them. The worst sort, she claimed, were those who were only interested in nursing as a means to meet young men. "It will be possible to flirt with officers during free time," they exclaimed, much to the chagrin of Stepanova, who viewed such desires as completely inappropriate. She was adamant about expressing a selfless desire to care for soldiers only, not engage in flirtatious behavior with officers. She was particularly disconcerted by those women who she believed entered wartime nursing in order to find a husband among the officers. "I'm sure I will be married at the front," Stepanova's cousin commented giddily to her before leaving to carry out medical service with a *letuchka*. Somewhat ironically, her cousin believed that in such a mobile frontline unit, the demands placed on her would be significantly less than those in a military hospital (a notion that belied the reality of frontline medical service).[1]

Shavli was the sight of heavy fighting during the early months of the war as a result of its close proximity to the German border, and after the German counterattack at Tannenberg, the area was evacuated.[2] In the ensuing confusion caused by a flood of refugees fleeing the region, Stepanova was separated from her parents and was taken in by a local military unit. She began working as a volunteer nurse for the unit, under the protection of some local aristocrats who knew her family. One of them, Baroness Knol', decided to take Stepanova with her when she left for Riga. There, she was given permission to serve in the main medical evacuation point through the intervention of Baron Knol', who used his connection with the chief physician of the unit, a doctor named Saksen. Stepanova was charged with overseeing the processing of the wounded and their dispatch to medical facilities in the interior of the empire. After serving in this capacity for several months and learning the practical duties involved with nursing, Saksen promised to promote her to the position of sister of mercy.

Stepanova served with more than a dozen other nurses at the Riga evacuation point, most of whom hailed from elite Saint Petersburg families. She remarked that at first, the women worked well together and were dedicated in their service. But she had very few good things to say about the men who served at the evacuation point and their relations with the women. In particular, she was appalled by what she believed to be the overly casual manner in which the doctors and officers interacted with the nurses, which she saw as completely inappropriate to their social status as young noblewomen. She was shocked when, sitting around the dining table, the male personnel engaged in ribald conversations, telling dirty jokes in the presence of the young ladies. Even worse, in Stepanova's eyes, was that the women did not protest such risqué conversation.

In fact, to her great vexation, she recalled that they "promoted it by asking questions, which made me blush for them." This only made matters worse, in her mind, encouraging the men to "act more freely and saucily every day" and leading to "flirtations, going out during free time and, what was worst of all, returning late at night." She related one episode with disgust, when several sisters had been socializing with officers and returned very late, completely drunk. Stepanova reasoned that "freedom and the absence of oversight could have been the cause of the depravity of the young girls." This behavior was increasingly disconcerting to her because rumors had begun to spread about the promiscuity of female medical workers. She was distraught that automobiles designated for medical service were labeled "nurse carriers," thought of as means by which sisters of mercy could engage in acquiring clientele for sexual commerce. She lamented that

> gradually, because of this [bad] behavior, the reputation of nurses had been so injured that it became somewhat shameful to wear a sister's uniform. Upon seeing nurses in uniform on the street, some officers would harass them, blowing kisses, grabbing at their waists. Obscene songs were created, unbelievable anecdotes were told with nurses as their sad heroines. Before, a highly respectable position, sisters became the "the talk of the town."

Indeed, the situation had deteriorated so much that when Stepanova was subjected to very real sexual harassment by a doctor (as described in chapter 6), many refused to believe that she was the victim. She was accused of flirting, leading him on, even getting him drunk with the intention of seducing him. The gossip that surrounded this episode "made life in the station unbearable" for Stepanova and led her to seek a transfer to another unit.[3]

THE "BAD REPUTATION" OF RUSSIAN WARTIME NURSES

In contrast to the positive patriotic images of sisters of mercy that predominated in public discourse and visual representation, a number of much more negative portrayals emerged during the course of the conflict. Although these representations are less well known in the modern memory of sisters of mercy, they were a significant factor in the image of sisters of mercy during the war. Such perceptions were not expressed in the patriotic press sources and were rare in those meant for widespread public consumption. Instead, they most often appeared in nonofficial, private, and even underground sources, and they circulated through society in the form of rumors, innuendos, personal correspondences and writings, and illicit images. The primary types of such representations can be seen as falling into two distinct but interrelated tropes. One focused on a critical portrayal of sisters of mercy who were perceived to be engaging in nursing not for altruistic, patriotic purposes but rather as self-serving, self-aggrandizing activities. The other focused on female sexuality and imagined wartime nursing merely as a means to access men and engage in promiscuous behavior. In this formulation, the positive label of "sisters of comfort" that had been used to describe the emotional and psychological support that nurses provided to wounded and dying men was applied pejoratively to implicate the women in prostitution. The presence of female medical personnel in the war zone was particularly troublesome when it came to issues of women's respectability. A number of sources reveal considerable anxiety over placing women, even as nurses, in the male sphere of war, where they would be accessible to thousands of men. Those critical of the way the tsarist government was prosecuting the war sometimes shifted the blame to the nurses themselves. Even a number of prowar commentators expressed concerns over the presence of women in the male sphere of war—concerns that were further heightened with regard to the sexual behavior of the nurses themselves. Yet this too can be seen as self-aggrandizement, because the sexual behavior was interpreted as something women desired for their own self-satisfaction.

In light of the important contribution of female nurses to the war effort, one that was officially appreciated and lauded, one might wonder why such negative associations arose. Previous attempts to explain their existence have simply linked them to revolutionary politics rather than examining them more carefully as representative of gendered wartime attitudes. Like the more sterile, passive prowar view presented in secondary literature, which misses much of the nuance of representation, the negative image of the wartime nurse has been oversimplified and even overstated by some scholars. For example, historians Orlando Figes and Boris Kolonitskii argue that it was these negative images that came to predominate among Russian troops by the end of the war, replacing positive images and completely devaluing and disparaging the sister of mercy. They assert that as the war dragged on, "front-line soldiers either looked upon the nurses ("sisters of comfort") as sex objects (an image reinforced by the tendency of Russia's wartime prostitutes to work the streets in nurses' uniforms) or else as useless women ("sisters without mercy") who rode in the staff cars ("nurse carriers") but had no medicine or other means of helping the soldiers. Any mention of nurses automatically gave rise to dirty jokes among the ranks."[4] In this formulation, nurses are depicted in the context of the antagonisms leading to the Russian Revolution of 1917, poised as representatives of the failing, uncaring, and out-of-touch aristocracy and tsarist regime, one that emanated from an atmosphere of lower-class resentment (coming specifically from the peasant soldiers) for elites who did not face the privations of war and seemed to even profit from the suffering of others.

Not only is it erroneous to suggest that such perceptions were ubiquitous and universal,[5] especially in light of all the positive associations with nurses, but grounding these negative views in explanations for the revolution is unsatisfactory. This is not to suggest that class antagonism is not an important component in understanding the "bad reputation" of nurses. True, the tone of many wartime sources changed considerably over the course of the war, even among those considered part of patriotic culture, and this shift was an important indicator of popular dissatisfaction that led to political upheaval in early 1917. Frustrations and class antagonisms that had long been accumulating in Russian society were certainly heightened, or at least made more visible, by certain dimensions of wartime nursing. As the conflict continued and the Russian population increasingly suffered under its strain, support for the war and, concomitantly, patriotic expressions of such support waned considerably. Posters, postcards, *lubki,* and even pictures and articles in the press less and less frequently featured heroic exploits of Russian victories (particularly because fewer such victories occurred as the war dragged on). Instead, focus shifted toward the human costs of the war, and cultural products began to include criticism of the way the war was being prosecuted. The association of nurses with the elite who seemed little affected by the hardships caused by the war and growing social and political tensions leading to the revolution should thus not be discounted completely. However, this can only partially account for the existence of conceptions of nurses as promiscuous sexual predators or self-serving opportunists. Working backward from the revolution to locate causation results in overlooking many of the more deeply rooted cultural factors that contributed to the image of nurses in Russian wartime society. An explanation centered on class antagonism and frustrations preceding the revolution fails to account for the fact that wartime nurses had suffered from accusations of sexual misconduct from their very first introduction in the zone of combat during the Crimean War. Similarly, it cannot explain why nurses in many of the other belligerent nations during World War I also acquired sullied reputations. A number of national cases, such as those of France, Germany, Great Britain, and Austria-Hungary, reveal animosity from both military and civilian quarters alike, often dividing wartime nurses into two categories: "real" or "good" nurses and "false" or "bad" nurses. The former entered wartime medical service as a result of the purest, most patriotic impulses to serve the suffering soldier in his time of need, while adhering to strict constraints on sexual behavior and displaying essentialist characteristics of caring and nurturing. The latter, by contrast, wanted only to advance themselves, receive accolades, or worse, engage in sexual adventure, and displayed blatantly unfeminine traits of aggression, ambition, and promiscuity. For example, as Margaret Darrow has demonstrated was the case in France, nurses were often seen in a similar light by the public and even by the male military establishment.[6] As Penny Summerfield has argued, "women's departure from the female sphere was considered redolent with risk: they were themselves sexually threatening to men; they incurred sexual danger from them."[7]

What seems more important, then, is to explore the specifically gendered context in which these images emerged, and to ask why in particular the actions of women would be questioned and disparaged. The views of self-aggrandizing and sexually promiscuous nurses that circulated in the Russian public imagination deserve to be analyzed more closely, viewed within the dynamic situation of the war itself, as well as *fin de siècle* Russian society. There is no doubt that during the conflict, concerns over the presence of women in the male sphere of war were heightened specifically in regard to their behavior. Indeed, such concerns existed long before this conflict. As indicated earlier, these kinds of assertions were heard frequently from the very inception of wartime nursing in Russia during the Crimean conflict, but such associations predate even that event, attached to the women labeled "camp followers" who performed a variety of services for the armed forces across time and place.

Further complicating matters is that a number of women actually engaged in commercial sex work while wearing clothing that resembled nursing uniforms. Yet rumors, speculation, and accusations of moral impropriety were not limited to those who used the uniform of the sister of mercy as a means to move about in the streets and engage in prostitution without arousing the suspicion of Russian officials. They extended into the actual nursing population itself. Accusations leveled against women who were believed to have enlisted in nursing as a result of selfish motives and the desire for recognition similarly have complex causes, with deeper roots than prerevolutionary class antagonisms. In many ways they reflect the apprehension present in Russian society associated with aggressive, ambitious women operating in public roles. Both disparaging views (those of opportunists and of sexual predators) and their intersection need to be examined in an attempt to discern how and why the wartime nurse was imagined in these decidedly negative ways. Indeed, they were by-products of the same set of circumstances of the war, which afforded women greater opportunity of action in the public sphere and, in turn, caused a great deal of anxiety in Russian society, as well as the same cultural conceptions about women that permeated both Russian military life and Russian society. The "bad reputation" of Russia's wartime nurses was thus reflective of heightened insecurities about women's activity in the male sphere and about women's respectability. These accusations stemmed from two sources: the culture of Russian nursing, which established strict standards of behavior for women, particularly with regard to sexuality, and the culture of Russian military life, which was infused with misogyny and suspicious of female intrusion into a hypermasculinized context.

The "Opportunists"

As indicated by Stepanova's memories, from the earliest calls for women to enlist in medical service, there were those who expressed suspicion of the true intentions of respondents. Public opinion was similarly highly critical of women who entered nursing services but were not always able, or willing, to live up to the rigorous demands placed on sisters of mercy. Particularly because wartime nursing was seen not only as an appropriate and patriotic means by which women could contribute to the national crisis, but also a prestigious and even elite occupation, the motives of some who wanted to become sisters of mercy were questioned. This is not altogether surprising, considering that a number of the women who became wartime nurses came from the upper echelons of the social elite, whose popular reputation was tinged with ideas of self-indulgence and callous lack of concern for public welfare. Wealthy aristocrats who had displayed little interest in serving national interests before the outbreak of war in 1914 were thus accused of being drawn to nursing for less than altruistic reasons.

The perception existed that a number of women, particularly those who hailed from the elite of Russian society, merely donned a uniform to benefit from the prestige associated with it, or because it was seen as fashionable, and undertook no hard work on behalf of wounded and ill soldiers. Thus, a central concern over the dedication of female nurses focused on the clothing worn by sisters of mercy. The nurse's uniform became highly fashionable, as a symbolic marker of female patriotism, prestige, and even privilege, during the war. Clothing, particularly fashion, has been noted by a number of cultural historians as significant to identity, status, and consciousness, particularly with regard to gender. As scholar Helena Goscilo has commented, fashion works to "signal social status" and "privileges image over character."[8] Nursing uniforms in particular worked to convey image in important ways, specifically, as Barton Hacker has indicated, that of patriotic duty and responsible citizenship. They not only served to distinguish "real" nurses from those with unofficial status, such as camp followers (who suffered from negative associations), but also "validated their claim to citizenship."[9] Undoubtedly, some who recognized the value associated with being a sister of mercy lacked the desire (or perhaps the fortitude) to carry out the difficult work of wartime nurse. They could, however, portray themselves favorably to society without actually performing significant service merely by donning the uniform of a sister of mercy. Thus, allegations that women were only superficially committed to the war effort circulated through Russian public opinion. These accusations may have been grounded in a real problem: those who were in no way authorized to wear Red Cross uniforms found ways to acquire them. In some cases, in the desire to appear as if they were contributing to the war effort, women appeared in public arenas dressed (at least partially) like sisters of mercy, even if they were not officially enlisted as nurses. This occurred despite the strict regulations of the Red Cross and its subordinate organizations concerning authorized wearing of the uniform. Khristina Semina described how, when she heard that the tsar would be visiting, the wife of the chief doctor of the local hospital—a woman who had no official role in medical work—asked if she could borrow Semina's uniform to wear during the royal procession. Both Semina and another doctor at the hospital insisted that this was impossible, as Red Cross regulations indicated that only those who possessed special permission from the Red Cross, having completed the proper coursework and certified as authentic sisters of mercy, were allowed to wear the uniform. But the chief doctor's wife paid no heed and continued to badger Semina until the latter finally relented and allowed her to borrow her white nurse's veil.

The "society lady" posturing as a nurse to improve her own standing was a particularly reviled image. The pages of a number of contemporary periodicals featured illustrations that mocked high-society women who seemed more concerned with their appearances than with the fate of the nation during its time of crisis. Again, the issue of clothing, and particularly fashion, is highly relevant. Criticisms were leveled against women for selfishly focusing on the latest dress styles and coiffures rather than acting in self-sacrificing, supportive ways for the war effort. One image that had originated in Great Britain appeared in several different illustrated publications in Russia, featuring a young nurse applying powder to her face, suggesting that she cared more about her appearance than her work as a nurse, and perhaps worse, had motivations of a more sexual nature for entering medical service (figure 8.1). The image was even adapted by a Russian artist and printed on the cover of the progressive illustrated women's journal *Zhenskoe Delo,* which was a strong champion of female wartime nursing (figure 8.2).

As in the case of wartime France, Russian observers often attempted to draw a clear line of distinction between "real" nurses, sisters of mercy, who were selfless and dedicated in their service to Russia's war-wounded, and those who were seen as disingenuous and motivated by selfish desires. Dr. S. K. Solov'ev, commander of the military medical units on the northern front, wrote extensively about the "categories" of nurses he encountered working in Red Cross establishments. While he described numerous women as hardworking and morally upright, he labeled others as self-serving socialites seeking aggrandizement and personal reward. Such lines were even drawn by wartime nurses themselves. Women who considered themselves "real" nurses denigrated others merely seeming to "act the part." Their criticism was often infused with issues of class and social status. Resentment was sometimes expressed for well-connected nurses serving in the rear, who were seen as not really performing much

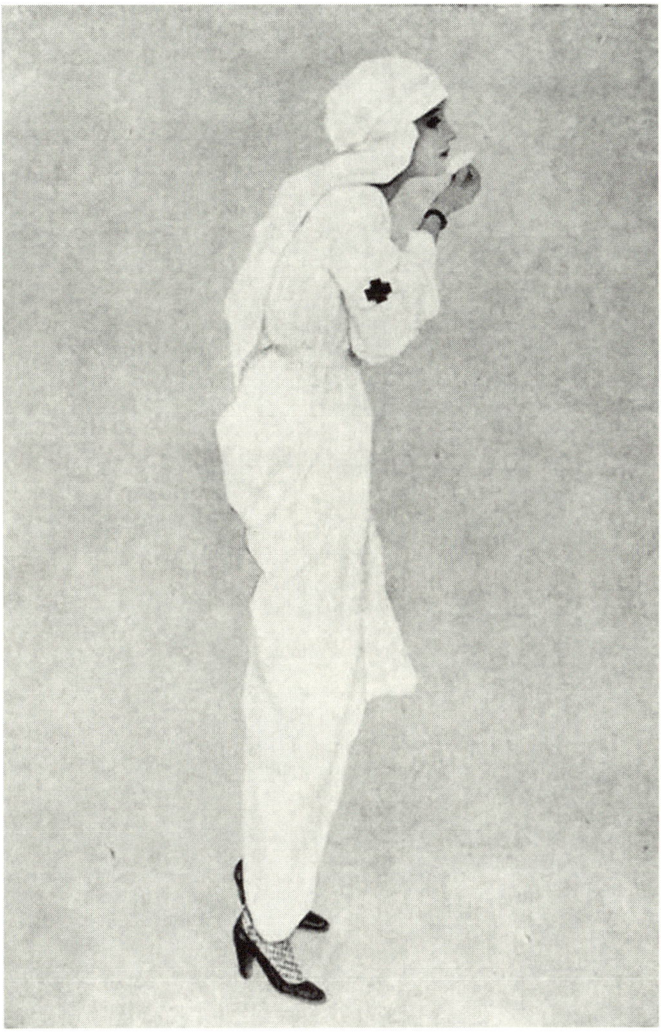

Figure 8.1. Disparaging image of nurse putting on makeup. "Sestrichka" [Little sister], *Solntse Rossii*, February 1916, 13.

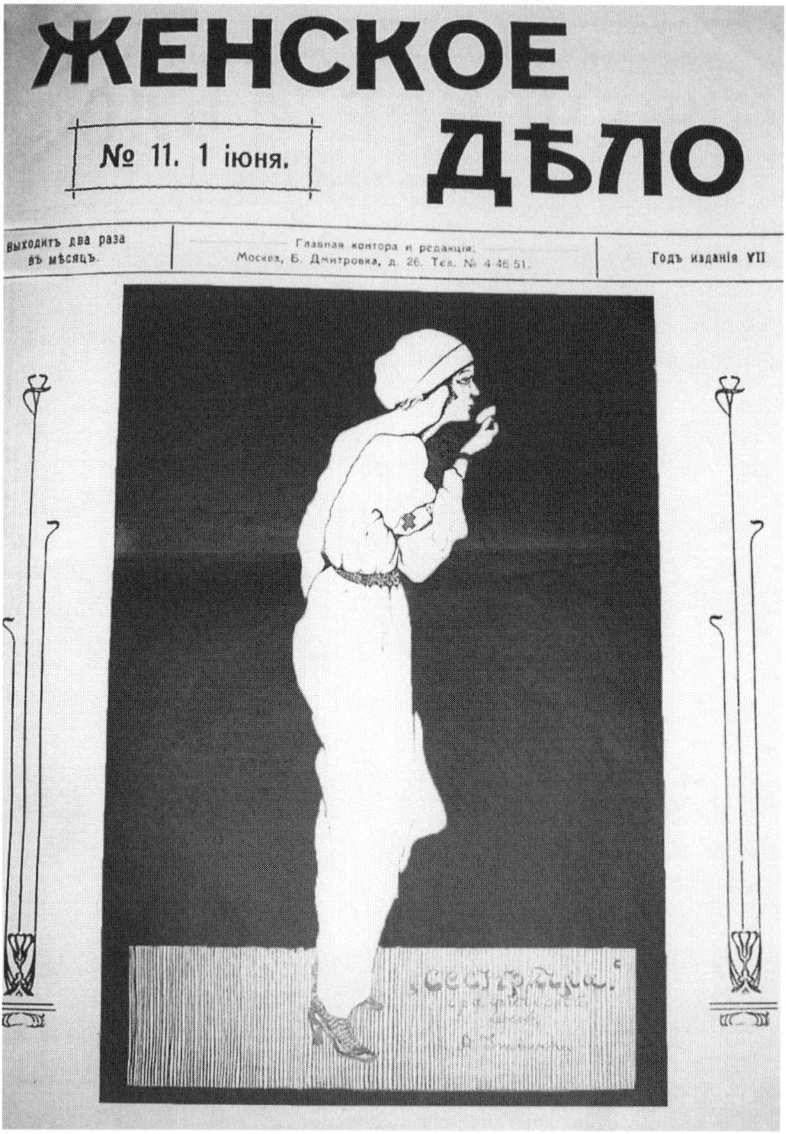

Figure 8.2. The same image reproduced on the cover of a progressive women's journal. "Sestrichka" [Little sister], *Zhenskoe Delo*, June 1, 1915, cover.

in the way of useful service. Nurses often expressed animosity toward, and worked to create distance between themselves and, those they considered to be less than committed to the cause. While working with a mobile hospital train at the front, Tat'iana Aleksinskaia encountered some society women with a Red Cross delegation visiting wounded men in a divisional hospital far behind the lines. She insisted that although they presented themselves as sisters, they did little to demonstrate that they actually carried out medical service. As a result, Aleksinskaia was irked by their presence and did not hide her scorn. "There were some ladies with them—society 'benefactresses' dressed in a mixture of their ordinary clothes and the uniform of the Sisters of Charity, with their bosoms adorned with medallions and figures," she chided, again indicating the importance of dress to the notion of "true" nursing. "I don't know why," she remarked, "but I felt a certain feeling of irritation against these ladies and their kind."[10] Farmborough echoed such sentiments when she encountered a group of sisters serving in the city of Minsk. She hesitated to even call them nurses; rather, she referred to them as "ladies who wore the uniform of Sisters" with "painted faces and long gold chains hanging down over the Red Cross on their breasts . . . befrilled and becurled." She could scarcely imagine such women performing the duties of a nurse at the front: "We tried to picture them out there where we had been: passing the long night hours in the open, buffeted by rain and wind; veiled with curtains of thick dust; wearing vermin-infested clothing for days on end; sleeping on benches, floors, under haystacks, on open fields; hunger stricken and thankful beyond measure for dried, black crusts."[11] Farmborough's comments not only reveal class antagonisms but also notions of respectability, considered essential for "true" nurses.

The distinction between nurses who served at the front and at the rear is a key component of the division between "true" and "false" sisters. Indeed, general public conceptions about the rear and the front are very important for understanding the representations of Russian nurses during World War I.[12] As Karen Petrone notes, the rear was often associated with corruption and immoral activity. Although scholars have yet to fully explore the extent to which such notions caused a ubiquitous rift between front and rear, a number of sources indicate the perception that those with money and influence avoided service and, worse, engaged in sexually promiscuous behavior on the home front. Moreover, the front and rear "were often cast in gendered terms with the front as the hardened and masculine arena and the rear as feminized, despised, and soft locale."[13] Although women assigned to medical facilities located on the home front often worked long hours in difficult conditions, there was a strong public perception that those who served in the rear faced considerably less arduous and dangerous conditions than their counterparts at the front. Securing a position in a rear medical establishment often could only be accomplished through status and connection, which was not available to all women. Umbrage over such privilege as well as a notion that these rear positions were secured through corruption, or worse, sexual impropriety, tainted the image of the rear nurse. The general impression was that certain elements of Russian society were not only unaffected by the great suffering that the war caused so many others but that they were actually benefitting in some way.

Particularly disconcerting to many observers was the sister of mercy who engaged in leisure activities while off duty. In rear areas, especially in larger towns and cities, nurses were often able to participate in forms of entertainment that were not available to those on the front. They could attend theater or opera performances, dine in restaurants, go to the movies, and engage in other forms of urban recreation. When they did so dressed in their uniforms, they often raised eyebrows, suspected of merely dressing the part rather than performing the hard labor associated with wartime medical service. P. Kukol' complained about this in a letter from Odessa to the Countess E. A. Uvarova in Moscow: "Sisters play tennis, luncheon, and dine in restaurants, and moreover, they always have flowers, and generally are inordinately elegant and cheerful. Throughout Galicia there is among medical personnel the air of a joyful picnicking and vulgar ostentation."[14] Even more unnerving to many observers were female nurses who were accompanied by male officers, leading to speculation about improper sexual relationships between them. Sisters of mercy were also criticized for being transported by automobile. When compared with others who only had horse-drawn carts at their disposal, these women were seen as selfishly taking advantage of access to privilege and comfort that others did not have. Perhaps more importantly, public perceptions that such cars were used for "joyriding" by sisters, rather than for official purposes associated with the care of the ill and wounded, were ubiquitous, so much so that these vehicles came to acquire the pejorative nickname *sestrovozy* ("sister carriers"). In some places, the Red Cross issued regulations prohibiting nurses from riding in automobiles. Again, the front/rear divide is important to these associations. Motorized vehicles were found much more frequently in urban settings, far behind the lines of the fighting. Thus, the nurses who were able to take advantage of such forms of transportation tended to be those that served in rear hospitals, where conditions were much less dangerous and considerably more comfortable. Such denigrations are also representative of antipathy toward the seeming lack of sufficient sacrifice being made by these women during the time of national crisis that was so burdensome for others, revealing growing social tensions. Nurses themselves were not immune to these images; they often internalized them within their own ranks, which could lead to enmity between sisters of different social backgrounds.[15]

Again, however, gender is particularly important in understanding the origins of accusations of self-aggrandizement, specifically, notions of culturally acceptable roles and behaviors for women. Criticisms leveled against nurses for engaging in social activities are specifically gendered. While officials expressed concern over the dissemination of sexually transmitted diseases when men engaged the services of prostitutes, male military personnel were not generally censured for engaging in social activities and seeking entertainment in an effort to relieve some of the pressures of combat life. If we recall the experience of the Crimean War, when women were first used in wartime medical services, significant opposition emerged as a result of male fears of female intrusion and authority. Male officials worried that women would attempt to meddle in their affairs, that they would seek to put an end to corruption and change the methods of service delivery. Some accused these women of being personally ambitious, seeking public roles for their own gain. As in the case of the Crimean War, male military and medical personnel during the First World War often found the assumption of such authority by women to be completely unacceptable. Particularly troublesome in gendered terms and indicative of a threat to patriarchy were women who tried to order male doctors around. Alon Rachamimov has demonstrated a similar dynamic with regard to Austro-Hungarian women who served as administrative nurses. These women were not assigned to auxiliary medical positions subordinate to male personnel but to positions of authority. They were given the task of reporting on the conditions of prisoners of war and ensuring their loyalty to the Austro-Hungarian government. Rachamimov reveals the considerable gendered tensions between male POWs and female administrative nurses. Men, not only those in medical service or in positions of military authority, but also many of the Austrians held as prisoners of war themselves—the very men for whom the administrative nurses had come to ensure humane treatment—often found it difficult to accept women in positions of power over them and reacted to their presence with indifference, sullenness, and even hostility. These views stand in stark contrast to POWs' perceptions of women serving in purely nursing capacities, who were subordinate to male doctors and military personnel. The latter were seen as a source of solace and comfort in their more traditional roles of caregivers and nurturers—roles that gave them no authority over men.[16]

In certain contexts, strength and even authority were highly valued in women. As scholars such as Vera Dunham have demonstrated, "'Russian womanhood' is remarkable in that there exists a perceptible motif" that "extols that coherence and strength of the woman in a historical sequence and in divergent class settings."[17] Russian literature is also replete with strong, independent heroines, women who possess moral superiority as well as the will and ability to act, set against male protagonists who are often indecisive and impotent.[18] However, Russian cultural expectations for women in the early twentieth century did not include positions of power and dominance in the public sphere. Even the strong woman was constrained within the patriarchal structure of Russian society, its positive aspects being limited to the context of the family and usually extending only to the eldest woman in the household. Outside of this context, as historian Cathy Frierson has noted, women who behaved in aggressive, independent ways were seen as disruptive forces, challenging traditional social structures and patriarchy.[19] When women pursued their own interests of self-preservation or development, they were vilified. The strength of women as portrayed in Russian literature was very often one expressed through the endurance of great suffering, rather than positive and heroic action.[20] The power and authority of women did not extend beyond the boundaries of familial concerns, and although their influence may have been felt indirectly through the men they reared or married, few women were able to become players in politics or other public affairs.

Not surprisingly in this cultural context, when women moved into wartime nursing and obtained positions of authority and leadership, there was considerable cultural backlash. This reaction was heightened by attempts to preserve the military as a hypermasculine sphere. Military officials were concerned that the presence of women in the war zone would compromise military security. Many believed that women were highly prone to gossip, rumormongering, and even traitorous behavior, activities that were obviously considered devastating to military ethos. Others expressed concern that women who already had been radicalized would use their positions as nurses, which gave them direct access to soldiers, to spread revolutionary or pacifist propaganda against the war. The fear that men would be "feminized," that is, weakened and unable to perform as soldiers, through contact with women led to a strong desire to keep women as far away from soldiers as possible. Many military men held a general notion that, as Joshua Sanborn has argued, "separation from women was necessary to achieve the proper military mindset."[21] Thus, the presence of any women in the war zone was a threat to the masculinity of the conflict, even if those women were there to help restore men to health.

THE "SISTER OF COMFORT"

The intrusion of women into the male space of war, along with the notion that many of the women there were engaging in sex work, combined to produce a particularly troublesome image of wartime nursing. In addition to the self-aggrandizing opportunist who benefited from her social position, connections, or corruption, a distinct trope of the sexually dissolute nurse spread through Russian popular imagination during the war. Despite efforts to desexualize the sister of mercy through her dress and conduct, the integrity of those who desired to enter this often dirty, dangerous, and even sordid affair was questioned, and rumors of nurses' loose morality circulated through Russian society in this conflict as it had in previous ones. In fact, during the First World War, the very term "sister of comfort," initially used to designate the positive emotional and psychological impact of wartime nurses' work, took on pejorative connotations of sexual impropriety. For some, only the desire for opportunities to engage in sexual promiscuity could explain the motivation of women to transgress into the masculine sphere of war. Most of these views emanated not from sources intended for public consumption; obviously the immoral nurse would be completely inconsistent with the patriotic image of the sister of mercy. As one might expect, unease about the presence of female nurses at the front, surrounded by men, often from detractors of the war and tsarist regime, was most often expressed in private sources, or those produced after the war. Yet, as with the case of the self-aggrandizing nurse, the trope of the licentious, sexually adventurous sister was not unique to the Great War, nor was it exclusive to Russia. Thus, it was not only the immediate circumstances of the war and the increasing dissatisfaction within Russian society that led to such imagery. Gendered expectations and assumptions concerning female behavior and war in general were essential components driving the creation of the wartime nurse's negative reputation.

In order to better understand the connections between such accusations, particularly those centered on the idea of nurses engaging in prostitution, it is necessary to establish the context with regard to sex work in Russia. Prostitution in imperial Russia was generally viewed as a social ill, although one that was nearly impossible to eliminate. As in many other European states, beginning in the mid-nineteenth century, the Russian government adopted the strategy of attempting to control and regulate the sex trade by controlling and regulating the women who engaged in it. This was largely a response to the spread of sexually transmitted diseases such as syphilis, which many public health officials worried were becoming epidemic in proportion.[22] But commercial sex work was also perceived as threatening to the social order, as Laura Engelstein has argued, because it "represented women's escape from patriarchal authority and from reproductive sex," specifically because it was seen as "a form of sexual activity that the family system did not control."[23] Regulation primarily took the form of issuing licenses, called "yellow tickets," to sex workers to allow them to ply their trade, or providing state licenses to officially sanctioned brothels, while forcing the women to submit to regular medical examinations to determine whether they were infected with venereal diseases and to be treated for these illnesses. By the turn of the twentieth century, however, many had come to regard government regulation as increasingly problematic for several reasons, not the least of which was that it had proven ineffective in stemming the dissemination of disease. This was largely due to the fact that no attempt was ever made (or thought possible) to police male clientele. Moreover, not all women who engaged in commercial sex work were "professional" prostitutes; many only occasionally did so out of economic necessity. Such occasional sex workers were very difficult to locate and monitor on a regular basis. As Engelstein has demonstrated, regulation functioned more like a "system for controlling women, not disease."[24]

By the outbreak of World War I, little had changed with regard to the official approach to prostitution. The central agency charged with oversight of issues concerning public health in Russia, the Ministry of Internal Affairs, had left regulation of commercial sex work largely to local authorities, who varied greatly in their methods.[25] Although some efforts to control and reduce it had been undertaken, including the closing of brothels in a number of cities along the front, the sex trade, as well as the spread of sexually transmitted illnesses, seems to have increased during the First World War.[26] This is not surprising, considering the chaos that the war brought about, including an almost complete breakdown in public health.

In many cases, the expansion of sex work was the result of the economic hardships caused by the war. Historian Peter Gatrell has noted the impact of the upheaval that forced millions of women into becoming homeless refugees, many of whom "turned to prostitution out of a desperate need to feed themselves and their dependents." Brothel owners and others who organized commercial sex were able to recruit from among the ranks of young women suffering from the economic recession during the war. As the war further loosened already eroding patriarchal and familial controls over women's sexuality by removing millions of fathers and other male authority figures from Russian homes, as well as separating families when they became refugees, some members of Russian society worried that this situation gave young women the opportunity to all too willingly follow paths of "debauchery."[27] Even soldiers' wives, known as *soldatki,* acquired reputations as prostitutes because of their economic vulnerability and lack of direct male supervision while their husbands were away performing military service. Once again, women who attempted to function independently were vulnerable to criticism and accusations of impropriety.

Similarly important is prostitution's long association with Russian military life. Soldiers and officers, separated from the civilian female population, sought out commercial sex workers to satisfy their sexual desires. Visiting a brothel was often seen as something of a "rite of passage" for newly inducted military servitors. Officially, however, military authorities frowned on prostitution, most significantly because the spread of sexually transmitted diseases was perceived as a serious threat to the health of soldiers. There was also considerable concern about the negative moral influence of sex workers. Women in general were seen as less than trustworthy by many in Russian society, but prostitutes had even more dangerous associations attached to them. Members of the male military establishment believed that sex workers were sources of treachery, spying, and other traitorous behavior. Brothels were often described as "hotbeds of propaganda" and were believed to be "infiltrated by German spies." In fact, some military commanders saw prostitution as closely linked to the problem of voluntary surrender during the Great War, convinced that sex workers "tried to 'implant ideas of desertion' into the heads of unwary soldiers."[28] The root of such views lies in the notion of the essential masculinity of warfare, one that desires to exclude female intrusion but stands at odds with the practical reality of warfare, which not only intersects with women in many ways but also relies on them to perform critical services.

Sex Work and Nurses

During the war, local authorities continued to use regulations that allowed them to round up and arrest women walking on the streets in an attempt to control and limit prostitution. The increased presence of military police heightened this problem and therefore proved to be a hindrance to sex workers attempting to attract clientele. As a result, in order to avoid drawing suspicion, some of these women seem to have used the mobility afforded to wearers of the Red Cross nursing uniform to engage in sex work. Because the sister of mercy of uniform carried with it a great deal of respect in Russian society, a nurse walking the streets initially aroused little attention. Over time, however, the disguise proved limited in its effectiveness. Instead of protecting the wearer from unwanted attention, the uniform began to raise suspicions. The press began to report instances in a number of cities along the front where women were found walking the streets wearing the uniforms of Red Cross sisters. These women apparently had no connection to the organization or medical services. One report in the Red Cross organ, *Vestnik Krasnago Kresta,* lamented that

> many frivolous creatures have begun to dress themselves in the uniform of the sister of mercy, and in this way to profane the sacred work of helping the suffering by looking for adventures in the streets. . . . The public has taken notice of this outrageous occurrence and have come to the [Red Cross] communities with all sorts of groundless rumors. . . . The majority of these "ladies," strolling with bandages for suspicious purposes, are just using the emblem of the Red Cross for their own personal, low goals.[29]

The use of language such as "frivolous creatures," "looking for adventures in the streets," and "strolling . . . for suspicious purposes" clearly indicates the fear that women were using nursing uniforms as a means to freely engage in prostitution.

Regulations pertaining to the wearing of Red Cross uniforms, however, proved insufficient to control unauthorized occurrences, leading the organization to take further measures. In a somewhat ironic move, considering the use of "yellow tickets" to regulate prostitution, the Red Cross began issuing special identification "tickets" (these were white) to nursing personnel and requiring them to present these documents to authorities on demand. Not only was this measure enacted in an attempt to hinder prostitutes from plying their trade in disguise, it was also a conscious effort to preserve the "honor" of the sister of mercy based on notions of sexual purity, which the Red Cross continued to insist was intact, by identifying and separating imposters. The implication was that "real" nurses would not engage in such immoral behavior. Indeed, the organization was careful to distinguish these women from those officially registered in medical services, who, they insisted, "are seldom seen on the streets, as they are too busy carrying out their highly humane work."[30] Such distinctions were inaccurate, however. In reality, the work of nurses was not always limited to the hospital or dressing station. As a result, they did appear in the streets wearing their uniforms often. In many cases, their official duties required them to transport patients from one location to another, to obtain supplies and equipment from other facilities, or to fulfill other responsibilities that required their public presence. It was when they entered such public spaces that eyebrows were raised. This was at least partially because the lines of respectability were distinctly drawn not only between the front and the rear but also for women and particularly sisters of mercy between the medical facility, where nurses carried out their "sacred work," and the street or other public spaces. When the sister of mercy left the protected sphere of the medical facility, her purpose became muddled in public opinion. Many had difficulty understanding why she would be present in such public areas, if her purpose was to attend to the needs of the wounded or ill soldier.

The Red Cross, nonetheless, took the threat posed to its image and that of the sister of mercy quite seriously, so much so that it established a "Commission for the Fight against the Misuse of the Name of the Sister of Mercy" as early as December 1914. This body did not merely attempt to distinguish between real sisters and those who impersonated them; it also laid at least some of the blame on the actions of actual nurses themselves. In a meeting held on December 15, the commission heard a report to the main administration of the Russian Red Cross about the "disapproved" behavior of sisters of mercy, and the measures that were being undertaken to "eliminate such phenomena." In particular, those present at the meeting were determined to remove from the ranks those women who had, in their view, "no right to wear the symbol of the Red Cross." The solution proposed was to ensure that only those that had been members of the *obshchiny* of the Red Cross and had undergone the vetting process through those organs would be designated as sisters of mercy.[31] Again, this was an impractical measure in a total war, which required the mobilization of vast numbers of individuals for medical service, many of whom had not passed through the Red Cross nursing communities, but rather were trained and assigned by other associations, such as the Zemgor union organizations.

Most troubling to the Russian public were nurses who appeared in public spaces in their uniforms, and in the company of men, in unofficial capacities. In an effort to curtail such incidences, the Red Cross issued an order that restricted the wearing of uniforms even for actual sisters of mercy to assigned work periods. As indicated in chapter 2, the authorities made it clear that "walking the streets or visiting entertainment establishments in the uniform of a sister of mercy is completely prohibited."[32] Thus, rather than attempting to control the behavior of the sisters themselves, a task the Red Cross may have found completely impractical, the organization opted to relieve themselves of such responsibility by forbidding women from wearing the Red Cross uniform while off duty. These measures seem to have been ineffective, as the problem continued through the end of the war. Nor did the attempt to separate "real" nurses, with the implication that they would not engage in sexually improper activity, from "real" prostitutes save Russia's wartime nursing from associations with moral impropriety. Not only did these measures fail to have their intended effect, but ultimately just the opposite occurred: rather than distinguishing the immoral "false" nurses from the pure "true" sisters, for some members of the Russian public, the former became largely indistinguishable from the latter, and the reputation of the wartime nurse because increasingly sullied.

This anxiety also stems from the fact that Russian nursing was, unlike that of some other nations, not a professionalized occupation but a charitable, voluntary activity with significant religious associations. Even the civilian women who became wartime sisters were required to adhere to the standards of behavior established by the quasi-religious communities of the Red Cross. As indicated previously, Russian sisters of mercy were supposed to be of the "highest moral caliber" and maintain respectability at all times. The standard of propriety had been set from the initial introduction of female nurses into the war zone during the Crimean War in an attempt to ensure that no sexual interaction with male personnel occurred. Although wartime nursing had come to be seen as an appropriate way for women to serve the nation in times of crisis, fears about their sexual conduct had not dissipated since they were first expressed in the middle of the nineteenth century.[33] When women who enlisted in nursing service failed to conform to the rigid standards of sexual propriety, their behavior became a point of contention. Very few of the women who became wartime nurses were members of religious communities or had any desire to be. A large number of the sisters of mercy were young women who, on entering wartime medical services, were immediately emancipated from the controlling atmosphere of domestic life, where their parents or other chaperones had watched their movements closely and limited the contact they had with members of the opposite sex. Indeed, as Stepanova has indicated, this kind of freedom was highly attractive to young women who chafed under such constraints and saw wartime nursing as a means of escape. It is clear that nursing often allowed them the opportunity to pursue relationships with men on their own terms. They could accept offers from male military and medical personnel to accompany them on outings, essentially to go on dates. For many, this was much too much freedom given to unmarried women, whose honor was still derived mostly from their sexual purity. The sight of young women on the arms of men strolling through the streets, attending concerts and theater performances, eating in restaurants, and in other public venues was disconcerting to many, who believed that given this kind of unfettered freedom, women would allow themselves to enter into sexual relations with the men. Moreover, as indicated in chapter 6, it is clear from the archival records indicating punishments meted out to those accused of "immorality" and "depraved behavior" that female nurses did indeed engage in intimate relationships with men, often male medical or military personnel. When they did, sisters of mercy ran afoul of strict expectations of sexual purity imposed on them by the code of conduct instituted by the Russian Red Cross. This opened the door not only to accusations of impropriety but also to prostitution, a line already blurred by social expectations that rooted female honor in chastity.

Not only was the nurse's sexual behavior to be strictly regulated; her very appearance was supposed to remove any suggestions of sexuality, intentionally concealing the feminine characteristics of her body. The Russian press expressed these concerns regarding the proper behavior and appearance of sisters of mercy. The illustration featured in the highly popular journal *Ogonek* in November 1915 reveals these anxieties, demonstrating the "proper" and "improper" ways for sisters of mercy to dress (figure 8.3). The captions indicate that if sisters of mercy only appeared as represented in the second examples rather than the first, the soldiers in their care could rest easier.

Concerns over the sexual respectability of Russian wartime nurses and the intersection of such concerns with clothing can be best understood within the context of a modernizing Russia. From the latter half of the nineteenth century, anxiety had been expressed not only over women's increasing public presence but also regarding their involvement in activities that contravened traditional notions of appropriate behavior for women, including consumerism and commercial activity. As historian Christine Ruane has demonstrated, even the act of shopping for fashionable clothing was seen by some as morally dangerous for women. In a book titled *Epidemic Insanity: Toward the Overthrow of the Yoke of Fashion,* published in 1914, "decorated military officer, journalist and self-appointed social commentator" Iulii Elets warned respectable women to steer clear of fashionable clothing shops, where unscrupulous store owners, dissolute saleswomen (who were also accused of being sex workers), and licentious customers of the demimonde colluded to seduce women into buying frivolous fashions that they then used to beguile their significant others. As Ruane argues, "all these women had abandoned appropriate 'female' behavior emphasizing modesty, restraint and self-sacrifice to participate in the world of commerce. Thus, a simple commercial transaction became, in the eyes of many commentators, a defiant and deviant expression of a woman's sexuality. In this sense any woman who participated in commercial activity was a *publichnaya zhenshchina,* a public woman who sold her body for men's pleasure."[34] If shopping in fashionable clothing stores was enough to arouse suspicions of prostitution among some observers, it seems a small step to extend such suspicions to women whose daily work required them to function in the

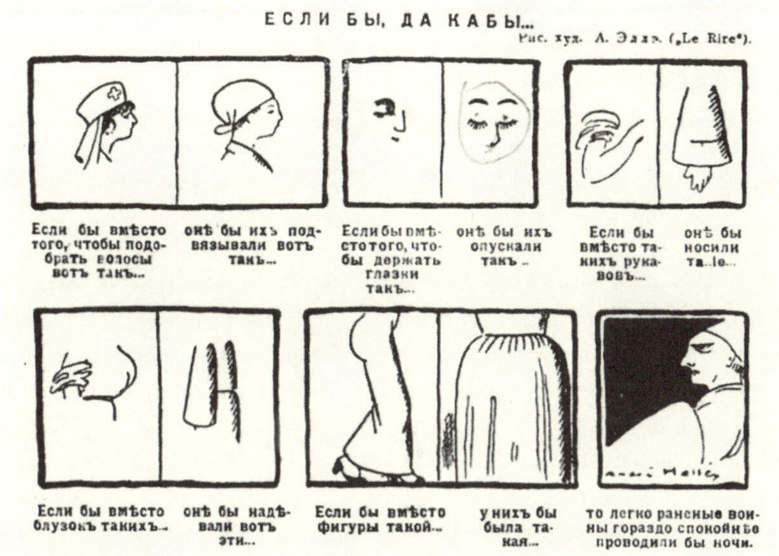

Figure 8.3. Depiction of "proper" and "improper" dress and comportment for nurses. "Esli by, da kaby . . . " [Yes, and if only . . .], *Ogonek*, November 8, 1915, 5.

public sphere and who came into direct contact with male bodies, often alone with those bodies. Thus, the appeal of nursing and wearing the nursing uniform as "fashionable" activity overlaps directly with public concerns about women's respectability. The uniform, which for so many was a symbol of self-sacrifice, modesty, and service, transformed into an indicator of immorality for others. The act of caring and nurturing taken out of the domestic context and applied to strange men further besmirched what was simultaneously seen as a noble and honorable activity for women. As such, wartime nursing presented a seemingly intractable paradox.

Accusations of improper decorum based on gender assumptions leveled against sisters of mercy should not be considered without the inclusion of class, however. While wartime nurses hailed from all social backgrounds, literacy and education requirements meant that the majority came from the middle and upper classes. But women who engaged in sex work were almost invariably from the lower ranks of Russian society. Notions of female sexual morality were considerably different for the working poor, who were often considered to be less respectable, than those applied to women of the comfortable middle and upper classes.

When middle- and upper-class women engaged in public work in close proximity to men and even in direct contact with male bodies, when they operated in a sphere dominated by men, one considered essentially masculine, their respectability was challenged and they risked being associated with other nonprivileged elements, women who were not accorded respectability because of their class. Moreover, there was considerable anxiety over the fact that the vast majority of the men with whom nurses came into contact were peasants and other members of the lower classes. Not only were their worries that nurses would behave in sexually inappropriate ways with such men; a number of members of the male military establishment expressed concern that nurses would become too sympathetic to the plight of the working classes through their interaction with such men in their care. As we have seen, nurses often heard their complaints concerning poor treatment at the hands of the officer corps (dominated by the upper classes), as well as about their difficult and troubled lives at home as a result of their social status. There was considerable worry that women would be radicalized by this exposure.[35] Moreover, these concerns reflected the deep-seated anxieties on the part of military officials and others who worried about the effect of the presence of women in what they believed should be a purely masculine space.

The result of this was dramatic. Public opinion, both military and civilian, about wartime nurses, which was overwhelmingly positive in many quarters, took on more negative associations. A report from an anonymous source in the 190th Ochakovskii Infantry Regiment on January 5 1915 to A. M. Ladyzhenskii in Moscow lamented on the entire state of medical services during the war. "Here no one is being healed, or it is that here they understand the word 'treatment' has nothing to do with it," the author complained. "Even in places and establishments where it was possible to receive actual treatment, because of the impertinence of doctors or because of other reasons, such care is not being carried out." The author included nurses in his protest but laid the blame equally on doctors, remarking that "in L'vov, the behavior of sisters is striking, as is, unfortunately, that of doctors." He went on to describe a common sight, "automobiles with red crosses and in them doctors and nurses riding around the town," and he claimed that "in general, the sisters that I saw here, all of them without exception, conducted themselves like prostitutes."[36] Future commander of the First Russian Women's Battalion of Death, Maria Bochkareva, when asking for permission to enlist as a soldier in a male regiment in 1915, rejected any suggestions that she should become a sister of mercy instead: "I had heard so many rumors about the women in the rear that I had come to despise them."[37] Similarly, Russian writer V. V. Rozanov, reflecting the idea that women became prostitutes as a result of their sexual desires, commented, "There is no doubt that some modest percent go in for prostitution and are intoxicated with it . . . passing along Nevskii, virtually in a massive gang, throwing their heads up, striding confidently . . . with a 'Take us! Take us!'—for 5 or a maximum of 10 rubles (the war, prices are rising)."[38] Here again, differentiations between the front and the rear are salient. As a result of the close association of the rear with corruption and depravity, it is not surprising that female medical personnel serving there were more likely to be viewed as sexually promiscuous than their counterparts at the front.

Even some of the strongest supporters of wartime nursing found it difficult to come to terms with unchaperoned, unattached women in such close proximity to large numbers of men. They complained that as the demand for female medical personnel increased, the caliber of individuals desiring to become nurses diminished. Dr. Solov'ev, commander of the military medical units on the northern front, who lamented the presence of self-promoting women, opined that many of them were of "dubious" character and displayed the most "immoral behavior." He was most disturbed by what he called the "worst category" of sisters of mercy: those who were nothing more than sexual predators looking for a captive audience in the sea of male military personnel. Solov'ev was particularly distraught that the Red Cross communities granted them the right to wear the honorable symbol of mercy as an equal member of the organization: the red cross on a field of white.

It is important to note, however, that many did not condemn all sisters of mercy but relegated their commentary to a "modest percent" who misbehaved. A number of observers believed that the sullied reputation of wartime nurses was undeserved, insisting that a few "bad apples" had contributed to creating a negative impression that was unreflective of the majority of sisters of mercy. The doctor under whom Nurse N. Chelakova worked commented that prior to meeting her, the nurses he had encountered were "of a different sort." Unlike Chelakova, who remained aloof and shunned the flirtatious advances of men, the doctor had observed only sisters "who loved and sought after male attention." After working with Chelakova and her fellow nurses, however, he changed his opinion.[39] Still others attempted to dismiss the negative associations altogether. General Alekei Brusilov, reflecting back on his wartime experiences in his memoirs, acknowledged that rumors of sexual impropriety had circulated in Russian society, but he dismissed them as "dirty-minded tittle-tattle" and attempted to counter the negative associations with nursing by lauding the self-sacrifice and hard work of the majority of sisters of mercy.[40] A soldier named Kolia, writing from the front in August 1915 to M. N. Shtiurmer in Moscow, insisted that nurses, like soldiers and officers, were "extraordinary people." "Many say otherwise about them," he remarked, "but it is mostly rubbish. Nurses are usually blamed if she [*sic*] chats with an officer or strolls with him on the street, but they forget what they endure when they work."[41]

Disparaging representations of wartime nurses also surfaced in images as well, although these are much more difficult to locate. They not only provide striking visualization of the rumors and innuendo that was expressed textually but further indicate the extent to which immoral associations with nursing transcended distinctions between front and rear, medical facility and public arena. These images were found in sources disseminated through illicit channels, certainly not reproduced in the periodical press or in sources intended for public distribution. Often they were circulated among soldiers at the front as picture postcards. They were often cartoonish but extremely graphic and suggestive. Those such as the postcards featured in figures 8.4 and 8.5 depict medical facilities as essentially brothels where male military personnel waited in line in highly aroused states to be "serviced" by female nurses. Such depictions also reveal nurses engaged in sexual activities with multiple men at once. The extent to which these were representative of commonly held attitudes about sisters of mercy, or whether they were merely indicative of male fantasies involving the women they most frequently came into contact with, is difficult to ascertain. Art historian Alexei Flegon, who reprinted these examples in his self-published work, suggested that these were used to "brighten the existence of men whose lives could be snuffed out at any moment."[42] Flegon's remarks, however, attribute such images with an innocuousness that is seemingly oblivious to more pernicious associations and their impact on the general reputation of nurses.

As indicated by Stepanova's account above, wartime sisters of mercy themselves were acutely aware of the spread of the "bad reputation" of nurses through the medical services, the military, and society in general. Her extensive commentary on the "bad" behavior of her fellow nurses was not the only voice among the nursing community to express such criticisms. But others recognized that those who misbehaved were

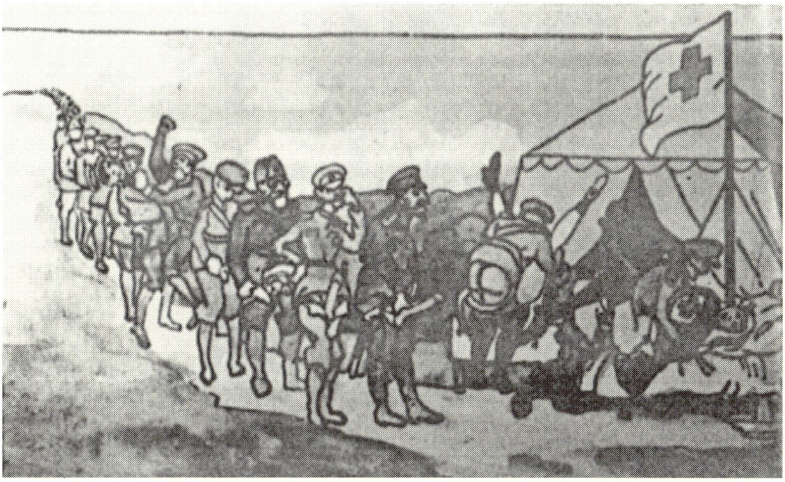

Figure 8.4. Postcard circulated among Russian troops featuring sexualized images of sisters of mercy. A. Flegon, *Eroticism in Russian Art* (London: Flegon, 1976).

greatly outnumbered by dedicated workers. They also realized, much to their chagrin, that despite the fact that these were in the minority, they did much damage to the public perception of nurses. The head nurse of Florence Farmborough's unit was extremely distraught by the gossip concerning women with less than honorable intentions who dressed as sisters of mercy, thereby tainting the reputation of nurses as a whole. Railing against the damage done, she exclaimed, "any woman under the patronage of an officer may put on our uniform and parade the streets with her painted cheeks. Half a dozen of these painted creatures are enough to ruin the reputation of all the Sisters at the front!" Farmborough also indicated that the image of sisters of mercy deteriorated after the October Revolution. As she traveled from the front to Moscow, she noted that "many disagreeable remarks were heard" from the soldiers on the train with her. "The fact that I was in Red Cross uniform seemed to make me a special target for criticism," she recalled.[43] However, such complaints, and specific references to sexual impropriety on the part of nurses, are relatively rare in the written records left behind by women who served during the war. While Aleksinskaia criticized women who seemed less than sincere and devoted to their work, she did not explicitly mention those who engaged in sexual misbehavior. In fact, Farmborough's and Chelakova's are the only published accounts that allude to these incidents. (Stepanova's memoirs were never published; they exist

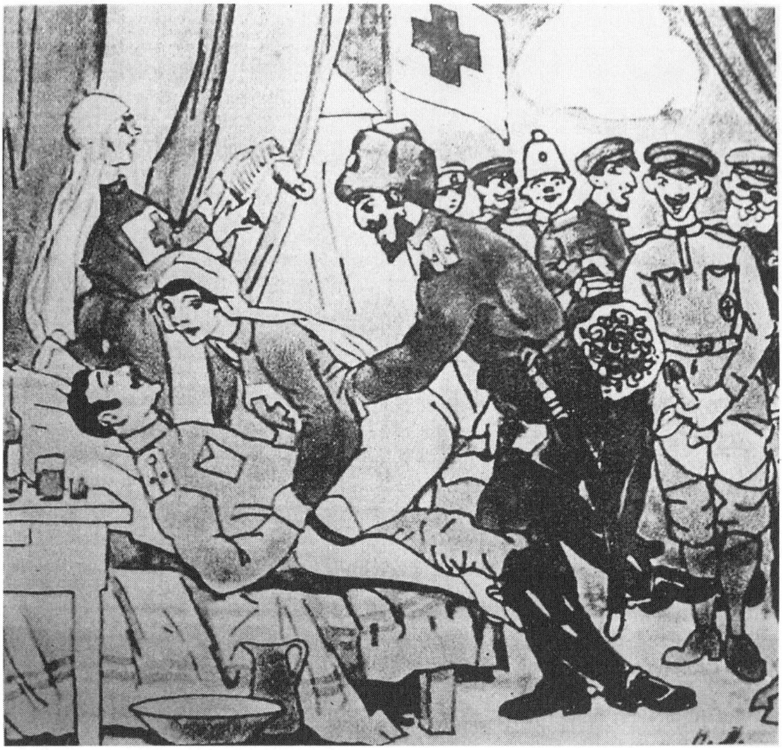

Figure 8.5. Postcard circulated among Russian troops featuring sexualized images of sisters of mercy. A. Flegon, *Eroticism in Russian Art* (London: Flegon, 1976).

solely in the form of a handwritten manuscript preserved in the Hoover Institution archives.)

CONCLUSIONS

Despite the modernization that Russia had experienced by the time of the outbreak of World War I, with regard to appropriate behavior, women were still held to expectations that required them to conform to traditional notions of sexual purity, submission to male authority, and selfless service to the family of the nation. As we have seen, this model of behavior was difficult for many nurses to emulate. When they failed to abide by these standards, they faced significant criticism and opened themselves up to attacks based on immorality, selfishness, and impudence.

As a result, wartime sisters of mercy earned a "bad reputation," which affected many of the women involved in medical service, regardless of their behavior. Negative images of nurses were used as sharp rebukes against those perceived as stepping outside the boundaries of acceptable behavior. The mere association of women with wartime nursing took on pejorative connotations in some circles as a result of the clash between the long-standing grasp of cultural traditions and the demands of modernization and total war. Some observers attempted to resolve this conflict by insisting on a separation of nurses into categories of "good" and "bad," "real" and "false," which were often synonyms for sexually "respectable" and "unrespectable." Such divisions also often corresponded to front and rear, whereby those in the rear were associated with corruption and immorality while those serving at the front were extolled. This may be partially attributed to the resentment of those suffering at the front for those who remained comfortably behind the lines, as well as to significant class antagonisms based on a view that the elite could escape both the duties and hardships of the war. Yet they also underlined a significant problem in accepting women's service.

In fact, accusations of self-aggrandizement and impropriety leveled against wartime nurses illustrate a central paradox of female wartime nursing, that of public versus private. Women in medical service exposed existing anxieties about the presence of women in the public domain and increasing opportunities for them to carry out public action. In doing so, they moved away from accepted notions of female selflessness in the domestic context, which grounded a woman's duties and responsibilities first and foremost in the family. Some of this concern was assuaged by imagining the nation as a family, but it was strained by the idea that women were not carrying out nursing service for purely selfless reasons—that they might personally gain from it. Furthermore, these concerns were exacerbated by the placement of female activity in what many perceived as the distinctly male sphere of war. They were even further heightened when the issue of female sexuality entered the picture. Nursing service, even in the rear, gave women access to thousands of men, which would lead to sexual activity that could only be used for pleasure or for monetary gain, as contrasted with "appropriate" sexual activity within consecrated marriage for the purposes of procreation.

The intersection of nursing and prostitution specifically points to the problem of accepting the notion that women's wartime nursing was acknowledged as public activity in "the field of state service," when one considers this within the context of the gendered formulation that associates the public sphere with lack of respectability for women. In fact, historian Laurie Bernstein argues that by regulating and licensing prostitution, the Russian government was "creating a category of 'public women' whose bodies were supposed to be available to clients, doctors, and policemen on demand."[44] The wartime nurse became something of a "public" woman, carrying out her service very visibly in the public sphere. That she was supposed to do so in a respectable manner presented a dilemma for society, particularly because she now came in direct contact with the bodies of strange men and did so in a context that was supposed to be free of female influence.

These were real concerns, precisely because the war did indeed lead to an increase in the public activity of women, some of which was of a sexual nature. One cannot ignore the fact that the chaos of the war coupled with the demands of total social mobilization created new opportunities for women to engage in relationships with men that might not have been available to them in peacetime society, including an expansion of commercial sex work. Although such expansion is indicative of the lack of other means of economic survival available to women resulting from the hardships created by the war, prostitution represented a serious threat to many in Russian society. It was more than just a nuisance, serving as a potential diversion of male attention away from military duty. It threatened the health of soldiers, through the spread of sexually transmitted diseases, thus potentially weakening the physical bodies of men at arms. Equally, if not more dangerous to many, sex work, and indeed, sexual contact with women, was perceived as having a tremendously negative moral effect and a weakening influence on men. These ideas were also applied to nurses, who similarly risked "feminizing" the military and introducing the opportunity for unwelcome sexual interaction. As such, women as both prostitutes and nurses presented a challenge to the masculinity of war, which was believed by many to be central for military success.

CONCLUSIONS

RUSSIAN WARTIME NURSING AFTER THE FEBRUARY REVOLUTION

The revolution that brought down the tsarist regime in February (old style) 1917 had little immediate impact on wartime nursing. In fact, in reading the documents of the Russian Society of the Red Cross, one can barely discern the massive political change that had occurred. Of primary concern was uninterrupted provision of medical services. However, while treatment continued, there was some confusion with regard to authority. Many of the officials at higher levels of the organization's administration wondered if they had the legitimacy to continue operating in their positions, considering that they had been appointed by the tsar or by his officials. A few even voluntarily removed themselves from their posts. Yet, for the most part, the organization maintained its functions.[1] The Zemstvo and Town Unions were similarly focused on ensuring that service provision continued without interruption, although political changes at the top of Russian government affected those organizations much less. It seems, however, that problems still plagued all of the agencies charged with caring for the ill and wounded, and despite the hopefulness created by the revolution, many of the issues they faced were still extremely daunting. Most significantly, the spread of epidemic diseases flowed unabated throughout the last year of the war.

The February Revolution did provide some momentum toward changing the nature of Russian nursing, specifically transforming it from a private, semireligious, charitable activity into professionalized service. Despite the obstacles and hindrances that impeded efficient provision of medical services, the roles performed by wartime nurses were essential for both the military and civilian populations of Russia during the Great War, leading many in Russian society to recognize the vital participation of these women in the war effort. After the February Revolution, when greater rights and freedoms were extended to the Russian population in general, an effort was made to regularize nursing service and give nurses rights and protections under the law. Women's participation in the war effort increased considerably during this period of renewed dedication to the war. The revolution gave a significant boost to women's organizations, which had been revitalized and expanding since the beginning of the war. These groups appealed to women throughout the country to devote their energies to helping the war effort. Progressive women's organizations such as the League for Women's Equality and the All-Russian Women's Union (Anna Shabanova's former Mutual Philanthropic Society) became increasingly involved in various war-related activities. Although Russian nursing remained a charitable, voluntary activity through the war, by 1917 many began to see the need for its transformation to professional service. The Union of Towns and the Union of Zemstvos established societies of sisters of mercy in an attempt to not only uniformly regulate nursing activity but also provide women in medical service with rights and protections, appropriate compensation, and benefits in return for their important work. Toward this aim, a Union of Russian Sisters of Mercy began to take shape in 1917. A number of prominent women lobbied the government to create a Women's War Work Commission within the Ministry of War. Established in July, the commission was headed by Olga Nechaeva, leader of the Russian Union of Women's Democratic Organizations, who herself had served as a sister of mercy during the war.[2] A proposal to relieve the massive shortages of medical personnel by calling on all women doctors under the age of forty-five for military service was submitted to the Ministry of War.[3] The Women's War Work Commission was placed under the authority of the main administration of the General Staff, and was charged with the task of preparing a report on the feasibility and possible ways of utilizing women's labor in the war effort. The commission submitted a proposal to the minister of war advocating the recruitment of women for medical service in the active army, at the front as well as in the rear, in mid-July.[4] Minister of war Kerensky approved the proposal and the Provisional Government ratified it on August 20.[5] The commission designated the formation of three women's reserve medical battalions, one each in Petrograd, Moscow, and

Kiev, and one women's medical reserve detachment in Kharkov. Recruitment for these units began in late August. In September the main administration of the General Staff approved the use of women as replacements for male medical personnel and accorded them the same rights as all servicemen.[6] In August, the First All-Union Congress of Sisters of Mercy was held in Petrograd as well. The congress moved to create a single organization in an attempt to consolidate the disparate efforts being undertaken by nurses throughout the country, the All-Russian Union of Sisters of Mercy (*Vserossisskii Soiuz Sester Miloserdiia*). As historian of Soviet nursing Susan Grant indicates, such an act signified "the first real attempt by Russian nurses to organize themselves on a national scale." The union was concerned with a variety of issues, including the rights of nurses and the standardization of their training, pay, and titles.[7] Despite these efforts, the union never managed to cohere into a viable organization, and it was disbanded and subsumed into the state administration of medical activities by the Bolsheviks in the 1920s. However, such efforts can be seen as setting the stage for the process of transformation to professionalization, one that would be completed after the October Revolution. In creating the state-directed nursing services that would come to characterize Soviet nursing, the Bolsheviks thus built on a series of precedents established during the war. Most importantly, it is vital to note the move away from its quasi-religious origins, which was not only as a result of Soviet rejection of religion but also heavily influenced by the influx of secularized women into nursing during the war. Although the Russian and later the Soviet Red Cross were not integrated into the international community of nursing, as a result of the war Russian nursing increasingly functioned as a secular public service, one that was crucial to prosecution of war. Indeed, no future conflicts were conducted without extensive involvement of women in medical service. More than eighty thousand women participated in the Russian Civil War between 1918 and 1921, the vast majority of them in medical capacities or other auxiliary functions.[8] Nearly one million Soviet women served in World War II, with more than half of them in medical service.[9] Thousands of women served in the Soviet war against Afghanistan beginning in 1979,[10] as well as in the post-Soviet Russian conflict in Chechnya.[11]

THE SIGNIFICANCE OF RUSSIAN NURSING DURING THE GREAT WAR

Perhaps the most salient conclusions reached as a result of in-depth investigation of wartime nursing in Russia during World War I are its paradoxes. On the surface, female medical service may seem consistent with efforts to retain or restore a traditional gender order because it was seen as passive and supportive to active, male warrior heroes. Thus, women's wartime nursing could have worked with the contemporary idea that the war would provide men with the opportunity to end what some scholars have argued was a perceived "crisis of masculinity."[12] Similarly, viewed as subordinate to male doctors and military officials, nurses could have buttressed conventional gender hierarchies, as an antidote to what others have argued was a prewar "crisis of patriarchy" for Russia.[13] Founded on notions that associated women with caring and compassion, sisters of mercy could have shored up essentialist conceptions of femininity. Instead, Russian wartime nursing served these purposes to a very limited extent, and in fact seemed to unsettle them to a greater measure. As Peter Gatrell has commented, "military nursing is the obvious example" of such disruption, as "the war also demonstrated female capacity to enter directly the military terrain, in ways that both liberated women and disturbed current convention."[14] It provided opportunities for women to engage in behaviors and activities beyond contemporary normative femininity and outside of traditional social structures and identities. Although wartime nursing did not radically subvert gendered dichotomies or break down imperial social structures, constrained as it was by social and cultural norms and values that limited the ability to affect change as well as the effectiveness of service delivery, it did present a number of challenges to both the gender and social order, even before the revolutions of 1917.

Russia's sisters of mercy thus demonstrate the limitations of conventional femininity and the permeability of sexual divisions of labor, blurring gendered boundaries as they engaged in dangerous, even violent roles, assumed leadership positions, and operated in spheres traditionally seen as off-limits to women. Women's actions also simultaneously obscured the separation between gendered conceptions of public and private spheres. Even when performing functions that were considered normatively feminine, they were carrying them out in distinctly masculine spaces, placed directly on the front rather than serving in the rear. Thus, they disrupted traditional notions of caring and nurturing by taking them out of their domestic context. Moreover, often the very characteristics associated with femininity that were valued in nurses were completely impractical, and in fact discouraged, in wartime medical service.

A close look at women's medical services in Russia during World War I also reveals that the common assumption that medical positions were less dangerous and better suited to women than combat is a fallacy. This challenges the "myth of the war experience," which assumes that war is an exclusively masculine phenomenon, defined by male combat experience. A scholarly investigation of wartime nursing takes account of the multiple ways that total war affects civilian populations as much as soldiering masses. While conventional wisdom often draws lines of demarcation between the active killing and dying of combat and the passive nurturance and support of nursing, in reality women's wartime medical service clouded such separations. Indeed, in many ways, the narratives of female medical personnel share many features with those of male combat personnel. At the same time, their experiences illuminate significant differences in the ways women and war intersected and interacted. As such, it serves as a corrective for previous studies that, as scholar Gail Braybon has pointed out, "choose to discuss 'women' as though all ages and classes went through a single, defining war experience."[15] In examining how female medical personnel participated in and were affected by the war, it becomes clear that gender, while salient, is not the only useful framework for analysis. In particular, class and social status were vitally important determinants for Russian sisters of mercy. Social position worked in significant ways to shape the experiences of female medical personnel, and the female staff of the civilian organizations engaged in wartime medical care often reflected the stratified nature of Russian society with clear divisions between the dominant and subordinate classes. Nurses' experiences also demonstrate the continued importance of traditional roles and old forms of social designation and, perhaps more importantly, personal connections based on status. Simultaneously, the war accentuated an increasing dynamism in social structures. Nurses' experiences expose the drawbacks of viewing Russian *soslovie* (estates) as rigid legal designations allowing little mobility and resistant to modernizing changes that placed increasing importance on class. They suggest that these categories were much less ossified and significantly adaptable to new conditions. Simultaneously, they indicate the extent to which such developments remained incomplete, as well as how wartime medical service was hampered by lingering trappings of imperial Russian politics, social structure, and culture. As a result, wartime nursing deepens our understanding of the impact of the First World War on Russia, beyond merely preparing the ground for the revolutions of 1917, focusing on the ways that the war created some new opportunities for action while attesting to the continued weight of existing social structures and identities.

A study of Russian wartime nursing also deepens our understanding of Russia's political development. As with social structure, nursing experience highlights the tremendous importance of a burgeoning modern civil society, while exposing problems impeding its growth and revealing important gendered aspects of this development. This process had begun in the late nineteenth century but was checked by an autocracy that greatly feared mass mobilization. Despite presence of ample desire, skill, resources, and initiative, imperial authorities were loath to relinquish responsibility to and were suspicious of private initiatives. Such problems reveal further the larger difficulties facing the country after enduring the extreme strain of the war. The conflict between military, governmental, and civilian authorities was particularly acute, hindering the nation's ability to effectively deliver necessary aid. Moreover, although opposed to such autocratic constraint, Russian liberals (not unlike those in the West) engaged in the war effort remained unable to utilize the full potential of civil society because, as Laura Engelstein has convincingly argued, "while insisting on expanded autonomy for men," they "persisted in their custodial attitude toward women."[16]

In particular, within the context of Russia's political history, the phenomenon of women's nursing during the Great War serves to further elucidate the processes associated with the development of Russian nationalism and patriotism, and to infuse gender into the argument. As Joshua Sanborn has indicated, wartime nurses are "crucial for a full understanding of Russian patriotism and nationalism."[17] The extent to which nationalism and patriotism were developed in Russia has long been a point of contention among historians. Yet since the inception of national military conscription in the 1870s, the Russian state worked to inculcate these ideals, believing them essential for the creation of effective armed forces. In this equation men, as citizens, were called to service by the state based on the notions of national duty. Women, by contrast, did not have such public citizenship. Instead, their service was a private one, to men (as their dependents) rather than to the state.[18] The onset of total war disrupted this formulation by thrusting women into public service. Nursing in particular represented the feminine ideal of patriotic duty during times of national crisis such as war, a national role to be fulfilled by women while men carried out their obligations to the state as soldiers. Their symbolic value, however, did not always match reality, which, as indicated above, often transcended and contradicted the traditional gender order. Thus it is important to examine the ways in which wartime nursing contributed to the development of Russian nationalism and patriotism and simultaneously transformed it. Women could display patriotism and hoped to demonstrate their worth as citizens by offering their services as nurses during the war. For some, however, this kind of public service raised significant anxieties based on gender, nationality, and religion. Removing women from the private sphere was particularly troublesome. Not only was there concern over the possible deleterious effects of public life on women, but fears over the possible negative influence of women on the masculine discipline and rigor of military life came to the fore. The wartime atmosphere was rife with rumors concerning spies, traitors, and saboteurs. Women were particularly susceptible to suspicions of treasonous behavior, as longstanding misogynistic notions of feminine "nature" associated women with failure to keep secrets, propensity for gossip, and general untrustworthiness. Factors such as ethnicity and religion were also highly influential. Concern over the growth of consciousness among non-Russians intensified worries over loyalty to the empire for those for whom Orthodoxy and Great Russian nationality were seen as litmus tests of patriotic fidelity. The Red Cross in particular expressed significant reluctance toward integration and continued its suspicion of minorities considered to be "politically unreliable." Despite a tremendous need for medical personnel, those who did not share these identities were often excluded from membership in the patriotic family of the empire and denied opportunity to serve in the same ways as those who did. Such restrictions on service further hindered Russia's ability to make efficacious use of its population in the crisis and indicate resistance to modern forms of comprehensive nationalism and citizenship.

As a result of this strong connection to ideas of citizenship, Russian wartime nursing is also extremely significant to the women's movement. The campaign for women's rights would see one of its greatest victories achieved during the course of the war: the extension of suffrage to women in July 1917 by the provisional government. The link between women's wartime service and feminist demands for greater rights and opportunities is readily apparent through the extensive support of nursing by progressive women. Feminists saw the war as an opportunity to demonstrate women's value to the state through war work, which they were convinced would be rewarded with civil, legal, and political rights. Moreover, many of the women who enlisted as nurses were themselves avowedly progressive in their views and often expressed ideas about their service in feminist terms. As historian Rochelle Ruthchild indicates, progressive women believed that the most appropriate way for women to serve the nation in its time of crisis was through "works of love and mercy."[19] Moreover, many of the women who became nurses during the war expressed overtly feminist views concerning the role of women in the public sphere and the need for legal change in the status of women in the nation. There is no doubt that the efforts of Russia's wartime nurses were considered central to the feminist movement's long-standing goals of suffrage and citizenship.

Scholarly analysis of Russia's wartime nurses also deepens our understanding of Russia's cultural history, particularly with regard to gender and sexuality, during the war. By examining the various conceptions of nurses that appeared in the public imagination, we are exposed to a wealth of diverse ideas. The examination presented herein works to correct the inadequacies in previous (relatively sparse) scholarship that addresses these images, which present a simple dichotomy, contending that nurses were perceived either as "good nurses" (angelic, secondary figures providing comfort to wounded men) or as "bad nurses" (self-serving, dissolute women seeking only opportunity for their own gain). On closer examination, it becomes clear that the representations of Russian nurses were extremely varied, complex, and ambiguous, with a number of important, nuanced, and unique representations lying between these poles. Even the prevalent positive public image of the Russian wartime nurse in prowar patriotic culture was not limited to traditional notions of nurses as passive providers of solace to heroic soldiers. The image of the nurse could be used to inspire service and loyalty to the empire, and even to represent Russia itself, making nurses significant as both abstract patriotic symbols and actual performers of civic duty. They also included depictions of nurses as strong, active, heroic figures, saviors of wounded men on the battlefield, as well as, at times, participants in the action on those battlefields. Simultaneously, they could be represented as victims of enemy violence requiring protection, used to inspire Russian men to take up their roles as defenders, but also serving as precautionary tales, highlighting the dangers associated with women operating in the war zone. Negative representations of wartime nurses, although less common, are also significant. In these portrayals, Russian sisters of mercy were seen as using the war for their own gain, by donning the prestigious nursing uniform while remaining safely in the rear and failing to carry out any real medical service. Other views depicted them as sex workers using proximity to captive male audiences to acquire clientele with whom to ply their trade. While such representations do serve to highlight class antagonisms that were significant factors leading to the 1917 revolutions, they are indicative of gender anxieties that arose with the greater freedom and opportunity afforded to women as a result of the war. They reflect more general concerns that had arisen in Russian society during the late nineteenth and early twentieth centuries, as women became increasingly visible in the public sphere and notions of appropriate behaviors and gender roles changed as a result of modernization.

Lastly, while this work presents an opportunity to integrate the Russian wartime sister of mercy into the general historiography of nursing during World War I, it also brings into sharp contrast the experiences of Russian nurses as compared to nurses from other belligerents. We can identify a number of similarities of experience in Russian and Western nursing and demonstrate how other national nursing experiences shared many features of Russian wartime medical service. Yet in many ways the experiences of Russian nurses, who often served directly on the front lines, were profoundly different from those of their Western counterparts, who served primarily in base hospitals far from the war zone. The highly mobile nature of the war on the eastern front, where it was extremely difficult to maintain stable lines of "front" and "rear," also deviates significantly from the very stationary type of medical service performed by most Western nurses. Indeed, as a result, Russian sisters of mercy were often subject to dangerous and difficult conditions very similar to those of combatants.

Russian nursing should also be differentiated from its Western counterpart in that by the time of the Great War, it had not developed into a professional occupation. Although the Western nations involved in the war all accepted volunteers to provide medical care, in many places, such as Great Britain and the United States, nursing had been professionalized in the nineteenth century. Russian sisters of mercy were closer to charity workers. The difference was not in terms of receipt of payment for services, because Russian sisters were paid, but rather in training, function, organization, and status of nurses. Even the highly trained permanent "staff" sisters of the Red Cross who had been part of the organization and practiced nursing prior to the outbreak of the war lacked the same kind of professional status as nurses in Great Britain and the United States. Because until the 1920s Russian nursing remained a semiprivate, charitable, and quasi-religious activity, nurses in that country did not have the benefit of organizations or associations that worked for the interests of nurses in nations where they were professionalized. However, the experiences of World War I helped lay the foundations for the professionalization of nursing during the Soviet period.

Ultimately, as this study indicates, the experiences of women who served Russia as wartime nurses during World War I deepen and broaden our understanding of that conflict considerably. And yet, while they transformed the temporary space of war in dynamic and important ways, the lasting effects of these experiences on Russian (soon to be Soviet) society are less pervasive. Despite the evidentiary experience of World War I that indicated multiple ways that gendered demarcations in both war and medical care were not possible or efficacious, efforts to maintain the exclusive masculinity of war and the femininity of nursing remained highly effective. War continued to be construed as a male sphere, with female mobilization into that sphere accepted only in times of exigency. The precedent established in World War I endured as the cultural norm. The crisis of war made women's participation in the conflict a temporarily acceptable feature of society but certainly not a desirable permanent one. Gendered divisions remained intact in the minds of most Soviet citizens, despite the realities of war. War and combat remained distinctly conceived as masculine, while nursing, even during war, retained its essentialist femininity. Indeed, medical care in general continued to be perceived of as a "natural" field for women in civilian life as well, whereby in the postwar period the majority of primary care physicians in the Soviet Union were women.

Thus, while the First World War gave women opportunities to act in the public sphere and engage in new kinds of behaviors, wartime nursing did not lead to a major reconceptualization of gender. Despite reservations concerning the ability of women to endure the rigors of war, and despite the detriments of essentialized traits such as emotionality, Russian society had come to view nursing as something specifically feminine, and necessary, even in the male zone of war. While war itself was still considered "men's work," nursing, even in wartime, was now considered "women's work," and respectable women's work at that. Men would fight on the battlefields and women would bind their wounds and care for them in medical facilities, the two activities perceived as worlds apart, but in proper balance, akin to the separation of public and private spheres in peacetime society. Such strict demarcations, however, were impossible to maintain, and thus society unwillingly breached the lines of separation of the gendered division of labor. This created a paradox in which the ideology of gender, which insisted on rigid dichotomies, was undermined and counteracted by the realities of war and wartime nursing. And it was this paradox, while insufficient to deter the use of women in wartime nursing capacities, that gave rise to significant anxieties and doubts that would plague wartime nursing. The inability of gendered ideology to match the realities of war and wartime nursing would remain unresolved. Perhaps nowhere was this paradox more apparent than in Russia during the Great War, where war and nursing intersected in ways that clearly indicated the inability to maintain gendered boundaries.

NOTES

INTRODUCTION

1. For more on women's activities, particularly in combat, during this war, see Laurie Stoff, *They Fought for the Motherland: Russia's Women Soldiers in World War I and the Revolution* (Lawrence: University Press of Kansas, 2006).

2. This included nurses serving in the Russian Society of the Red Cross as well as in organizations "under the flag" of the Red Cross such as the All-Russian Union of Zemstvos (local government organs) and All-Russian Union of Towns. Rossiiskii Gosudarstvennyi Voenno-Istoricheskii Arkhiv (hereafter RGVIA) fond (f.) 12651, opis (op.) 3, delo (d.) 456, list (l.) 71.

3. Women also served as doctors, with the number of female physicians increasing significantly during the war.

4. Margaret H. Darrow, "French Volunteer Nursing and the Myth of War Experience in World War I," *American Historical Review* 101, no. 1 (February 1996): 81.

5. George L. Mosse, *Fallen Soldiers: Reshaping the Memory of the World Wars* (New York: Oxford University Press, 1990).

6. See, for example, Kimberly Jensen, *Mobilizing Minerva: American Women in the First World War* (Urbana: University of Illinois Press, 2008); Margaret Darrow, *French Women and the First World War: War Stories of the Home Front* (New York: Berg, 2000); Susan Grayzel, *Women and the First World War* (London: Pearson, 2002); Gail Braybon, *Women Workers in the First World War* (London: Routledge, 1989); the essays on World War I in Margaret Higonnet, Jane Jenson, Sonya Michel, and Margaret Weitz, eds., *Behind the Lines: Gender and the Two World Wars* (New Haven, Conn.: Yale University Press, 1987); Lettie Gavin, *American Women in World War I: They Also Served* (Boulder: University Press of Colorado, 2006); Janet Watson, "Khaki Girls, VADs, and Tommy's Sisters: Gender and Class in First World War Britain," *International History Review* 19 (February 1997): 32–51; Henriette Donner, "Under the Cross: Why V.A.D.s Performed the Filthiest Task in the Dirtiest

War: Red Cross Women Volunteers, 1914–1918," *Journal of Social History* 30, no. 3 (Spring 1997): 687–704.

7. In the Soviet Union the memory of World War I was not cultivated as it was in places such as Great Britain or France; in fact, for Russians the conflict is often thought of as the "forgotten" or "unknown war." See Aaron Cohen, "Oh, That! Myth, Memory, and World War I in the Russian Emigration and the Soviet Union," *Slavic Review* 62 (Spring 2003): 69–86; Daniel Orlovsky, "Velikaia voina i rossiiskaia pamiat," in N. N. Smirnov et al., eds., *Rossiia i pervaia mirovaia voina: Materialy mezhdunarodnogo kollokviuma* (Saint Petersburg, 1999). Historian Karen Petrone, however, in her book *The Great War in Russian Memory* (Bloomington: Indiana University Press, 2012), demonstrates that "the absence of official commemoration did not mean the absence of war memory itself." In addition to Petrone's valuable contribution, a number of studies have recently emerged focusing on Russia's experience in this conflict as part of a concerted effort to restore Russia's place in the study of the Great War. Most notably, currently in progress is an international collaborative effort working to produce a multivolume series on Russia's experiences in World War I, which will be titled *Russia's Great War and Revolution* and will consist of more than twenty individual books dedicated to various aspects of the conflict in Russia.

8. Jane Marcus, "Corpus/Corps/Corpse: Writing the Body in/at War," in H. M. Cooper, A. A. Munich, and S. M. Squier, eds., *Arms and the Woman: War, Gender and Literary Representation* (Chapel Hill: University of North Carolina Press, 1989), 135.

9. Works that explore Russian women's roles in the conflict are rare, and there is, as of yet, no comprehensive scholarly work devoted to Russian women and World War I. Those that focus on women in nursing activities specifically are indeed scant. Some scholars of nursing have engaged with Russian subject matter to a limited extent, but few have engaged with wartime nursing as a subject of scholarly inquiry. See, for example, Christine Hallett, "Russian Romances: Emotionalism and Spirituality in the Writings of 'Eastern Front' Nurses, 1914–1918," *Nursing History Review* 17 (2009): 102–128, but her analysis is limited to two Englishwomen serving as nurses in Russia and one Anglo-Russian woman. Elizabeth Murray discusses the nursing profession in Russia and the Soviet Union in "Russian Nurses: From the Tsarist Sister of Mercy to the Soviet Comrade Nurse: A Case Study of Absence of Migration of Nursing Knowledge and Skills," *Nursing Inquiry* 11 (2004): 130–137, but her analysis does not include the period of World War I. To date, the only published scholarly work that engages specifically with Russia's wartime nurses of World War I is my own: Laurie Stoff, "The 'Myth of the War Experience' and Russian Wartime Nursing in World War I," *Aspasia: The International Yearbook of Central, Eastern, and Southeastern European Women's and Gender History* 6 (2012): 96–116.

10. For example, John F. Hutchinson's work examining public health in Russia between 1890 and 1918 (including the war years) is myopic in its exclusive concern with physicians, making scarce mention of the nurses who carried out much of the actual care during the war. See John F. Hutchinson, *Politics and Public Health in Revolutionary Russia, 1890–1918* (Baltimore, Md.: Johns Hopkins University Press, 1990). Although a collection of essays (edited by Hutchinson and Susan G. Solomon) on health and society in Russia in the late nineteenth and early twentieth centuries prominently features the image of a nurse on its cover, specifically a prerevolutionary sister of mercy, the text contains only one brief mention of nurses, and this in the context of the process of phasing out feldshers (doctors' assistants) in the 1920s under the Soviet government. See Susan G. Solomon and John F. Hutchinson, eds., *Health and Society in Revolutionary Russia* (Bloomington: Indiana University Press, 1990).

11. These include N. A. Beliakova, *Sestry miloserdiia Rossii* (Saint Petersburg, 2005); N. N. Blokhina, "Moskovskie obshchiny sester miloserdiia v XIX—nachale XX veka," *Problemy sotsial'noi gigieny, zdravookhraneniia i istorii meditsiny* 5 (1997): 52–54; V. P. Romaniuk, V. A. Lapotnikov, and Ia. A. Nakatis, *Istoriia sestrinskogo dela v Rossii* (Saint Petersburg: SPbGMA, 1998). A number of these studies emerge from the religious community, seeking to highlight the importance of the Russian nursing tradition in its religious and charitable context. As a result, although they are valuable sources of information, they are not always as objective as one would hope, in many cases portraying the women who served as nurses as saintly "guardian angels." See, for example, L. A. Karpycheava, "Kto takie *sestry miloserdiia?* Ot istoricheskoi etimologii k sovremennomu kontekstu," *Pravoslavnyi Letopicets Sankt-Peterburga* 24 (2005): 11–28; A. V. Posternak, *Ocherki po istorii obshchin sester miloserdiia* (Moscow: Izdatel'stvo Sviato—Dimitrievskoe uchilishche sester miloserdiia, 2001).

12. See, for example, Peter Gatrell, *A Whole Empire Walking: Refugees in Russia during World War I* (Bloomington: Indiana University Press, 1999), and Joshua Sanborn, *Imperial Apocalypse: The Great War and the Destruction of the Russian Empire* (Oxford: Oxford University Press, 2014).

13. Hallett, "Russian Romances," 102.

14. Scholars have long considered the gendered implications of the Great War to be of primary importance. The debate over the impact of the war on gender roles covers a range of arguments, from an emancipatory experience for women to one that solidified the sexual division of labor and restored patriarchy. More recently, scholarship has moved to presenting more nuanced interpretations of the ways that war and gender intersected. See, for example, Arthur Marwick, *The Deluge: British Society and the First World War* (London: Bodley Head, 1965), which presents the war as liberating for women. Others

such as Joanna Bourke, *Dismembering the Male: Men's Bodies, Great Britain, and the Great War* (Chicago: University of Chicago Press, 1996), and Billie Melman, ed., *Borderlines: Genders and Identities in War and Peace, 1870–1930* (New York: Routledge, 1998), present more nuanced and ambivalent pictures of the gendered implications of the conflict. Those such as Erika Kuhlman's *Reconstructing Patriarchy after the Great War: Women, Gender, and Postwar Reconciliation between Nations* (New York: Palgrave Macmillan, 2008) explore the ways the war actually further restricted women.

15. "Introduction" in Melman, *Borderlines*, 6.

16. For the myth of the war in Russian emigration, see Cohen, "Oh, That!" 69–86.

CHAPTER 1. CONTEXT AND CONTROVERSY

1. Tat'iana Aleksandrovna Varnek, typeset, "Vospominaniia 1912–1922," Hoover Institution Archives, Box 1, 1–2. All translations from Russian are by the author unless otherwise noted.

2. Ibid., 2.

3. Ibid., 3–4.

4. Adele Lindenmeyr, "Public Life, Private Virtues: Women in Russian Charity, 1762–1914," *Signs: Journal of Women in Culture and Society* 18, no. 3 (Spring 1993): 563–565.

5. Robert A. Rothstein, "Songs of Women Warriors and Women Who Waited," in Helena Goscilo and Yana Hashamova, eds., *Embracing Arms: Cultural Representations of Slavic and Balkan Women in War* (Budapest: Central University Press, 2012), 180.

6. Karpycheava, "Kto takie *sestry miloserdiia?*"

7. Murray, "Russian Nurses," 131.

8. Rose Glickman, "The Peasant Woman as Healer," in Barbara Evans Clements, Barbara Alpern Engel, and Christine D. Worobec, eds., *Russia's Women: Accommodation, Resistance, Transformation* (Berkeley: University of California Press, 1991), 148–162.

9. Jeanette E. Tuve, *The First Russian Women Physicians* (Newtonville, Mass.: Oriental Research Partners, 1984), 46.

10. Barbara Alpern Engel, *Women in Russia, 1700–2000* (Cambridge: Cambridge University Press, 2004), 65, 112.

11. See nineteenth-century works on women in Russia such as Vitalii Shul'gin, *O sostoianii zhenshchin v Rossii do Petra Velikago: Istoricheskoe issledovanie* (Kiev, 1850).

12. Romaniuk et al., *Istoriia sestrinskogo dela v Rossii*, 35.

13. Posternak, *Ocherki po istorii sester miloserdiia*, 28.

14. Karpycheava, "Kto takie *sestry miloserdiia?*"
15. Posternak, *Ocherki po istorii sester miloserdiia,* 29.
16. Karpycheava, "Kto takie *sestry miloserdiia?*"
17. Posternak, *Ocherki po istorii sester miloserdiia,* 62.
18. Barton C. Hacker, "Women and Military Institutions in Early Modern Europe: A Reconnaissance," *Signs* 6, no. 4 (Summer 1981): 643–644.
19. Yuri Bessonov, "Russian Nurses after the Crimean War: Bureaucracy and Prejudice against Nurses," *RN Journal of Nursing,* http://www.rnjournal.com/journal_of_nursing/russian_nurses_after_the_crimean_war.htm.
20. John C. Curtiss, "Russian Sisters of Mercy in the Crimea, 1854–1855," *Slavic Review* 25, no. 1 (1966): 84.
21. Quoted in Posternak, *Ocherki po istorii sester miloserdiia,* 62–63.
22. Iurii E. Khechikov, *Angely-Khraniteli: Stranitsy istorii Otechestva* (Moscow: RIA DIUM, 1996), 22.
23. Quoted in Curtiss, "Russian Sisters of Mercy," 85.
24. Florence Nightingale to Lady Canning, September 9, 1855, quoted in Sue M. Goldie, ed., *"I Have Done My Duty": Florence Nightingale in the Crimean War, 1854–56* (Iowa City: University of Iowa Press, 1987), 154.
25. Curtiss, "Russian Sisters of Mercy," 85.
26. M. Sokolov and F. Kiiakovskii, quoted in Bessonov, "Russian Nurses after the Crimean War."
27. Kh. Ia. Giubbenet, quoted in Posternak, *Ocherki po istorii sester miloserdiia,* 63.
28. Curtiss, "Russian Sisters of Mercy"; Murray, "Russian Nurses."
29. Murray, "Russian Nurses," 132.
30. Bessonov, "Russian Nurses after the Crimean War."
31. Pirogov, as quoted in O. L. Leikinda, *Blagotvoritel'nost' v Rossii: Istoricheskie i sotsial'no-ekonomicheskie issledovaniia* (Saint Petersburg: Liki Rossii, 2003), 311–318. http://www.omophor.ru/articles/istoriya-obshchin sester-miloserdiya.
32. Bessonov, "Russian Nurses after the Crimean War."
33. Ibid.
34. Romaniuk et al., *Istoriia sestrinskogo dela v Rossii,* 62. The authors misidentify the founder of the International Committee of the Red Cross and the author of the Geneva Convention as Andre Dudan.
35. D. Mikhialov, *Krasnyi Krest i sestry miloserdiia v Rossii i za-granitsei* (Petrograd-Kiev: Knigoizdatel'stvo "Sotrudnik," 1914), 88–91.
36. Romaniuk et al., *Istoriia sestrinskogo dela v Rossii,* 63.
37. As part of his general reforming efforts, and inspired by the example of women's medical activities in the Crimean War, Tsar Alexander II granted women legal access to higher medical education in 1856. Many flocked to the newly opened courses. In 1865 Varvara Kashevarova-Rudneva became the first woman

doctor of medicine. Alexander rescinded this order in 1863, after a number of female medical students were linked with burgeoning radical and revolutionary movements. Only Kashevarova-Rudneva was allowed to continue to completion. See Tuve, *First Russian Women Physicians,* 48–49. This did not deter other Russian women seeking to become doctors, a number of whom went abroad to complete their medical degrees at foreign universities. Once again, the Russian government reacted with anxiety to this expatriate activity as a result of the association of female medical students with radical politics, and it recalled all Russian students studying abroad. To satisfy liberal demands for increased opportunities for women's education in the 1870s, the Russian government opened non–degree-granting "higher courses" for women that allowed hundreds to complete medical training and become midwives, *feld'sheristy,* pharmacists, and woman-doctors (*zhenschina-vrachy*—a designation inferior to male doctors). Professionalization would also prove difficult for female doctors, who could not be legally admitted to the Table of Ranks, effectively denying them the right to serve in state medical institutions. See Christine Johanson, "Autocratic Politics, Public Opinion, and Women's Medical Education during the Reign of Alexander II, 1855–1881," *Slavic Review* 38, no. 3 (September 1979): 426–443.

38. Quoted in Johanson, "Autocratic Politics," 441.

39. Quoted in Christine Johanson, *Women's Struggle for Higher Education in Russia, 1855–1900* (Kingston, Ont.: McGill–Queen's University Press, 1987), 10.

40. Khechikov, *Angely-Khraniteli,* 30.

41. Iu. N. Ivanova, *Khrabreishche iz prekrasnykh: Zhenshchiny Rossii v voinakh* (Moscow: Rossiiskaia Politicheskaia Entsiklopediia, 2002), 28.

42. Ivanova, *Khrabreishche iz prekrasnykh,* 31, 29.

43. Khechikov, *Angely-Khraniteli,* 30.

44. Romaniuk et al., *Istoriia sestrinskogo dela v Rossii,* 68.

45. Khechikov, *Angely-Khraniteli,* 22.

46. Posternak, *Ocherki po istorii sester miloserdiia,* 103–104.

47. Khechikov, *Angely-Khraniteli,* 34.

48. Kh. D. Alcheevskii, quoted in Posternak, *Ocherki po istorii sester miloserdiia,* 104.

49. Ivanova, *Khrabreishche iz prekrasnykh,* 29.

50. Posternak, *Ocherki po istorii sester miloserdiia,* 108.

51. Ivanova, *Khrabreishche iz prekrasnykh,* 31.

52. Posternak, *Ocherki po istorii sester miloserdiia,* 108.

53. Military nursing opponent Tolstoi now became minister of internal affairs, and he and his reactionary cohort of statesmen, such as Procurator of the Holy Synod Konstantin Pobedonostsev, were adamant about keeping women relegated to traditional roles. See Johanson, "Autocratic Politics," 442.

54. Samuel C. Ramer, "Feldshers and Rural Health Care in the Early Soviet Period," in Solomon and Hutchinson, *Health and Society in Revolutionary Russia*, 123.

55. Khechikov, *Angely-Khraniteli*, 36–37.

56. Ivanova, *Khrabreishche iz prekrasnykh*, 52–53.

57. Khechikov, *Angely-Khraniteli*, 40.

58. Posternak, *Ocherki po istorii sester miloserdiia*, 150.

59. Raymond Spear, *Report on the Russian Medical and Sanitary Features of the Russo-Japanese War to the Surgeon-General, U.S. Navy* (Washington, D.C.: Government Printing Office, 1906), 17.

60. Ivanova, *Khrabreishche iz prekrasnykh*, 55.

61. Posternak, *Ocherki po istorii sester miloserdiia*, 149.

62. Barton C. Hacker, "Reformers, Nurses, and Ladies in Uniform: The Changing Status of Military Women (c. 1815–c. 1914)," in Barton C. Hacker and Margaret Vining, eds., *A Companion to Women's Military History* (Leiden, Netherlands: Koninklijke Brill, 2012), 165.

63. Posternak, *Ocherki po istorii sester miloserdiia*, 151.

64. L. M. Vasilevskii, *Po sledam voiny: vpechatleniia voennago vracha* (Petrograd: Tip. Imp. Nikolaev. Voen. Akad., 1916), 38.

65. P. Kaufman, quoted in Posternak, *Ocherki po istorii sester miloserdiia*, 151.

66. Spear, *Russo-Japanese War*, 11–12.

67. Romaniuk et al., *Istoriia sestrinskogo dela v Rossii*, 77.

68. Varnek, "Vospominaniia," 4–5.

69. Bianca Schönberger, "Motherly Heroines and Adventurous Girls: Red Cross Nurses and Women Army Auxiliaries in the First World War," in Karen Hagemann, ed., *Home/Front—Military, War, and Gender in Twentieth-Century Germany* (Oxford: Berg, 2002), 88.

70. John VanR. Hoff, "The Soldier Nurse," *American Journal of Nursing* 11, no. 5 (February 1911): 342.

71. Darrow, "French Volunteer Nursing," 86.

CHAPTER 2. MOBILIZING MEDICAL SERVICE

1. Khristina Semina, *Tragediia russkoi armii pervoi velikoi voiny 1914–1918 gg.: Zapiski sestry miloserdiia kavkazkogo fronta*, 2 vols. (New Mexico: privately published, 1963), 1:1–11, 35, 44–62, 84–87, 96–101, 130–139.

2. Hutchinson, *Politics and Public Health*, 110.

3. Tsentral'noe Statisticheskoe Upravlenie, Otdel Voennoi Statistiki, *Rossiia v mirovoi voine, 1914–1918 goda (v tsifrakh)* (Moscow: Tipografia M.K.Kh. imeni F. Ia. Lavrova, 1925), 25, 99.

4. Schönberger, "Motherly Heroines," 89.

5. Darrow, *French Women and the First World War*, 140–141.

6. Kimberly Jensen, "A Base Hospital Is Not a Coney Island Dance Hall: American Women Nurses, Hostile Work Environment, and Military Rank in the First World War," *Frontiers: A Journal of Women Studies* 26, no. 2 (2005): 208.

7. Aeleah Soine, "The Relation of the Nurse to the Working World: Professionalization, Citizenship, and Class in Germany, Great Britain, and the United States before World War I," *Nursing History Review* 18 (2010): 52.

8. Donner, "Under the Cross," 704.

9. Gavin, *American Women in World War I*, 44.

10. Grayzel, *Women and the First World War*, 38–39.

11. Darrow, *French Women and the First World War*, 139.

12. Grayzel, *Women and the First World War*, 39–40.

13. Joshua Sanborn, *Drafting the Russian Nation: Military Conscription, Total War, and Mass Politics, 1905–1925* (DeKalb: Northern Illinois University Press, 2003), 96.

14. Taking issue with traditional notions that tsarist Russia was a prime of example of a failed, or in Antonio Gramsci's words, a "primordial and gelatinous" civil society, scholars have demonstrated that Russia did possess some aspects of civil society as indicated by the presence of a multitude of voluntary organizations. See, for example, Joseph Bradley, "Subjects into Citizens: Societies, Civil Society, and Autocracy in Tsarist Russia," *American Historical Review* 107, no. 4 (October 2002): 1096. Bradley argues that "despite the fact that the autocracy was suspicious of an autonomous civil society, in the later eighteenth and nineteenth centuries Russians did create a public sphere and an associational life based on the model of the European enlightenment." Gramsci, quoted in Joseph Bradley, *Voluntary Associations in Tsarist Russia: Science, Patriotism, and Civil Society* (Cambridge, Mass.: Harvard University Press, 2009), 3. Those such as Aaron Cohen have argued, "one cannot deny that Imperial Russia had a functioning civil society mobilized to conduct tasks in a public sphere made up of mass media, commercial culture, and nongovernmental institutions by the early twentieth century." See Aaron Cohen, *Imagining the Unimaginable: World War, Modern Art, and the Politics of Public Culture in Russia, 1914–1917* (Lincoln: University of Nebraska Press, 2008), 7. More cautious in her analysis, taking into account the tremendous resistance from the Russian autocracy to such efforts, Laura Engelstein promotes a more tempered view. "The state," she argues, "was indeed powerful and strictly patrolled the social landscape, suspicious of any force outside its control. Yet tsars could not rule entirely as they pleased, but contended with public opinion, if only on a limited scale. Society was not formless." See Laura Engelstein, "The Dream of Civil Society in Tsarist Russia: Law, State,

and Religion," in Nancy Bermeo and Philip Nord, eds., *Civil Society before Democracy: Lessons from Nineteenth-Century Europe* (Lanham, Md.: Rowman & Littlefield, 2000), 24.

15. Sanborn, *Drafting the Russian Nation,* 97.

16. Paul P. Gronsky, *The War and the Russian Government: The Central Government* (New Haven, Conn.: Yale University Press, 1929), 26–27. These imperial family members included the Empress Alexandra (Nicholas II's wife), who served as president of the Supreme Council for the Care of Soldiers' Families, and of Families of the Wounded and Dead, with her sister, Grand Duchess Elizabeth, and her eldest daughter, Grand Duchess Ol'ga, serving as vice presidents. The Committee for the Temporary Relief of War Sufferers was formed under the direction of the Grand Duchess Tatiana (another of the tsar's daughters) to provide assistance to the large numbers of refugees created by the war. Another organ, the Romanov Committee, was assigned the task of aiding children of soldiers as well as those who had become orphaned by the fighting. Although it experienced a near complete hiatus from legislative activity during the war, the Duma responded to the central government's goal of alleviating the suffering of the Russian population by establishing a Provisional Committee of the Duma for the Relief of the Wounded and Sick Soldiers and War Sufferers. The committee established hospitals and medical units both at the front and in the rear.

17. Quoted in Hutchinson, *Politics and Public Health,* 111.

18. Ibid.

19. William Gleason, "The All-Russian Union of Towns and the All-Russian Union of Zemstvos in World War I: 1914–1917," PhD diss., Indiana University, 1972, 1.

20. Hutchinson, *Politics and Public Health,* 112, 116, 121, 127–142.

21. Nicholas Astrov, *The War and the Russian Government: The Municipal Government and the All-Russian Union of Towns* (New Haven, Conn.: Yale University Press, 1929), 171–172.

22. Prince Georgi V. L'vov, *The Russian Union of Zemstvos* (London: P. S. King & Sons, 1917), 6. Indeed, it was these local organizations, along with the army, that gained the most authority in the crisis of the war, despite the tsarist government's attempts to enhance its centralized power.

23. Hutchinson, *Politics and Public Health,* 110–111.

24. Laura Engelstein, *The Keys to Happiness: Sex and the Search for Modernity in Fin-de-Siècle Russia* (Ithaca, N.Y.: Cornell University Press, 1992).

25. Choi Chatterjee and Karen Petrone, "Models of Selfhood and Subjectivity: The Soviet Case in Historical Perspective," *Slavic Review* 67, no. 4 (Winter 2008): 984–985.

26. Circular from the Main Directorate of the Russian Society of the Red Cross (hereafter ROKK) to the district and local committees and the com-

mittees and fiduciary councils of the communities of sisters of mercy of the Society, September 4, 1914. RGVIA f. 12674, op. 2, d. 1, 1. 54. Previously, nursing courses lasted from eight months to a year.

27. Romaniuk et al., *Istoriia sestrinskogo dela v Rossii,* 77–78.

28. RGVIA, f. 12651, op. 3, d. 456, 1. 71. This included nurses serving in the Russian Society of the Red Cross as well as in organizations "under the flag" of the Red Cross, such as the Union of Zemstvos and Union of Towns.

29. Preliminary Report of the Mobilization Council of the ROKK, October 16, 1914, RGVIA f. 12651, op. 3, d. 346, 1. 388.

30. Mikhailov, *Krasnyi Krest,* 78.

31. Varnek, "Vospominaniia," 4.

32. "O naznachenii zhenshchin-vrachei v peredovye otriady," *Vestnik Krasnago Kresta* 2 (February 1915): 530.

33. For this view, see Alfred Meyer, "The Impact of World War I on Russian Women's Lives," in Clements et al., *Russia's Women,* 220.

34. The most common bases for these kinds of rejections were issues of nationality or religion, which will be explored in the next chapter.

35. Rossisskoe Obshchestvo Krasnago Kresta, *Sbornik glavneishikh kasaiushikhsia i glavneishikh tsirkuliarov Glavnago Upravleniia nazvannago obshchestva* (Petrograd: Gosudarstvennaia tipigrafiia, 1917), 109.

36. "Otchet doktora meditsny S. K. Solov'ev, zaveduiuvaiushchii meditsinkoi chastiu severnom front," RGVIA, f. 12674, op. 1, d. 10, 1. 370–371, 375.

37. Circular from the Main Directorate of the ROKK to the District and Regional administrations, September 4, 1914, RGVIA f. 12675, op. 2, d. 1, 1. 55.

38. D. Mikhailov, *Spravochnaia kniga po voenno-sanitarnomu delu: Prakticheskoe rukovodstvo dlia voennykh vrachei i deiatelei po voenno-sanitarnoi chasti* (Petrograd-Kiev: Knigoizdatel'stvo "Sotrudnik," 1915), 6.

39. "Vysochiaishie utverzhdennoe polozhenie Admiralteistsvo-Soveta," *Vestnik Krasnago Kresta,* January 1915, 6.

40. "Otchet doktora meditsny S. K. Solov'ev," 374–377; "Zhurnal #14, 24 Okt. 1914," in *Zhurnal zacedaniia ispolnitel'nago biuro Vserossiiskogo Gorodskogo Soiuza, 1914 g.* (Moscow: Vserossiskii Gorodskii Soiuz, 1914), 1.

41. Excerpt from Orders of the Main Administration of the Russian Society of the Red Cross to the armies of the Northern Front, November 28, 1916, RGVIA f. 12675, op. 2, d. l, 1. 92.

42. Circular from the Main Directorate of the ROKK, March 28, 1917, RGVIA f. 12675, op. 2, d. 1, 1. 216.

43. "Zhurnal #14, 24 Okt., 1914," 1.

44. Mikhialov, *Krasnyi Krest,* 88.

45. Ibid., 89.

46. "Otchet doktora meditsny S. K. Solov'ev," 374–377.

47. Ibid.

48. M. V. Rodzianko, *The Reign of Rasputin: An Empire's Collapse*, trans. Catherine Zvegintzoff (Gulf Breeze, Fla.: Academic International Press, 1973), 112, 116.

49. Kseniia Iureva, *Rasskazy: sestry miloserdiia* (Göttingen, 1948), 2–3.

50. Lidiia Zakharova, *Dnevnik sestry miloserdiia (na peredovykh pozitsiakh)* (Petrograd: Izdatel'stvo Biblioteka "Velikoi Voiny," 1915), 111.

51. Sophie Botcharsky and Florida Pier, *The Kinsmen Know How to Die* (New York: William Morrow, 1931), 29. Because of the variable transliterations from the Cyrillic alphabet, the spelling of names in source citations may differ from those used in the text.

52. Varnek, "Vospominaniia," 7, 8, 10.

53. Rodzianko, *Reign of Rasputin,* 116.

54. Telegram from Warsaw: Concerning military conditions: To: General Volkov, ZAPADOKREST, Nov. 19, 1914, RGVIA f. 12651, op. 3, d. 370, 1. 19.

55. "Otchet doktora meditsny S. K. Solov'ev," 370–371.

56. Session #3 of the Mobilization Committee of ROKK, October 27, 1916, RGVIA f. 12651, op. 3, d. 418, 1. 154.

57. Fedor Stepun, *Byvshee i nesbyvsheesia,* 2nd ed. (Saint Petersburg: Aleteiia, 2000), 284.

58. Telegram from Warsaw, to the Main Administration of the ROKK in Petrograd, November 30, 1914, RGVIA f. 12651, op. 3, d. 370, 1. 90.

59. Telegram from Petrograd, Main Administration of the ROKK, to Warsaw, December 1, 1914, RGVIA f. 12651, op. 3, d. 370, 1. 93.

60. Telegram from Warsaw, to the Main Administration of the ROKK in Petrograd, December 29, 1914, RGVIA f. 12651, op. 3, d. 370, 1. 224.

61. Violetta Thurstan, *A Text Book of War Nursing* (London: G. P. Putnam's Sons, 1917), xvi. A number of foreign observers made note of the serious deficiencies in medicine, equipment, and basic supplies that plagued Russian medical units.

62. Untitled report, Gosudarstvennyi Arkhiv Rossiiskoi Federatsii (hereafter GARF), f. 102 Departament politsii Ministerstva vnutrennykh del. Piatoe otdelenie osobogo otdela departamenta politsii (sekretnaia chast'), op. 265, d. 1042, 1. 135.

63. Botcharsky and Pier, *Kinsmen Know How to Die,* 24–25.

64. Semina, *Tragediia russkoi armii,* 1:34.

65. Botcharsky and Pier, *Kinsmen Know How to Die,* 8–9.

66. See Hutchinson, *Politics and Public Health.*

67. N. Chelakova, "Iz zapisok sestry miloserdiia," *Novoe Russkoe Slovo,* (June 16, 1969): 4.

68. Zakharova, *Dnevnik sestry miloserdiia,* 82–84.

69. Hutchinson, *Politics and Public Health,* 111.

70. The interaction between female nursing personnel and male medical personnel (particularly military) will be explored in greater depth in chapter 6.

71. See the Records of the Press Bureau of the Main Administration of the Red Cross, RGVIA f. 12651, op. 10, and the Journal of Sessions of the Mobilization Committee of the Russian Society of the Red Cross, RGVIA f. 12651, op. 3, for numerous examples of these requests.

72. Session #20 of the Mobilization Committee of the ROKK, July 7, 1916, RGVIA f. 12651, op. 3, d. 416, 1. 251.

73. Session of the Mobilization Committee of ROKK, December 10, 1915, RGVIA f. 12651, op. 3, d. 373, 1. 156.

74. "O nedopustimosti otkaza sestep miloserdiia rabotat' v zaraznykh gospitaliakh," Circular from the Main Administration of the Russian Society of the Red Cross to the District and Local Administrations, April 15, 1916, RGVIA f. 12675, op. 2, d. 1, 1. 72.

75. Chelakova, "Iz zapisok sestry miloserdiia," 4.

76. Ibid.

77. Records of the meetings of the Mobilization Department under the Main Administration of the ROKK, Journal No. 26, October 6, 1916, RVGIA f. 12651, op. 3, d. 418, 1. 105.

78. See Rossisskoe Obshchestvo Krasnago Kresta, *Sbornik glavneishikh.*

79. Urgent secret message to the Saint George's Community of the Red Cross, Petrograd, from the Chief Doctor of Polotskii Mobile Field Hospital No. 3, December 22, 1914, RGVIA f. 12651, op. 3, d. 370, 1. 364.

80. The Journal of Sessions of the Mobilization Committee of the Russian Society of the Red Cross, RGVIA f. 12651, op. 3, contains hundreds of documents pertaining to this problem.

81. Session #15 of the Mobilization Committee of ROKK, June 16, 1916, RGVIA f. 12651, op. 3, d. 416, 1. 208.

82. Session #9 of the Mobilization Committee of ROKK, February 4, 1916, RGVIA f. 12651, op. 3, d. 414, 1. 104.

83. Session #12 of the Mobilization Committee of ROKK, February 6, 1916, RGVIA f. 12651, op. 3, d. 414, 1. 115.

84. "Otchet doktora meditsny S. K. Solov'ev," 383–384.

85. "Pravila noshcheniia formy ses. mil. i litsami zhenskago sanitarnogo personala ROKK," RGVIA f. 12675, op. 2, d. 1, 1. 61.

86. Resolution of the Trustee of the Committee of the Omsk Community of the Red Cross from January 3, 1915, RGVIA f. 12651, op. 3, d. 373, 1. 5, #19.

87. Session #13 of the Mobilization Committee of ROKK, March 18, 1917, RGVIA f. 12641, op. 3, d. 452, 1. 130.

88. "O zloupotreblenii zvaniem sester miloserdiia," *Vestnik Krasnago Kresta,* March 1915, 917–918. The intersections between sexual promiscuity, prostitution, and wartime nursing will be further explored in chapter 8.

CHAPTER 3. CLASS AND SOCIAL STATUS IN RUSSIAN WARTIME NURSING

1. Tatiana Alexinsky, *With the Russian Wounded,* trans. Gilbert Cannan (London: T. F. Unwin, Ltd., 1916), 1.

2. As indicated in chapter 1, the Russian imperial government did not allow women to study at the medical-surgical academies after 1863, and women could not receive the professional rank of physician but instead attended Women's Higher Medical Courses, completion of which conferred on the graduate the designation of "woman-doctor." This title denied women physicians the same professional status and privileges as male doctors. See Tuve, *First Russian Women Physicians*; Johanson, *Women's Struggle for Higher Education.*

3. Alexinsky, *With the Russian Wounded,* 26.

4. Ibid., 10–13.

5. Boris Kolonitskii, *Tragicheskaia erotika: Obrazy imperatorskoi sem'i v gody Pervoi mirovoi voiny* (Moscow: Novoe literaturnoe obozrenie, 2010), 251; Marie, Grand Duchess of Russia, *Education of a Princess* (London: Viking, 1930).

6. Quoted in Richard Stites, *The Women's Liberation Movement in Russia: Feminism, Nihilism, and Bolshevism, 1860–1930* (Princeton, N.J.: Princeton University Press, 1991), 279.

7. Vanda Kazimirovna Stepanova, holograph, "Zapiski velikoi voiny 1914–1918 gg.," Box 1, Hoover Institution Archives, Collection No. 22175, 53.

8. Photograph and caption, *Iskry,* November 9, 1915, 347.

9. Photograph and caption, *Iskry,* February 22, 1915, 59.

10. Photograph and caption, *Stolitsa i usadba,* no. 83–88 (1917), 20. Skrydlova went on to join Maria Bochkareva's First Russian Women's Battalion of Death when it was formed in May 1917, serving as the commander's adjutant.

11. General Basil Gourko, *War and Revolution in Russia, 1914–1917* (New York: Macmillan, 1919), 206.

12. Aleksandra Tolstaia, *Doch'* (Moscow: Vagrius, 2000), 228.

13. Photograph and caption, *Niva,* November 8, 1914, 869.

14. Photograph and caption, *Iskry,* September 21, 1914, 293; photograph and caption, *Sol'ntse Rossii,* September 8, 1916, 10.

15. "Zhenshchiny i voina," *Zhenskii Vestnik,* no. 12 (1914), 267.

16. Botcharsky and Pier, *Kinsmen Know How to Die.*

17. Varnek, "Vospominaniia," 1–3.

18. Stepanova, "Zapiski velikoi voiny," 53.

19. Quoted in Engel, *Women in Russia,* 129.

20. Zakharova, *Dnevnik sestry miloserdiia.*

21. Photograph and caption, *Vestnik Krasnago Kresta,* no. 2 (January 1915): 189.

22. Grand Duchess Marie, *Education of a Princess,* 188.

23. Varnek, "Vospominaniia," 5.

24. See RGVIA f. 12651, op. 3, d. 417, 418, 420, 451, and 452, Journal of Sessions of the Mobilization Committee of the Russian Society of the Red Cross, 1916, for numerous examples of such requests.

25. Such a view has been promoted in works such as Stites, *Women's Liberation Movement.*

26. Records of the meetings of the Mobilization Department under the main administration of the Russian Society of the Red Cross, Journal No. 14, October 6, 1916, RVGIA f. 12651, op. 3, d. 418, 1. 102.

27. "Iz dvenika sestry miloserdia," *Vestnik Krasnago Kresta,* no. 1 (January 1915): 230.

28. Florence Farmborough, *With the Armies of the Tsar: A Nurse at the Russian Front in War and Revolution, 1914–1918* (New York: Cooper Square, 2000).

29. Mary Britnieva, *One Woman's Story* (London: Arthur Barker, 1936), 11.

30. Violetta Thurstan, *Field Hospital and Flying Column: Being the Journal of an English Nursing Sister in Belgium and Russia* (London: G. P. Putnam's Sons, 1915), 125.

31. Meriel Buchanan, *The City of Trouble* (New York: Charles Scribner's Sons, 1918), 31.

32. The perceptions of the empress that circulated in Russian society are explored in-depth in Kolonitskii, *Tragicheskaia erotica.*

33. "Sestra miloserdiia—Bulgarskaia poddaniia," *Vestnik Krasnago Kresta,* no. 2 (February 1915): 552.

34. "Otkaz v priem vracha-avtriitsa," *Vestnik Krasnago Kresta,* no. 2 (February 1915): 552.

35. The issue of citizenship existing in an autocracy can be problematic, if citizenship is defined as a set of rights and obligations granted to individual legal members of a state. While subjects of the Russian autocracy had many obligations, they had few rights as individuals (women even less so than men). However, citizenship rarely contains a balance of rights and obligations (especially for women, even in democracies during this period), and thus in Russia citizenship emphasized obligations more heavily. See Eric Lohr, "The Ideal Citizen and Real Subject in Late Imperial Russia," *Kritika: Explorations in Russian and Eurasian History* 7, no. 2 (Spring 2006): 173–194.

36. Nancy F. Cott, "Marriage and Women's Citizenship in the United States, 1830–1934," *American Historical Review* 103, no. 5 (1998): 1442.

37. Maureen Healy, "Becoming Austrian: Women, the State, and Citizenship in World War I," *Central European History* 35, no. 1 (2002): 1–35.

38. "Italianka-Russkaia sestra miloserdiia," *Vestnik Krasnago Kresta,* no. 1 (January 1915): 213.

39. Grand Duchess Elena Pavlovna, quoted in Murray, "Russian Nurses," 132.

40. Sanborn, *Drafting the Russian Nation,* 116.

41. Eric Lohr, "The Russian Army and the Jews: Mass Deportation, Hostages, and Violence during World War I," *Russian Review* 60 (2001): 404.

42. See Journal of Sessions of the Mobilization Committee of the Russian Society of the Red Cross, RGVIA f. 12651, op. 3 and op. 10, within multiple *delo* (files) indicating documents concerned with individual applications by Jewish women for permission to be granted the title of "sister of mercy" by the Red Cross.

43. Journal of Sessions of the Mobilization Committee of the Russian Society of the Red Cross, November 14, 1915, RGVIA f. 12651, op. 3, d. 373, l. 52.

44. Telegram to Grigorii Antonovich Blokh from L. Perets, March 2, 1916, RGVIA, f. 12651, op. 10, d. 25, l. 193.

45. Sanborn, *Drafting the Russian Nation,* 116–124.

46. Lohr, "Russian Army and the Jews," 404.

47. See the Journal of Sessions of the Mobilization Committee of the Russian Society of the Red Cross, RGVIA f. 12651, op. 3.

48. *Voina i evrei,* no. 1 (1915): 8, 11. I would like to thank Melissa Stockdale for directing me to this source.

49. *Voina i evrei,* no. 4 (1915): 8–9.

50. *Voina i evrei,* no. 8 (1915): 9.

51. *Voina i evrei,* no. 1 (1915): 7, 12.

52. *Voina i evrei,* no. 8 (1915): 4.

53. *Voina i evrei,* no. 6 (1915): 3.

54. *Voina i evrei,* no. 3 (1915): 3–16.

55. *Voina i evrei,* no. 5 (1915): 8.

56. M. N. Vasilevich, *Polozhenie russkikh plennykh v Germanii i otnoshennie Germanstev k nasileniiu zaniatykh imi oblastei Tsarstva Polskago i Litvy* (Petrograd, 1917), 206–208.

57. "V lazarete Vilenskoi obshchiny," *Voina i evrei,* no. 1–14 (1915): 8.

58. The personnel of local government organizations that were part of the Union of Zemstvos and Union of Towns were notoriously anti-tsarist, but they worked hard to serve the Russian people. See Hutchinson, *Politics and Public Health.*

59. Valentina Kostyleva, "Nashi Amazonki," *Zhenskaia Zhizn',* October 1914, 24.

60. Stepanova, "Zapiski velikoi voiny," 13.

61. Tolstaia, *Doch'*, 226–227.

62. George A. Lensen, trans. and ed., *War and Revolution: Excerpts from the Letters and Diaries of the Countess Ol'ga Poutiatine* (Tallahassee, Fla.: Diplomatic Press, 1971).

63. Thurstan, *Field Hospital and Flying Column,* 125.

64. Chelakova, "Iz zapisok sestry miloserdiia," *Novoe Russkoe Slovo* (June 12, 1969): 4.

65. Stites, *Women's Liberation Movement,* 279.

66. Alexinsky, *With the Russian Wounded,* 11.

67. Zakharova, *Dnevnik sestry miloserdiia,* 11.

68. Tolstaia, *Doch'*, 227.

69. Linda Edmondson, *Feminism in Russia, 1900–1917* (Stanford, Calif.: Stanford University Press, 1984), 158.

70. As translated by Stites in *Women's Liberation Movement,* 283, taken from *Zhenskoe delo,* August 15, 1915, 1–2.

71. "Voina," *Zhenskii Vestnik,* September 1914, 173.

72. Alexinsky, *With the Russian Wounded,* 11.

73. V. V. Brusianin, *Voina, zhenshchiny i deti* (Petrograd: Kinoizdatel'stvo "Mlechny Put'," 1917), 61.

74. Grand Duchess Marie, *Education of a Princess,* 172, 187.

75. Buchanan, *City of Trouble,* 121.

76. Gourko, *War and Revolution in Russia,* 206.

77. Chelakova, "Iz zapisok sestry miloserdiia," 4.

78. Botcharsky and Pier, *Kinsmen Know How to Die,* 29.

79. Tolstaia, *Doch'*, 230.

80. Britnieva, *One Woman's Story*, 26.

81. Botcharsky and Pier, *Kinsmen Know How to Die.*

82. Stepanova, "Zapiskii velikoi voiny," 60–62, 67.

83. Varnek, "Vospominaniia," 9.

84. S. Ansky, *The Enemy at His Pleasure: A Journey through the Jewish Pale of Settlement during World War I,* trans. and ed. Joachim Neugroschel (New York: Henry Holt, 2002), 86.

85. Chelakova, "Iz zapisok sestry miloserdiia," 4.

86. Alexinsky, *With the Russian Wounded,* 101.

87. Semina, *Tragediia russkoi armii,* 1:35, 44–62, 84–87, 96–101, 130–139.

88. Varnek, "Vospominaniia," 16–17.

89. See, for example, the memoirs of Tatiana Aleksinskaia, Lidiia Zakharova, and Florence Farmborough.

90. The dangerous conditions of wartime nursing at the front, and parallels to male combat experience, will be explored in greater detail in chapter 4.

91. Farmborough, *With the Armies of the Tsar,* 148–149.

92. Zakharova, *Dnevnik sestry miloserdiia,* 35.

93. Watson, "Khaki Girls," 32–51.

94. Varnek, "Vospominaniia," 5–7.

95. The term "baba" was a somewhat derogatory word loosely translated as "broad" or "wench" and was almost always applied to women of the lower classes.

96. Varnek, "Vospominaniia," 6–7.

97. Tolstaia, *Doch'*, 230.

98. Dmitrii A. Furmanov, *Dnevnik (1914–1915–1916)* (Moscow: Moskovskii Rabochii, 1929), 25–26. I would like to thank Karen Petrone for directing me to this source.

99. Stites, *Women's Liberation Movement,* 279; Varnek, "Vospominaniia," 13.

100. Gourko, *War and Revolution in Russia,* 206.

101. Semina, *Tragediia Russkii armii,* 1:11, 16.

102. Tolstaia, *Doch'*, 230.

103. "Otchet doktora meditsny S. K. Solov'ev, zaveduiuvaiushchii meditsinkoi chastiu severnom front," RGVIA, f. 12674, op. 1, d. 10, 11. 383–384.

104. Buchanan, *City of Trouble*, 120.

105. Semina, *Tragediia Russkii armii,* 1:103.

106. Botcharsky and Pier, *Kinsmen Know How to Die,* 31.

107. Tolstaia, *Doch'*, 230.

108. Botcharsky and Pier, *Kinsmen Know How to Die,* 25.

109. B. Radonich, *Dnevnik sestry miloserdiia prozhivshei v Germanskom plenu bez malago 4 mesiatsa* (Petrograd: Biblioteka "Vechernago vremeni," 1915), 4.

110. Alexinsky, *With the Russian Wounded,* vi, 149.

CHAPTER 4. BLURRED BOUNDARIES. GENDER AND RUSSIAN WARTIME NURSING EXPERIENCE

1. Farmborough, *With the Armies of the Tsar*, 19–22.

2. Ibid., 27–30.

3. Ibid., 33, 36.

4. Some of the information and ideas presented in this chapter were originally published in Stoff, "Myth of the War Experience."

5. Margaret Higonnet, "Introduction," in Margaret Higonnet, ed., *Lines of Fire: Women Writers of World War I* (New York: Plume, 1999), xxii.

6. Margaret Higonnet, "Introduction," in Margaret Higonnet, ed., *Nurses at the Front: Writing the Wounds of the Great War* (Boston: Northeastern University Press, 2001), xiii.

7. Gavin, *American Women in World War I*, 43–66.

8. Christine Hallett has catalogued the numerous serious dangers Western nurses faced in wartime medical service. See Hallett, *Containing Trauma: Nursing Work in the First World War* (Manchester: Manchester University Press, 2009), 209–214.

9. A number of scholars of Russian women have noted this significant difference from the Western tradition. See, for example, Elizabeth A. Wood, *The Baba and the Comrade: Gender Politics in Revolutionary Russia* (Bloomington: Indiana University Press, 1997); Engelstein, *Keys to Happiness*.

10. Thurstan, *Text Book of War Nursing*, 22–23.

11. Farmborough, *With the Armies of the Tsar,* 152, 21.

12. Semina, *Tragediia russkoi armii,* 1:11.

13. N. I. Vladimirsteva, "Iz vospominaniia sestry miloserdiia F. N. Slepchenko," *Otechestvennye arkhivi* 6 (1994): 60.

14. Semina, *Tragediia russkoi armii,* 1:35.

15. Leonid Andrusov, as quoted by Joshua Sanborn, *Imperial Apocalypse: The Great War and the Destruction of the Russian Empire* (New York: Oxford University Press, 2014), 150. Many thanks to the author for allowing me to see an advance copy of the manuscript.

16. George L. Mosse, "Two World Wars and the Myth of the War Experience," *Journal of Contemporary History* 21, no. 4 (October 1986): 493.

17. Samuel Hynes, *The Soldiers' Tale: Bearing Witness to a Modern War* (New York: Penguin, 1997), 45–48.

18. Thurstan, *Field Hospital and Flying Column*, 133.

19. Chelakova, "Iz zapisok sestry miloserdiia," *Novoe Russkoe Slovo* (June 13, 1969): 8.

20. Stepanova, "Zapiskii velikoi voiny," 14.

21. Alexinsky, *With the Russian Wounded,* 30, 151.

22. Chelakova, "Iz zapisok sestry miloserdiia," *Novoe Russkoe Slovo* (June 17, 1969): 4.

23. Zakharova, *Dnevnik sestry miloserdiia,* 112.

24. Farmborough, *With the Armies of the Tsar,* 128.

25. Botcharsky and Pier, *Kinsmen Know How to Die*, 33.

26. *Vestnik Krasnago Kresta,* no. 1 (January 1915): 209; *Vestnik Krasnago Kresta* no. 5 (May 1915): 1860.

27. Botcharsky and Pier, *Kinsmen Know How to Die*, 64.

28. Reports to the Main Directorate of the Russian Society of the Red Cross from various command personnel of the armies of the Northern Front, RGVIA, f. 12675, op. 2, d. 2; Reports in *Vestnik Krasnago Kresta,* 1915–1916; Reports in *Vserossiskii Zemskii Soiuz pomoshchi bol'nym i ranenym voinam: Izvestiia Glavnogo Komiteta,* 1914–1916.

29. For more on women soldiers, see Stoff, *They Fought for the Motherland.* A fuller examination of representations of nurses in Russian culture during the war is provided in chapters 7 and 8.

30. A. A. Brussilov, *A Soldier's Notebook, 1914–1918* (London: Macmillan, 1930), 190.

31. See *Niva, Ogonek, Rech', Iskry, Voina,* 1914–1915.

32. "Sestra miloserdiia-geroi," *Niva,* April 11, 1915, 3.

33. Chelakova, "Iz zapisok sestry miloserdiia," *Novoe Russkoe Slovo* (June 18, 1969): 4.

34. Sanborn, *Drafting the Russian Nation,* 149.

35. Stoff, *They Fought for the Motherland,* 32.

36. Sanborn, *Drafting the Russian Nation,* 149.

37. See *Vestnik Krasnago Kresta,* 1914–1917.

38. Varnek, "Vospominaniia," 29.

39. Farmborough, *With the Armies of the Tsar,* 237–246.

40. Zakharova, *Dnevnik sestry miloserdiia,* 133–170.

41. "Lechenie Sester Miloserdiia," *Vestnik Krasnago Kresta,* no. 3 (March 1915): 912–913.

42. Tolstaia, *Doch',* 242.

43. Radonich, *Dnevnik sestry miloserdiia.*

44. Lensen, *War and Revolution,* 29.

45. Ol'ga Aleksandrovna Romanova, "Pisma c fronta Velikoi kniagina Ol'ga Aleksandrovnyi k plemiannitsam, Velikim Kniazhnam Ol'ge, Tat'iane, Marii i Anastasii, 1914 25 Avgusta g. Rovna," in N. K. Zvereva, ed., *Avgusteishie sestry miloserdiia* (Moscow: Veche, 2006), 257.

46. Zakharova, *Dnevnik sestry miloserdiia,* 46.

47. Farmborough, *With the Armies of the Tsar,* 148–149.

48. Varnek, "Vospominaniia," 9.

49. Zakharova, *Dnevnik sestry miloserdiia,* 26–27.

50. Semina, *Tragediia russkoi armii,* 1:30.

51. Zakharova, *Dnevnik sestry miloserdiia,* 33.

52. Chelakova, "Iz zapisok sestry miloserdiia," *Novoe Russkoe Slovo* (June 16, 1969): 4.

53. Chelakova, "Iz zapisok sestry," *Novoe Russkoe Slovo* (June 19, 1969): 9.

54. Botcharsky and Pier, *Kinsmen Know How to Die,* 26.

55. Alexinsky, *With the Russian Wounded,* 149.

56. Furmanov, *Dnevnik,* 40.

57. Botcharsky and Pier, *Kinsmen Know How to Die,* 10. Additional commentary on the effect of amputations on nurses is included in chapter 5.

58. The extent to which the war actually served such a purpose has been contested by those such as Mosse, *Fallen Soldiers.*

59. Ia. Okunev, *Na peredovykh pozitsiiakh, Na peredovykh pozitsiiakh: Boevyia vpechatleniia* (Petrograd, n.d.), 83, quoted in and translated by Petrone, *Great War in Russian Memory,* 88–89.

60. Sanborn, *Drafting the Russian Nation,* 111–112.

61. Vladimir Paduchov, *Zapiski nizhnego china 1916 god* (Moscow, 1931), 14, quoted in and translated by Joshua Sanborn, "Unsettling the Empire: Violent Migrations and Social Disaster in Russia during World War I," *Journal of Modern History* 77 (June 2005): 298.

62. Sanborn, *Drafting the Russian Nation,* 103.

63. Chelakova, "Iz zapisok sestry miloserdiia," *Novoe Russkoe Slovo* (June 16, 1969): 4.

64. Varnek, "Vospominaniia," 20.

65. Farmborough, *With the Armies of the Tsar,* 22.

66. Britnieva, *One Woman's Story*, 11.

67. Zakharova, *Dnevnik sestry miloserdiia,* 137–138.

68. Chelakova, "Iz zapisok sestry miloserdiia," 4.

69. Grand Duchess Marie, *Education of a Princess*, 187.

70. Romanova, "Pisma c fronta Velikoi," 257.

71. Thurstan, *Field Hospital and Flying Column,* 133.

72. Scholar George Mosse led this challenge, but others have concurred. See, for example, Mosse, *Fallen Soldiers*; Eric J. Leed, *No Man's Land: Combat and Identity in World War I* (Cambridge: Cambridge University Press, 1979).

73. Photograph and caption, *Niva,* January 10, 1915, 30.

74. Farmborough, *With the Armies of the Tsar,* front cover and frontispiece photograph.

75. Zakharova, *Dnevnik sestry miloserdiia,* 20, 73, 95.

76. Lensen, *War and Revolution,* 82.

77. Farmborough, *With the Armies of the Tsar,* 150.

78. Tolstaia, *Doch'*, 239, 245.

79. Semina, *Tragediia russkoi armii,* 1:31.

80. Tricia Starks, "*Papirosy,* Smoking, and the Anti-Cigarette Movement," in Tricia Starks and Matthew Romaniello, eds., *Tobacco in Russian History and Culture: From the Seventeenth Century to the Present* (New York: Routledge, 2009), 138.

81. "Otchet doktora meditsiny S. K. Solov'ev, zaveduiuvaiushchii meditsinkoi chastiu severnom front," RGVIA f. 12674, op. 1, d. 10, 1, 396.

82. The grand duchess had gone through the shortened training course and had served less than a month in the Red Cross before her appointment as head nurse.

83. See the memoirs of Grand Duchess Maria Pavlovna, Sofia Bocharskaia, and Aleksandra Tolstaia, among others.

84. Grand Duchess Marie, *Education of a Princess,* 187–188.

85. Alexinsky, *With the Russian Wounded,* 10.

86. Chelakova, "Iz zapisok sestry miloserdiia," 4.

87. "E. P. Samsonova," *Zhenshchina i voina,* March 5, 1915, 5–6.

88. Alexinsky, *With the Russian Wounded,* 13.

89. For more on these individuals, see Stoff, *They Fought for the Motherland,* 23–52.

90. Elena Gromova, "Sestra miloserdiia Rimma Ivanova. 115 let c dnia rozhdeniia," *Stavropol'skaia Pravda,* June 1, 2009. http://pda.stapravda.ru

/20090701/sestra_miloserdiya_rimma_ivanova_115_let_so_dnya_rozh deniya_38465.html.

91. Ibid. Ivanova's legacy will be discussed further in chapter 7.

92. Farmborough, *With the Armies of the Tsar,* 238, 242.

CHAPTER 5. PSYCHOLOGICAL WARFARE

1. Zakharova, *Dnevnik sestry miloserdiia* (1915), 5–11.
2. Ibid., 20–22.
3. Ibid., 24–29.
4. Kostyleva, "Nashi Amazonki," 24.
5. Botcharsky and Pier, *Kinsmen Know How to Die*, 46–47, italics added.
6. Chelakova, "Iz zapisok sestry miloserdiia," *Novoe Russkoe Slovo* (June 18, 1969): 4.
7. This concept will be explored more fully in chapter 7.
8. Hallett, *Containing Trauma*, 161.
9. Higonnet, "Introduction," *Nurses at the Front*, xvii.
10. Romanova, "Pisma c fronta Velikoi," 256.
11. Botcharsky and Pier, *Kinsmen Know How to Die,* 11–12, 218.
12. Tolstaia, *Doch',* 228.
13. Farmborough, *With the Armies of the Tsar,* 22.
14. Ibid., 119, 41–42, 102.
15. Thurstan, *Field Hospital and Flying Column,* 165–166.
16. "Sestry," *Vestnik Krasnago Kresta,* no. 2 (February 1915): 598.
17. Farmborough, *With the Armies of the Tsar,* 130–131.
18. Britnieva, *One Woman's Story,* 19.
19. Zakharova, *Dnevnik sestry miloserdiia,* 52.
20. Ibid., 98–99, 110–111, 113.
21. "Sestry," *Vestnik Krasnago Kresta,* 598.
22. Ernst Jünger, as quoted in Hynes, *Soldiers' Tale*, 68.
23. "Sestry," *Vestnik Krasnago Kresta*, 598.
24. Furmanov, *Dnevnik*, 20, 32.
25. Christopher Schultz, "The Self Separated from Violence: Spectacle, Material Appropriation, and Voices of Resistance on the Western Front, 1914–18," *Canadian Journal of History* 46 (Winter 2011): 568.
26. Chelakova, "Iz zapisok sestry miloserdiia," *Novoe Russkoe Slovo* (June 17, 1969): 4.
27. Farmborough, *With the Armies of the Tsar.*
28. Zakharova, *Dnevnik sestry miloserdiia,* 51–52.
29. Thurstan, *Field Hospital and Flying Column,* 172–173.
30. Ibid., 136.

31. Chelakova, "Iz zapisok sestry miloserdiia," *Novoe Russkoe Slovo* (June 14, 1969): 4.

32. Margaret R. Higonnet, "Authenticity and Art in Trauma Narratives of World War I," *Modernism/Modernity* 9, no. 1 (2002): 91–107.

33. There is extensive literature on the psychological effects of the war on soldiers in the West, particularly in Great Britain. See, for example, Leed, *No Man's Land*; Elaine Showalter, *The Female Malady: Women, Madness, and English Culture, 1830–1980* (London: Virago, 1987); Laurinda Stryker, "Mental Cases: British Shellshock—Politics of Interpretation," in Gail Braybon, ed., *Evidence, History and the Great War: Historians and the Impact of 1914–1918,* 3rd ed. (New York: Berghahn, 2008).

34. Jan Plamper, "Fear: Soldiers and Emotion in Russian Military Psychology," *Slavic Review* 68, no. 2 (Summer 2009): 261.

35. Paul Wanke, *Russian/Soviet Military Psychiatry, 1904–1945* (New York: Routledge, 2005), 30.

36. Plamper, "Fear," 261. See also Irina Sirotkina, "The Politics of Etiology: Shell Shock in the Russian Army, 1914–1918," in Angela Brintlinger and Ilya Vinitsky, eds., *Madness and the Mad in Russian Culture* (Toronto: University of Toronto Press, 2007), 117–129.

37. Showalter, *Female Malady*, 173.

38. Stryker, "Mental Cases," 156.

39. Laura L. Philips, "Gendered Dis/ability: Perspectives from the Treatment of Psychiatric Casualties in Russia's Early Twentieth-Century Wars," *Social History of Medicine* 20, no. 2 (August 2007): 334.

40. Sirotkina, "Politics of Etiology," 119–120, 127.

41. A. S. Preobrazhenskii, *Materialy k voprosu o dushevnykh zabolevaniiakh voinov i lits, prichastnykh k voennym deistviiam v sovremenoi voine* (Petrograd, 1917), 79–80.

42. Ibid., 155–156.

43. Thurstan, *Field Hospital and Flying Column,* 136–137.

44. Botcharsky and Pier, *Kinsmen Know How to Die,* 9.

45. Chelakova, "Iz zapisok sestry miloserdiia," 6.

46. Alexinsky, *With the Russian Wounded,* 1.

47. Botcharsky and Pier, *Kinsmen Know How to Die,* 10.

48. Tolstaia, *Doch'*, 231.

49. Farmborough, *With the Armies of the Tsar,* 220.

50. Britnieva, *One Woman's Story,* 35.

51. Wilfred Owen, "Dulce et Decorum Est," in *The Oxford Book of War Poetry,* ed. John Stallworthy (Oxford: Oxford University Press, 1988), 189.

52. Britnieva, *One Woman's Story,* 35.

53. Varnek, "Vospominaniia," 7.

54. Chelakova, "Iz zapisok sestry miloserdiia," 6.

55. Santanu Das, "'The Impotence of Sympathy': Touch and Trauma in

the Memoirs of the First World War Nurses," *Textual Practice* 19, no. 2 (2005): 239.

56. Vasilevskii, *Po sledam voiny,* 64; Stanley Washburn, *On the Russian Front in World War I: Memoirs of an American War Correspondent* (New York: Robert Speller & Sons, 1939), 113.

57. Higonnet, "Authenticity and Art," 92.

58. Quoted in Hynes, *Soldiers' Tale,* 56–57.

59. Plamper, "Fear," 262.

60. Ernst Jünger, *Storm of Steel* (New York: Penguin, 2004), 8.

61. Dmitrii Os'kin, *Zapiski soldata* (Moscow: Federatsiia, 1929), 274–276.

62. V. Dmitriev, *Dobrovolets: Vospominaniia o voine i plene* (Moscow: Gosizdat, 1929), 18.

63. Zakharova, *Zapiski sestry miloserdiia,* 54.

64. Semina, *Tragediia russkoi armii,* 1:44.

65. Quoted in Lessen, *War and Revolution,* 31.

66. Chelakova, "Iz zapisok sestry miloserdiia," *Novoe Russkoe Slovo* (June 17, 1969): 4.

67. L. N. Voitolovskii, *Po sledam voiny: Pokhodnye zapiski. 1914–1917* (Leningrad: Izdatel'stvo Pisatelei, 1925), 69, translated by and quoted in Plamper, "Fear," 260.

68. Zakharova, *Dnevnik sestry miloserdiia,* 110, 112.

69. Chelakova, "Iz zapisok sestry miloserdiia," *Novoe Russkoe Slovo* (June 14, 1969): 6.

70. Britnieva, *One Woman's Story*, 21–22.

71. Quoted in Hynes, *Soldiers' Tale,* 67.

72. Farmborough, *With the Armies of the Tsar,* 158–159.

73. Furmanov, *Dnevnik,* 20–21.

74. Chelakova, "Iz zapisok sestry miloserdiia," *Novoe Russkoe Slovo* (June 17, 1969): 4.

75. Farmborough, *With the Armies of the Tsar,* 43.

76. Preobrazhenskii, *Materialy k voprosu,* 156–157.

77. Catherine Merridale, "The Collective Mind: Trauma and Shell-Shock in Twentieth-Century Russia," *Journal of Contemporary History* 35, no. 1 (2000): 41.

78. Alexinsky, *With the Russian Wounded,* 109.

79. Tolstaia, *Doch',* 235.

80. Botcharsky and Pier, *Kinsmen Know How to Die*, 46, 217–218.

81. Zakharova, *Dnevnik sestry miloserdiia,* 116, 150–151.

82. Kati Dadeshkeliani, *Princess in Uniform,* trans. Arthur Ashton (London: G. Bell & Sons, 1934), 96, 97. Dadeshkeliani maintained her male guise for the remainder of the war, however, and continued to function successfully in this role, serving in a medical capacity until mid-1917. One might wonder why she did not just reveal her true sexual identity and enlist as a sister of mercy, but undoubtedly the male guise afforded the princess a much

greater range of opportunities and freedom than acting as a woman could have given her.

83. *Vestnik Krasnago Kresta,* 1915–1916.

84. Materials on the activities of the ROKK gathered for publication in the press. Report #272, January 9, 1915, RGVIA f. 12651, op. 10, d. 23, l. 363; Report #270, January 8, 1915, RGVIA f. 12651, op. 10, d. 23, l. 367; Report #704, March 28, 1915, RGVIA f. 12651, op. 10, d. 24, l. 59.

85. Semina, *Tragediia russkoi armii,* 2:57.

86. Furmanov, *Dnevnik,* 21.

CHAPTER 6. WOMEN AND MEN AT WAR. RELATIONS AND PERCEPTIONS

1. Chelakova, "Iz zapisok sestry miloserdiia," *Novoe Russkoe Slovo* (June 13, 1969): 3.

2. Ibid.

3. Chelakova, "Iz zapisok sestry miloserdiia,"*Novoe Russkoe Slovo* (June 14, 1969): 6.

4. Chelakova, "Iz zapisok sestry miloserdiia,"*Novoe Russkoe Slovo* (June 16, 1969): 4.

5. Ibid.

6. Zakharova, *Dnevnik sestry miloserdiia,* 177.

7. Botcharsky and Pier, *Kinsmen Know How to Die,* 8.

8. Darrow, "French Volunteer Nursing," 80–106.

9. Petrone, *Great War in Russian Memory*, 18.

10. Darrow, "French Volunteer Nursing," 81.

11. As quoted in Sanborn, *Imperial Apocalypse,* 145.

12. Zakharova, *Dnevnik sestry miloserdiia,* 156.

13. As quoted in N. D. Sudavtsov, "Geroina, protivopastavivshaia tevtonskoi zabronirovanmoi sile svoiu velikuiu liubiashchuiu dushu russkoi zhenshchiny," *Voenno-istoricheskii zhurnal*, no. 3 (2002): 47.

14. Alexinsky, *With the Russian Wounded,* 133–135.

15. Ibid., 141–158.

16. Ibid., 106.

17. Zakharova, *Dnevnik sestry miloserdiia,* 21.

18. Botcharsky and Pier, *Kinsmen Know How to Die,* 7.

19. Farmborough, *With the Armies of the Tsar,* 22.

20. A. Ul'ianov, *Liubov sil'nee vrazhdy: rasskazy sestry miloserdiia iz poslednei voiny* (Iaroslav: Tipografiia K. F. Nekrasova, 1915), 5.

21. Alexinsky, *With the Russian Wounded,* 62, 113–114.

22. Tolstaia, *Doch',* 228.

23. Zakharova, *Dnevnik sestry miloserdiia,* 45.

24. Botcharsky and Pier, *Kinsmen Know How to Die,* 27.

25. Alexinsky, *With the Russian Wounded,* 62.

26. Zakharova, *Dnevnik sestry miloserdiia,* 76.

27. Allison Scardino Belzer, *Women and the Great War: Femininity under Fire in Italy* (New York: Palgrave Macmillan, 2010), 99.

28. Chelakova, "Iz zapisok sestry miloserdiia," *Novoe Russkoe Slovo* (June 17, 1969): 4.

29. Farmborough, *With the Armies of the Tsar*, 46.

30. Tolstaia, *Doch'*, 229.

31. Botcharsky and Pier, *Kinsmen Know How to Die,* 14.

32. Stepanova, "Zapiski velikoi voiny 1914–1918 gg.," 62, 64, 67.

33. Alexinsky, *With the Russian Wounded,* 60.

34. Tolstaia, *Doch'*, 227.

35. Vasilii Shul'gin, *Poslednii ochevidets*, 260–261.

36. Alexinsky, *With the Russian Wounded,* 127.

37. Farmborough, *With the Armies of the Tsar*, 345.

38. Varnek, "Vospominaniia," 15.

39. Tolstaia, *Doch'*, 229.

40. Botcharsky and Pier, *Kinsmen Know How to Die,* 13.

41. Zakharova, *Dnevnik sestry miloserdiia,* 22, 133–134.

42. Vladimirsteva, "Iz vospominaniia sestry miloserdiia F. N. Slepchenko," 60.

43. Varnek, "Vospominaniia," 20, 12–13.

44. Botcharsky and Pier, *Kinsmen Know How to Die*, 24–25.

45. *Vestnik Krasnago Kresta,* February 1915, 728.

46. Varnek, "Vospominaniia," 10–11.

47. Stepanova, "Zapiski velikoi voiny 1914–1918 gg.," 58.

48. Alexinsky, *With the Russian Wounded,* 10.

49. Varnek, "Vospominaniia," 9.

50. Stepanova, "Zapiski velikoi voiny 1914–1918 gg.," 63–64.

51. Tolstaia, *Doch'*, 245.

52. Sanborn, *Drafting the Nation,* 146.

53. Jünger, *Storm of Steel*, 314.

54. Furmanov, *Dnevnik,* 21–23.

55. Sanborn, *Drafting the Nation,* 159–160.

56. Secret message to the Main Administration of the Red Cross from the Chief of Staff of the Dvinsk Military District, Department of the Military Sensor, November 6, 1914. RGVIA f. 12674 op. 1, d. 7, 1. 4.

57. Secret message from the Chief of Staff of the Dvinsk Military District, Department of the Military Sensor, to the Main Commission of the Society of the Red Cross with the armies of the Northwestern Front, November 12, 1914. RGVIA f. 12674 op. 1, d. 7, 1. 1.

58. O. D. Ul'ianova, "Maria Il'inichna Ul'ianova," in M. I. Ul'ianova, *O V. I. Lenine i sem'e Ul'ianovkh* (Moscow: Izdat. Polit. Liter., 1989), 26.

59. Message to the Main Military-Sanitary Inspector from the Assistant of the Supreme Head of the Sanitation and Evacuation Section, March 24, 1916, RGVIA f. 12651, op. 2, d. 547, 1. 2.

60. Message from the Assistant of the Supreme Head of the Sanitary and Evacuation Section, September 2, 1916, RGVIA f. 12651, op. 2, d. 547, 1. 12; Message to the Mobilization Department (n.d.), RGVIA f. 12651, op. 2, d. 547, 1. 15.

61. Alexinsky, *With the Russian Wounded,* 10.

62. Obzor perliustrirovannykh pisem 1914–1915, GARF, f. 102, op. 265, d. 1042, 1. 135.

63. Session #21 of the Mobilization Committee of ROKK, July 7, 1916, RGVIA f. 12651, op. 3, d. 416, 1. 251.

64. Session #17 of the Mobilization Committee of ROKK, July 14, 1916, RGVIA f. 12651, op. 3, d. 416, 1. 267.

65. Session #3 of the Mobilization Committee of ROKK, October 27, 1916, RGVIA f. 12651, op. 3, d. 418, 1. 154.

66. Session #11 of the Mobilization Committee of ROKK, March 18, 1916, RGVIA f. 12651, op. 3, d. 452, 1. 130.

67. Varnek, "Vospominaniia," 7.

68. Stepanova, "Zapiski velikoi voiny 1914–1918 gg.," 53.

69. "Otchet doktora meditsny S. K. Solov'ev, zaveduiuvaiushchii meditsinkoi chastiu severnom front," RGVIA f. 12674, op. 1, d. 10, 11. 386–389, 396.

70. Urgent secret message to the Saint George's Community of the Red Cross, Petrograd, from the Chief Doctor of Polotskii Mobile Field Hospital No. 3, December 22, 1914, RGVIA f. 12651, op. 3, d. 370, 1. 364.

71. Farmborough, *With the Armies of the Tsar,* 229–230.

72. Alexinsky, *With the Russian Wounded,* 95, 97, 98.

73. Furmanov, *Dnevnik*, 25–26.

74. Ibid., 27.

75. Copy of a letter to Aleksei Alekseivich from Baroness (?), Correspondence with the Main Authority of the ROKK on the Northwestern Front, f. 12651, op. 3, d. 370, 1. 370.

76. Session #38 of the Mobilization Committee of ROKK, June 17, 1917, RGVIA f. 12651, op. 3, d. 452, 1. 311.

77. Varnek, "Vospominaniia," 7–9.

78. Chelakova, "Iz zapisok sestry miloserdii," *Novoe Russkoe Slovo* (June 14, 1969): 6.

CHAPTER 7. IMAGINING SISTERS. REPRESENTATIONS OF WARTIME NURSES IN RUSSIAN POPULAR CULTURE

1. *Geroiskii podvig Sestry Miloserdiia Elizavety Bychkovoi* (Moscow: Tipographiia "Nashe Slovo," 1914), 3–7.
2. Ibid., 8.
3. Ibid., 9–10.
4. Ibid., 11.
5. Jeffrey Brooks, *When Russia Learned to Read: Literacy and Popular Literature, 1861–1917* (Princeton, N.J.: Princeton University Press, 1985).
6. Karen Petrone, "Family, Masculinity, and Heroism in Russian War Posters of the First World War," in Melman, *Borderlines*, 98.
7. Hubertus F. Jahn, *Patriotic Culture in Russia during World War I* (Ithaca, N.Y.: Cornell University Press, 1995), 4.
8. Ibid.
9. Ernest Gellner, *Nations and Nationalism* (Ithaca, N.Y.: Cornell University Press, 1983), 7.
10. Stephen Norris, *A War of Images: Russian Popular Prints, Wartime Culture, and National Identity, 1812–1945* (DeKalb: Northern Illinois University Press, 2006), 8, 9.
11. With some notable exceptions, including Josh Sanborn's work, as well as that of Peter Gatrell and Boris Kolonitskii.
12. Jahn, *Patriotic Culture in Russia,* 42.
13. Engel, *Women in Russia,* 129.
14. The negative portrayals of Russian sisters of mercy will be explored more fully in the next chapter.
15. Victoria Bonnell, *Iconography of Power: Soviet Political Posters under Lenin and Stalin* (Berkeley: University of California Press, 1997), 66.
16. Victoria Bonnell, "Representations of Women in Early Soviet Political Art," *Russian Review* 50, no. 3 (July 1991): 269.
17. Edmondson, *Feminism in Russia,* 158.
18. "Khronika zhenskago dela," *Zhenskoe Delo,* August 1, 1914, 22.
19. E. A. Klodt, "Na peredovykh positsiakh," *Zhenskoe Delo,* October 15, 1914, front cover.
20. "Odna iz mnogikh," *Vestnik Krasnago Kresta,* no. 2 (February 1915): 598.
21. Kolonitskii, *Tragicheskaia erotika,* 251–252.
22. Ibid., 253–254.
23. *Letopis' Voiny,* November 15, 1914, 205.
24. A high-society publication catering to Russia's elite, roughly equivalent to *Town and Country.*
25. O. Liatkovaskaia, "Sestra," *Ogonek,* January 4, 1915, 3.

Я вчера еще была усталая,
Никому ненужная, унылая . . . Жизнь творить давно уж перестала я,
Прокляла свою судьбу постылую . . . А сегодня мне светло и сладостно!
На руке моей повязка белая,
И туда, смерть, легко и радостно,
Я иду покорная и смелая . . . Просвистят над нами пули шалые,
Упадут ряды бойцов несметные,
И кресты сестер, багрово-алые
Замелькают ласково-приветные . . . Я, как мать, склонюсь над умирающим,
Дам ему всю ласку неизжитую.
И зажгусь сама огнем пылающим,
Никому ненужная, забытая,
Если смерть придет, умру спокойная.
Ведь и я цвела любовью братскую,
И теперь, наверное, достойна я
Лечь в могилу общую солдатскую . . .

26. L. M. Brailovskii, "Kukly v pol'zu detei, sirot voinov" (Moscow: T-vo koropechatni A. A. Levenson, 1914), color, 14" x 19". Hoover Institution Poster Collection, RU/SU 79.

27. "Moskva-ranenym," *Iskry,* November 30, 1914, 374. http://www.odin-fakt.ru/iskry.

28. "Zina Kotliarova. Volodia Shenfein," *Iskry,* August 31, 1914, 271.

29. "Pomogite zhertvam voiny. Mariupol.' Malenkiia prodavshchitsi v den' flazhkov 31-go avgusta," *Iskry,* September 21, 1914, 295.

30. "Malen'kiia sborshchitsy Fatima i Mariam Ishukovy," *Iskry*, December 14, 1914, 386.

31. D. Berdakin, "Sestry-Uteshchitel'nitsy," *Zhenskaia Zhizn',* October 7, 1914, 9. Perhaps ironically, this term would be used later in the war to describe nurses as prostitutes.

32. Jahn, *Patriotic Culture in Russia,* 21.

33. S. Mikheev, "Sestra Miloserdiia," *Novyi Satirykon,* September 25, 1914, 10:

У нее коричневое платье,
Белый фартук с символом Христа,
Ее вера—радостно проста:
Все вокруг—ее родные братья . . . В сердце боль, но точно боль ответа

На давно отцветшую любовь . . . Все привычно . . . Стены лазарета,
И бинты, и даже эта кровь . . . Перед ней все новые утраты,
И она встречает их шутя,
Лишь порою, выйдя из палаты,
Вдруг заплачет горько, как дитя! . . .

34. "Zhenshchina i Voina," *Zhenskaia Zhizn'*, October 7, 1914, 8.

35. Berdakin, "Sestry-Uteshchitel'nitsy," 9.

36. Sanborn, *Drafting the Russian Nation*, 147.

37. N. D. Alekseev, "V polevom gospitale . . . " (Moscow: Tipo-litografiia Chelnokova, 1914–1916?), color, 22" x 16". Hoover Institution Poster Collection, RU/SU-32.

38. Khristofor Shukhman, *Liubov Sestry Miloserdiia, ili mat' pod pul'iami i bombami* (Moscow: Tipografia "Lomonosov," 1915), iiv–viii.

39. Argus, "Kogda muzhchiny na fronte, vot gde vashe mesto, zhenshchiny!" (Russkoe Obshchestvo Pechatnogo Dela, n.d.), black and white, 25" x 36". Hoover Institution Poster Collection, RU/SU 1107.

40. I. Simov, "Geroiskii podvig sestry miloserdia . . . " (Moscow: T-vo Tipolitografiia I. M. Mashitova, 1914–1917), color, 17" x 23". Hoover Institution Poster Collection, RU/SU 353.

41. The contrast with the negative images of wartime nurses often associated with the rear will be developed in chapter 8.

42. Brusianin, *Voina, zhenshchiny i deti*, 61.

43. See *Vestnik Krasnago Kresta*, 1914–1916.

44. "Sestra Miloserdiia—geroi," *Niva*, April 11, 1915, 3.

45. "M. F. Kokh," *Letopis' Voiny*, November 29, 1914, 248.

46. *Letopis' Voiny*, November 21, 1915, 1062.

47. *Letopis' Voiny*, April 23, 1916, 1414.

48. A. Lavrov, untitled (Moscow: Nikol'skaia Obshchina R. O. Krasnago Kresta, n.d.), Helsinki University Slavonic Library (digitized image courtesy of Boris Kolonitskii).

49. P. Petrov, "Podvig Sestry E. P. Korkinoi" (Moscow: Litografiia T-va. I. D. Sytina, 1915), color, various sizes. Hoover Institution Poster Collection, RU/SU 322.

50. "Spasenie znameni. Gruppa M. Dillov (Patrioticheskaia vystavka kartin v Petrograd)," *Niva*, June 6, 1915, 442.

51. "Metamorfozy: Doma u na fronte" or "The Sketch," *Sinii Zhurnal*, November 25, 1916, 6.

52. Many members of the Russian public even accepted women who engaged directly in combat by becoming soldiers. For more public perception of women soldiers, see Stoff, *They Fought for the Motherland*, chapter 7.

53. As described in chapter 4. Iu. N. Khristinin, "Ne radi nagrad, no radi tokmo rodnogo narodu," *Voenno-Istoricheskii Zhurnal* 1 (1994): 92–93.

54. Ibid.; Sanborn, *Drafting the Russian Nation,* 149.

55. Vladimir Rogoza, "Pochemu Rimmu Ivanovu nazyvali Rossiskoi Zhannoi d'Ark?" *Shkola Zhizny, Posnavitel'nyi Zhurnal,* February 24, 2008. http://shkolazhizni.ru/archive/0/n-12952/.

56. Denise Youngblood, "Fade to Black: The Russian 'Bourgeois' Film Industry during War and Revolution," in Murray Frame, Boris Kolonitskii, Steven G. Marks, and Melissa K. Stockdale, eds., *Russian Culture in War and Revolution, 1914–22, Book 1: Popular Culture, the Arts, and Institutions* (Bloomington: Slavica Publishers of Indiana University, 2014), 85.

57. Norris, *War of Images,* 160–161.

58. B. V. Kudinov, "Nemetskiia zverstva. Zverstva kotoryia . . . ," (Moscow: Tipo-lit. T. D. Br. Evdokimy, 1914–1917?), color, 17" x 24". Hoover Institution Poster Collection, RU/SU 355.

59. A. A., "Zverstvo v Kalishe. Kalishskie sobytiia . . . " (Moscow: Tipo-Litografiia Relnokova, 1914–1917?), color, 14" x 22". Hoover Institution Poster Collection, RU/SU 448.

60. N. D. Alekseev, "Zverstvo nemstev" (publisher unknown, 1914–1917?), color, 16" x 22". Hoover Institution Poster Collection, RU/SU 445.

61. "Nevinnaia zhertva v rukakh kul'turnykh palachei" (Moscow: Tipo-lit. E. F. Chelnokova, 1914–1918?), color, 15" x 20". Hoover Institution Poster Collection RU/SU 334.

62. Prosvieshchennye varvary . . . " (Moscow: Litografiia t-va I. D. Sytina, 1915), copy #97, color, 17" x 22". Hoover Institution Poster Collection, RU/SU 382.

63. Jahn, *Patriotic Culture in Russia,* 165.

64. Valentina Kostyleva, "Zhenshchina, sem'ia, and voina," *Zhenskaia Zhizn',* September 1914, 28.

65. For more on this, see Vera S. Dunham, "The Strong Woman Motif," in *The Transformation of Russian Society,* ed. Cyril Black (Cambridge, Mass.: Harvard University Press, 1960), 459–483.

66. For fuller discussions of this concept, see Sanborn, *Drafting the Nation;* Petrone, "Family, Masculinity, and Heroism."

CHAPTER 8. "SISTERS OF COMFORT" AND "SISTERS WITHOUT MERCY"

1. Stepanova, "Zapiski velikoi voiny 1914–1918 gg.," 14.

2. The Battle of Tannenberg was the first major battle of the Great War on the eastern front. Despite an earlier victory at the Battle of Gumbinnen, Rus-

sian forces were completely routed during the German counterattack, leading to the destruction of the Russian Second Army after being entirely encircled by German forces.

3. Stepanova, "Zapiski velikoi voiny 1914–1918 gg.," 59, 65–67.

4. Orlando Figes and Boris Kolonitskii, *Interpreting the Russian Revolution: The Language and Symbols of 1917* (New Haven, Conn.: Yale University Press, 1999), 24.

5. Figes and Kolonitskii provide two examples of disparaging remarks made by soldiers about nurses. Their commentary, extrapolated out to include all nurses, is actually focused primarily on the image of Empress Alexandra. See ibid., 24.

6. Darrow, *French Women and the First World War.*

7. Penny Summerfield, "Gender and War in the Twentieth Century," *International History Review* 19, no. 1 (February 1997): 8.

8. Helen Goscilo, "Keeping A-Breast of the Waist-Land: Women's Fashion in Early Nineteenth-Century Russia," in *Russia—Women—Culture*, ed. Helen Goscilo and Beth Holmgren (Bloomington: Indiana University Press, 1996), 32.

9. Hacker, "Reformers, Nurses, and Ladies in Uniform," 137–188.

10. Alexinsky, *With the Russian Wounded,* 70–71.

11. Farmborough, *With the Armies of the Tsar,* 150.

12. As indicated in the previous chapter, although nursing in general was associated with the rear, many female medical personnel actually served very close to or at the front, and indeed, divisions between the front and rear were very difficult to maintain as a result of the constantly fluctuating battle lines on the eastern (Russian western) front.

13. For a fuller discussion of gendered and negative associations of the rear as compared to the front, see chapter 3 of Petrone's *Great War in Russian Memory*; quotation on 85–86.

14. "Obzor Perliustrirorovannykh pisem 1914–1915 gg.," GARF, f. 102, op. 265, d. 1042, l. 135. Department of the Police of the Ministry of Internal Affairs. Fifth Section (Secret), "Perliustratsii," 1889–1917.

15. See chapter 3 for specific examples of class antagonism between nurses.

16. Alon Rachamimov, "'Female Generals' and 'Siberian Angels': Aristocratic Nurses and the Austro-Hungarian POW Relief," in Nancy M. Wingfield and Maria Bucur, eds., *Gender and War in Twentieth-Century Eastern Europe* (Bloomington: Indiana University Press, 2006), 22–46.

17. Dunham, "Strong Woman Motif," 462.

18. See Barbara Heldt, *Terrible Perfection: Women and Russian Literature* (Bloomington: Indiana University Press, 1987), for examination of such characters.

19. Cathy A. Frierson, *Peasant Icons: Representations of Rural People in*

Late Nineteenth Century Russia (New York: Oxford University Press, 1993), 167–168.

20. Dunham, "Strong Woman Motif," 468.

21. Sanborn, *Drafting the Russian Nation,* 160.

22. Barbara Alpern Engel, "St. Petersburg Prostitutes in the Late Nineteenth Century: A Personal and Social Profile," *Russian Review* 48, no. 1 (January 1989): 21–44.

23. Engelstein, *Keys to Happiness*, 41.

24. Laura Engelstein, "Morality and the Wooden Spoon: Russian Doctors View Syphilis, Social Class, and Sexual Behavior, 1890–1905," *Representations* no. 14 (Spring 1986): 195.

25. Laurie Bernstein, "Yellow Tickets and State-Licensed Brothels: The Tsarist Government and the Regulation of Urban Prostitution," in Susan G. Solomon and John F. Hutchinson, eds., *Health and Society in Revolutionary Russia* (Bloomington: Indiana University Press, 1990), 45–65.

26. Laurie Bernstein, *Sonia's Daughters: Prostitutes and Their Regulation in Imperial Russia* (Berkeley: University of California Press, 1995), 294.

27. Peter Gatrell, "The Epic and the Domestic: Women and War in Russia," in Braybon, *Evidence, History, and the Great War*, 208.

28. Sanborn, *Drafting the Russian Nation*, 160.

29. "O zloupotreblenii zvaniem sester miloserdiia," *Vestnik Krasnago Kresta,* no. 3 (March 1915): 917–918.

30. Ibid., 917.

31. Commission for the Fight against the Misuse of the Name of Sister of Mercy, January 20, 1915, RGVIA f. 12651, op. 10, d. 23, 1. 336.

32. "O zloupotreblenii zvaniem sester miloserdiia," 918.

33. Curtiss, "Russian Sisters of Mercy," 84–100.

34. Christine Ruane, "Clothes Shopping in Imperial Russia: The Development of a Consumer Culture," *Journal of Society History* 28, no. 4 (Summer 1995): 773–774.

35. Secret documents sent to the Main Authority of the Society of the Red Cross for the Armies of the North-Western Front, RGVIA, f. 12674 op. 1 d. 7, 11. 1–4.

36. "Obzor Perliustrirorovannykh pisem 1914–1915 gg."

37. Maria Botchkareva, *Yashka: My Life as Peasant Officer and Exile* (New York: Frederick A. Stokes, 1919), 74.

38. V. V. Rozanov, *Poslednie list'ia. Poslednie list'ia 1916 god. Poslednie list'ia 1917 god. Voina 1914 goda i russkoe vozrozhdenie* (Moscow: Respublika, 2000), 181–185.

39. Chelakova, "Iz zapisok sestry miloserdiia," *Novoe Russkoe Slovo* (June 13, 1969): 8.

40. Brusilov, *Soldier's Notebook,* 190.

41. "Obzor Perliustrirorovannykh pisem 1914–1915 gg."

42. A. Flegon, *Eroticism in Russian Art* (London: Flegon, 1976), 214–215.

43. Farmborough, *With the Armies of the Tsar*, 151, 345.

44. Bernstein, *Sonia's Daughters,* 3.

CONCLUSIONS

1. See documents of the Russian Society of the Red Cross, RGIVA, f. 12651 Main Directorate of the Russian Society of the Red Cross (op. 1–13).

2. *Russkie vedomosti,* June 16, 1917, 4.

3. *Russkii invalid,* May 7, 1917, 3.

4. From the Commission on Women's Labor Conscription to the Minister of War, July 18, 1917, RGVIA, f. 2000, op. 2, d. 1557, 1. 83, 1. 91.

5. From the Minister of War to the Provisional Government, RGVIA, f. 2000, op. 2, d. 1557, 1. 84; Resolution of the Provisional Government, RGVIA, f. 2000, op. 2, d. 1557, 1. 85.

6. Report of the Commission on Women's Labor Conscription to the Chief of the General Staff, Sept. 11, 1917, RGVIA, f. 2000, op. 2, d. 1557, 1. 169.

7. Susan Grant, "Nursing in Russia and the Soviet Union, 1914–1941: An Overview of the Development of a Soviet Nursing System," *Bulletin of the UK Association for the History of Nursing* 2 (2012): 22–23.

8. Ann Eliot Griese and Richard Stites, "Russia: Revolution and War," in Nancy Loring Goldman, ed., *Female Soldiers: Combatants or Noncombatants? Historical and Contemporary Perspectives* (Westport, Conn.: Greenwood, 1982).

9. Reina Pennington, *Wings, Women, and War: Soviet Airwomen in World War II Combat* (Lawrence: University Press of Kansas, 2001).

10. Mohammad Yahya Nawroz and Lester W. Grau, "The Soviet War in Afghanistan: History and Harbinger of Future War?" *Military History,* September/October 1995, http://fmso.leavenworth.army.mil/documents/waraf.htm.

11. Carlotta Gall and Thomas de Waal, *Chechnya: Calamity in the Caucasus* (New York: New York University Press, 1998).

12. See, for example, Mosse, *Fallen Soldiers*; Higonnet et al., *Behind the Lines*; Darrow, *French Women and the First World War.*

13. For examples of this, see Sanborn, *Drafting the Russian Nation*; Petrone, "Family, Masculinity, and Heroism," 95–119.

14. Gatrell, "Epic and the Domestic," 202.

15. Gail Braybon, "Introduction," in *Evidence, History and the Great War*, 15.

16. Engelstein, *Keys to Happiness*, 422.

17. Sanborn, *Drafting the Russian Nation,* 146.

18. For a fuller articulation of this argument as it applied in France, see Darrow, "French Volunteer Nursing," 80–106.

19. Rochelle Ruthchild, *Equality and Revolution: Women's Rights in the Russian Empire, 1905–1917* (Pittsburgh, Penn.: University of Pittsburgh Press, 2010), 215.

BIBLIOGRAPHY

PRIMARY SOURCES

Archives

Gosudarstvennyi Arkhiv Rossiiskoi Federatsii
(GARF, State Archive of the Russian Federation), Moscow

F. 102 Department of the Police of the Ministry of Internal Affairs. Fifth Section (Secret)

Hoover Institution Library and Archives, Stanford University, Stanford, California

American National Red Cross Papers, Boxes 180–181
Pamphlet Collection
Poster Collection
Stepanova, Vanda Kazimirovna. Papers
Varnek, Tat'iana Aleksandrovna, "Vospominaniia 1912–1921," Box 1, 1–2
Von Etter, Maria. Papers 1895–1915
Vrangel, Mariia Dmitrievna (Box 19–20) File 13, Folder 40, Box 37

Rossiiskii Gosudarstvennyi Voenno-Istoricheskii Arkhiv
(RGVIA, Russian State Military-Historical Archive), Moscow

F. 12651 Main Directorate of the Russian Society of the Red Cross (op. 1–13)
F. 12656 Separate Commission of the Russian Society of the Red Cross for Evacuation of the Ill and Wounded in the Moscow Military District (op. 1)
F. 12674 Directorate of the Main Commission of the Russian Society of the Red Cross under the Armies of the Northwestern front (op. 1–5)
F. 12675 Directorate of the Main Commission of the Russian Society of the Red Cross under the Armies of the Northern front (op. 1–8)
F. 12676 Directorate of the Main Commission of the Russian Society of the Red Cross under the Armies of the Western front (op. 1–10)

F. 12677 Directorate of the Main Commission of the Russian Society of the Red Cross under the Armies of the Southern front (op. 1)

Periodicals

Damskii Mir
Izvestii Glavnogo Komiteta: Vserossiiksii Soiuz Pomoshchi Bol'nym i Ranenym Voinam
Iskry
Izvestii Vserossiiskago Soiuza Gorodov
Mir Zhenshchiny
Niva Novyi Satirykon
Ogonek
Petrogradskii Listok
Rech'
Russkiia Vedemosti
Russkoe Slovo
Sinii Zhurnal
Solntse Rossii
Stolitsa i Usadba
Vestnik Krasnago Kresta
Voina
Voina i Evrei
Zhenskaia Zhizh'
Zhenskoe Delo
Zhenskii Vestnik
Zhenshchina i Voina
Zhurnal dlia Koziaek

Personal and Contemporary Accounts

Aleksinskaia, Tatiana. *Zhenshchina v voine i revoliutsii.* Petrograd, 1917.

Alexinsky, Tatiana. *With the Russian Wounded.* Translated by Gilbert Cannan. London: T. F. Unwin, Ltd., 1916.

Ansky, S. *The Enemy at His Pleasure: A Journey through the Jewish Pale of Settlement during World War I.* Translated and edited by Joachim Neugroschel. New York: Henry Holt, 2002.

Bazilevich, M. P. *Polozhenie Russkikh plennykh v Germanii i otnoshenie Germantsev k naseleniu zaniatykh imi oblastei tsarstva Pol'skago i Litvy.* Petrograd, 1917.

Bogdanov, Aleksandr. *Voina i zhenshchina.* Petrograd, 1914.

Botcharsky, Sophie, and Florida Pier. *The Kinsmen Know How to Die (Being a Narrative of the Personal Experiences of a Red Cross Sister on the Russian Front).* New York: William Morrow, 1931.

Botchkareva, Maria. *Yashka: My Life as Peasant, Soldier, and Exile* (as told to Isaac Don Levine).. New York: Frederick A. Stokes, 1919.
Britnieva, Mary. *One Woman's Story.* London: Arthur Barker, 1936.
Brusianin, V. V. *Voina, zhenshchiny i deti.* Petrograd: Kinoizdatel'stvo "Mlechny Put'," 1917.
Brussilov, A. A. *A Soldier's Note-book, 1914–1918.* London: Macmillan, 1930.
Buchanan, Meriel. *The City of Trouble.* New York: Charles Scribner's Sons, 1918.
Chelakova, N. "Iz zapisok sestry miloserdiia." *Novoe Russkoe Slovo* (June 13–18, 1969): 4–8.
Dadeshkeliani, Kati. *Princess in Uniform.* Translated by Arthur Ashton. London: G. Bell & Sons, 1934.
Dmitriev, V. *Dobrovolets: Vospominaniia o voine i plene.* Moscow: Gosizdat, 1929.
Dorr, Rheta Childe. *Inside the Russian Revolution.* New York: Macmillan, 1917.
Farmborough, Florence. *With the Armies of the Tsar: A Nurse at the Russian Front in War and Revolution, 1914–1918.* New York: Cooper Square, 2000.
Fedorchenko, Sof'ia. *Narod na voine. Frontovyia zapisi.* Kiev: Izdanie Izdatel'skago Podotdela, 1917; Moscow: Sovietskii Pisatel', 1990.
Furmanov, Dmitrii A. *Dnevnik (1914–1915–1916).* Moscow: Moskovskii Rabochii, 1929.
Geroiskii podvig Sestry Miloserdiia Elizavety Bychkovoi. Moscow: Tipographiia "Nashe Slovo," 1914.
Gourko, General Basil. *War and Revolution in Russia, 1914–1917.* New York: Macmillan, 1919.
Hoff, John VanR. "The Soldier Nurse." *American Journal of Nursing* 11, no. 5 (February 1911): 342–346.
Iureva, Kseniia. *Rasskazy: sestry miloserdiia.* 2 vols. Göttingen, 1948.
Jünger, Ernst. *Storm of Steel.* New York: Penguin, 2004.
Kostyleva, Valentina. "Nashi Amazonki." *Zhenskaia Zhizn',* October 1914.
Lessen, George Alexander, ed. *War and Revolution: Excerpts from the Letters and Diaries of the Countess Olga Poutiatine.* Tallahassee, Fla.: Diplomatic Press, 1971.
L'vov, Prince Georgi V. *The Russian Union of Zemstvos.* London: P. S. King & Sons, 1917.
Marie, Grand Duchess of Russia. *Education of a Princess.* London: Viking, 1930.
Mikhailov, D. *Karmannyi meditsinskii spravochnik dlia voennykh feldsherov, sester i bratev miloserdiia, samaritian i samaritianok, voennykh farmatsevtov, veterinarnykh feldsherov, feldsherskikh uchenikov, voennykh sanitarov i dezinfektorov.* Petrograd: Knigoizdatel'stvo "Sotrudnik," 1915.

———. *Krasnyi Krest i sestry miloserdiia v Rossii i za-granitsei.* Petrograd-Kiev: Knigoizdatel'stvo "Sotrudnik," 1914.

———. *Spravochnaia kniga po voenno-sanitarnomu delu: Prakticheskoe rukovodstvo dlia voennykh vrachei i deiatelei po voenno-sanitarnoi chasti.* Petrograd-Kiev: Knigoizdatel'stvo "Sotrudnik," 1915.

Nikoforov, S. I. *Zhenshchiny geroi na voine, ili Znai nashikh bab!* Odessa, 1914.

Ocherk deiatelnosti Petrogradskoi oblastnoi organizatsii Vserossiiskago soiuza gorodov za pervyi god voiny. Petrograd, 1917.

Os'kin, Dmitrii. *Zapiski soldata.* Moscow: Federatsiia, 1929.

Owen, Wilfred. "Dulce et Decorum Est." In *The Oxford Book of War Poetry,* edited by John Stallworthy, 189. Oxford: Oxford University Press, 1988.

Pirogovskii s"ezd vrachei i predstavitelei organizatsii zemstv i gorodov. Petrograd, 1916.

Preobrazhenskii, A. S. *Materialy k voprosu o dushevnykh zabolevaniiakh voinov i lits, prichastnykh k voennym deistviiam v sovremenoi voine.* Petrograd, 1917.

Radonich, B. *Dnevnik sestry miloserdiia: prozhivshe: v germanskom plenu: bez malago 4 mesiatsa.* Petrograd: Biblioteka "Vecherniago vremeni," 1915.

Rodzianko, Mikhail. *The Reign of Rasputin.* Translated by Catherine Zvegintzoff. Gulf Breeze, Fla.: Academic International Press, 1973.

Romanoff, Alexandra. "An Appeal from Russia: An Open Letter to American Nurses." *American Journal of Nurses* 2, no. 3 (1922): 226–229.

Romanova, Ol'ga Aleksandrovna. "Pisma c fronta Velikoi kniagina Ol'ga Aleksandrovnyi k plemiannitsam, Velikim kniazhnam Ol'ge, Tat'iane, Marii i Anastasii." In *Avgusteishie sestry miloserdiia*, edited by N. K. Zvereva, 255–284. Moscow: Veche, 2006.

Rossisskoe Obshchestvo Krasnago Kresta, Sbornik glavneishikh kasaiushikhsia i glavneishikh tsirkuliarov Glavnago Upravleniia nazvannago obshchestva. Petrograd: Gosudarstvennaia tipigrafiia, 1917.

Rozanov, V. V. *Poslednie list'ia. Poslednie list'ia 1916 god. Poslednie list'ia 1917 god. Voina 1914 goda i russkoe vozrozhdenie.* Moscow: Respublika, 2000.

Sbornik glavnieishikh, kasaiushchikhsia deiatel'nosti Rossiiskago Obshchestva Krasnago Kresta zakonopolozhenii i glavneishikh deistvuiushchikh tsirkuliarov Glavnago Upravleniia nazvannogo obshchestva. Saint Petersburg, 1914.

Semina, Khristina. *Tragediia russkoi armii pervoi velikoi voiny 1914–1918 gg.: Zapiski sestry miloserdiia kavkazskogo fronta.* 2 vols. New Mexico: privately published, 1963.

Shukhman, Khristofor. *Liubov Sestry Miloserdiia, ili mat' pod pul'iami i bombami.* Moscow: Tipografia "Lomonosov," 1915.

Shul'gin, Vasilii. *Poslednii ochevidets: Memuary. Ocherki. Sny.* Moscow: OLMA-PRESS Zveznyi mir, 2002.

Shul'gin, Vitalii. *O sostoianii zhenshchin v Rossii do Petra Velikago: Istoricheskoe issledovanie.* Kiev, 1850.

Spear, Raymond. *Report on the Russian Medical and Sanitary Features of the Russo-Japanese War to the Surgeon-General, U.S. Navy.* Washington, D.C.: Government Printing Office, 1906.

Stepun, Fedor. *Byvshee i nesbyvsheesia.* 2nd ed. Saint Petersburg: Aleteiia, 2000.

———. *Iz pisem praporshchika artillirista.* Prague: Plamia, 1926.

Thurstan, Violetta. *Field Hospital and Flying Column: Being the Journal of an English Nursing Sister in Belgium and Russia.* London: G. P. Putnam's Sons, 1915.

———. *A Text Book of War Nursing.* London: G. P. Putnam's Sons, 1917.

Tolstaia, Aleksandra. *Doch'.* Moscow: Vagrius, 2000.

Tsentral'noe Statisticheskoe Upravlenie, Otdel Voennoi Statistiki. *Rossiia v mirovoi voine, 1914–1918 goda (v tsifrakh).* Moscow: Tipografia M.K.Kh. imeni F. Ia. Lavrova, 1925.

Ul'ianov, A. *Liubov sil'nee vrazhdy: rasskazy sestry miloserdiia iz poslednei voiny.* Iaroslav: Tipografiia K. F. Nekrasova, 1915.

Varnek, T., M. Bocharnikova, and Z. S. Mokievskaia-Zubok. *Dobrovolitsy: sbornik vospominanii.* Moskva: Russkii put', 2001.

Vasilevich, M. N. *Polozhenie russkikh plennykh v Germanii i otnoshennie Germanstev k nasileniiu zaniatykh imi oblastei Tsarstva Polskago i Litvy.* Petrograd, 1917.

Vasilevskii, L. M. *Po sledam voiny: vpechatleniia voennago vracha.* Petrograd: Tip. Imp. Nikolaev. Voen. Akad., 1916.

Vladimirsteva, N. I. "Iz vospominaniia sestry miloserdiia F. N. Slepchenko." *Otechestvennye arkhivi* 6 (1994): 58–72.

Voitolovskii, L. *Po sledam voiny: pokhodnye zapiski. 1914–1917.* Leningrad: Izdatel'stvo Pisatelei, 1925.

Vospominaniia vrachei Iulii A. Kviatkovskoi i Marii P. Rashkovich i kratkiia biografii N.A. i S. P. Doroshevskikh. Paris, 1937.

Vyrubova, Anna. *Memories of the Russian Court.* New York: Macmillan, 1923.

Washburn, Stanley. *On the Russian Front in World War I: Memoirs of an American War Correspondent.* New York: Robert Speller & Sons, 1939.

Zakharova, Lidiia. *Dnevnik sestry miloserdiia (na peredovykh pozitsiiakh).* Petrograd: Izdatel'stvo biblioteka "Velikoi Voiny," 1915.

Zhurnal zasedaniia ispolnitel'nago biuro Vserossiiskogo Gorodskogo Soiuza, 1914 g. Moscow: Vserossiskii Gorodskii Soiuz, 1914.

Zververa, N. K., ed. *Avgusteishie sestry miloserdiia.* Moscow: Veche, 2006.

Secondary Sources

Astrov, Nicholas. *The War and the Russian Government: The Municipal Government and the All-Russian Union of Towns.* New Haven, Conn.: Yale University Press, 1929.

Beliakova, N. A. *Sestry miloserdiia Rossii.* Saint Petersburg, 2005.

Belzer, Allison Scardino. *Women and the Great War: Femininity under Fire in Italy.* New York: Palgrave Macmillan, 2010.

Bermeo, Nancy, and Philip Nord, eds. *Civil Society before Democracy: Lessons from Nineteenth-Century Europe.* Lanham, Md.: Rowman & Littlefield, 2000.

Bernstein, Laurie. *Sonia's Daughters: Prostitution and Their Regulation in Imperial Russia.* Berkeley: University of California Press, 1995.

———. "Yellow Tickets and State-Licensed Brothels: The Tsarist Government and the Regulation of Urban Prostitution." In Solomon and Hutchinson, 45–65.

Bessonov, Yuri. "Russian Nurses after the Crimean War: Bureaucracy and Prejudice against Nurses," *RN Journal of Nursing,* http://www.rnjournal.com/journal_of_nursing/russian_nurses_after_the_crimean_war.htm.

Blokhina, N. N. "Moskovskie obshchiny sester miloserdiia v XIX—nachale XX veka." *Problemy sotsial'noi gigieny, zdravookhraneniia i istorii meditsiny* 5 (1997): 52–54.

Bonnell, Victoria. *Iconography of Power: Soviet Political Posters under Lenin and Stalin.* Berkeley: University of California Press, 1997.

———. "Representations of Women in Early Soviet Political Art." *Russian Review* 50, no. 3 (July 1991): 267–288.

Bourke, Joanna. *Dismembering the Male: Men's Bodies, Great Britain, and the Great War.* Chicago: University of Chicago Press, 1996.

Bradley, Joseph. "Subjects into Citizens: Societies, Civil Society, and Autocracy in Tsarist Russia." *American Historical Review* 107, no. 4 (October 2002): 1094–1123.

———. *Voluntary Associations in Tsarist Russia: Science, Patriotism, and Civil Society.* Cambridge, Mass.: Harvard University Press, 2009.

Braybon, Gail, ed. *Evidence, History and the Great War: Historians and the Impact of 1914–1918.* 3rd ed. New York: Berghahn, 2008.

———. *Women Workers in the First World War.* London: Routledge, 1989.

Brooks, Jeffrey. *When Russia Learned to Read: Literacy and Popular Literature, 1861–1917.* Princeton, N.J.: Princeton University Press, 1985.

Brower, Daniel. *Estate, Class, and Community: Urbanization and Revolution in Late Tsarist Russia.* Pittsburgh, Penn.: University of Pittsburgh Press, 1983.

Chatterjee, Choi, and Karen Petrone. "Models of Selfhood and Subjectivity: The Soviet Case in Historical Perspective." *Slavic Review* 67, no. 4 (Winter 2008): 967–986.

Clements, Barbara Evans, Barbara Alpern Engel, and Christine D. Worobec, eds. *Russia's Women: Accommodation, Resistance, Transformation.* Berkeley: University of California Press, 1991.

Cohen, Aaron. *Imagining the Unimaginable: World War, Modern Art, and the Politics of Public Culture in Russia, 1914–1917*. Lincoln: University of Nebraska Press, 2008.

———. "Oh, That! Myth, Memory, and World War I in the Russian Emigration and the Soviet Union." *Slavic Review* 62 (Spring 2003): 69–86.

Cott, Nancy F. "Marriage and Women's Citizenship in the United States, 1830–1934." *American Historical Review* 103, no. 5 (1998): 1440–1474.

Crofton, Eileen. *The Women of Royaumont: A Scottish Women's Hospital on the Western Front*. East Linton, U.K.: Tuckwell, 1997.

Curtiss, John. "Russian Sisters of Mercy in the Crimea, 1854–1855." *Slavic Review* 25, no. 1 (1966): 84–100.

Darrow, Margaret. "French Volunteer Nursing and the Myth of War Experience in World War I." *American Historical Review* 101, no. 1 (February 1996): 80–101.

———. *French Women and the First World War: War Stories of the Home Front*. New York: Berg, 2000.

Das, Santanu. "'The Impotence of Sympathy': Touch and Trauma in the Memoirs of First World War Nurses." *Textual Practice* 19, no. 2 (2005): 239–262.

Donner, Henriette. "Under the Cross: Why V.A.D.s Performed the Filthiest Task in the Dirtiest War: Red Cross Women Volunteers, 1914–1918." *Journal of Social History* 30, no. 3 (Spring 1997): 687–704.

Dunham, Vera S. "The Strong Woman Motif." In *The Transformation of Russian Society*, edited by Cyril Black, 459–483. Cambridge, Mass.: Harvard University Press, 1960.

Edmondson, Linda. *Feminism in Russia, 1900–1917*. Stanford, Calif.: Stanford University Press, 1984.

Engel, Barbara. "St. Petersburg Prostitutes in the Late Nineteenth Century: A Personal and Social Profile." *Russian Review* 48, no. 1 (January 1989): 21–44.

———. *Women in Russia, 1700–2000*. Cambridge: Cambridge University Press, 2004.

Engelstein, Laura. "The Dream of Civil Society in Tsarist Russia: Law, State, and Religion." In Bermeo and Nord, 23–41.

———. *The Keys to Happiness: Sex and the Search for Modernity in Fin-de-Siècle Russia*. Ithaca, N.Y.: Cornell University Press, 1992.

———. "Morality and the Wooden Spoon: Russian Doctors View Syphilis, Social Class, and Sexual Behavior, 1890–1905." *Representations* no. 14 (Spring 1986): 169–208.

Figes, Orlando, and Boris Kolonitskii. *Interpreting the Russian Revolution: The Language and Symbols of 1917*. New Haven, Conn.: Yale University Press, 1999.

Flegon, A. *Eroticism in Russian Art.* London: Flegon, 1976.

Freeze, Gregory. "The *Soslovie* (Estate) Paradigm and Russian Social History." *American Historical Review* 91, no. 1 (February 1986): 11–36.

Frierson, Cathy A. *Peasant Icons: Representations of Rural People in Late Nineteenth Century Russia.* New York: Oxford University Press, 1993.

Gall, Carlotta, and Thomas de Waal. *Chechnya: Calamity in the Caucasus.* New York: New York University Press, 1998.

Gatrell, Peter. "The Epic and the Domestic: Women and War in Russia." In Braybon, *Evidence,* 198–215.

———. *Russia's First World War: A Social and Economic History.* Harlow, U.K.: Pearson, 2005.

———. *A Whole Empire Walking: Refugees in Russia during World War I.* Bloomington: Indiana University Press, 1999.

Gavin, Lettie. *American Women in World War I: They Also Served.* Boulder: University Press of Colorado, 2006.

Gellner, Ernest. *Nations and Nationalism.* Ithaca, N.Y.: Cornell University Press, 1983.

Gleason, William. "The All-Russian Union of Towns and the All-Russian Union of Zemstvos in World War I: 1914–1917." PhD dissertation, Indiana University, 1972.

———. "The Zemstvo Union and World War I." In *The Zemstvo in Russia,* edited by Terrence Emmons and Wayne S. Vucinich, 365–382. Cambridge: Cambridge University Press, 1982.

Glickman, Rose. "The Peasant Woman as Healer." In Clements et al., 148–162.

Goldie, Sue M., ed. *"I Have Done My Duty": Florence Nightingale in the Crimean War, 1854–56.* Iowa City: University of Iowa Press, 1987.

Goscilo, Helen. "Keeping A-Breast of the Waist-Land: Women's Fashion in Early Nineteenth-Century Russia." In *Russia—Women—Culture,* edited by Helen Goscilo and Beth Holmgren, 31–63. Bloomington: Indiana University Press, 1996.

Grant, Susan. "Nursing in Russia and the Soviet Union, 1914–1941: An Overview of the Development of a Soviet Nursing System." *Bulletin of the UK Association for the History of Nursing* 2 (2012): 21–33.

Grayzel, Susan. *Women and the First World War.* London: Pearson, 2002.

———. *Women's Identities at War: Gender, Motherhood, and Politics in Britain and France during the First World War.* Chapel Hill: University of North Carolina Press, 1999.

Griese, Ann Eliot, and Richard Stites. "Russia: Revolution and War." In *Female Soldiers: Combatants or Noncombatants? Historical and Contemporary Perspectives,* edited by Nancy Loring Goldman. Westport, Conn.: Greenwood, 1982.

Gromova, Elena. "Sestra miloserdiia Rimma Ivanova. 115 let c dnia rozhdeniia," *Stavropol'skaia Pravda,* June 1, 2009, http://pda.stapravda.ru

/20090701/sestra_miloserdiya_rimma_ivanova_115_let_so_dnya_rozhdeniya_38465.html.

Gronsky, Paul P. *The War and the Russian Government: The Central Government.* New Haven, Conn.: Yale University Press, 1929.

Hacker, Barton C. "Reformers, Nurses, and Ladies in Uniform: The Changing Status of Military Women (c. 1815–c. 1914)." In *A Companion to Women's Military History,* edited by Barton C. Hacker and Margaret Vining, 137–188. Leiden, Netherlands: Koninklijke Brill, 2012.

———. "Women and Military Institutions in Early Modern Europe: A Reconnaissance." *Signs* 6, no. 4 (Summer 1981): 643–644.

Hagemann, Karen, ed. *Home/Front—Military, War, and Gender in Twentieth-Century Germany.* Oxford: Berg, 2002.

Hallett, Christine. *Containing Trauma: Nursing Work in the First World War.* Manchester, U.K.: Manchester University Press, 2009.

———. "Russian Romances: Emotionalism and Spirituality in the Writings of 'Eastern Front' Nurses, 1914–1918." *Nursing History Review* 17, no. 1 (January 1, 2009): 102–128.

Harris, Kristy. "In the 'Grey Battalion': Launceston General Hospital Nurses on Active Service in World War I." *Health and History* 10 (2008): 21–40.

Healy, Maureen. "Becoming Austrian: Women, the State, and Citizenship in World War I." *Central European History* 35, no. 1 (2002): 1–35.

Heldt, Barbara. *Terrible Perfection: Women and Russian Literature.* Bloomington: Indiana University Press, 1987.

Higonnet, Margaret. "Authenticity and Art in Trauma Narratives of World War I." *Modernism/Modernity* 9, no. 1 (2002): 91–107.

———, ed. *Lines of Fire: Women Writers of World War I.* New York: Plume, 1999.

———, ed. *Nurses at the Front: Writing the Wounds of the Great War.* Boston: Northeastern University Press, 2001.

Higonnet, Margaret, Jane Jenson, Sonya Michel, and Margaret Weitz, eds. *Behind the Lines: Gender and the Two World Wars.* New Haven, Conn.: Yale University Press, 1987.

Hutchinson, John. *Champions of Charity: War and the Rise of the Red Cross.* Boulder, CO: Westview, 1996.

———. *Politics and Public Health in Revolutionary Russia, 1890–1918.* Baltimore: Johns Hopkins University Press, 1990.

Hynes, Samuel. *The Soldiers' Tale: Bearing Witness to a Modern War.* New York: Penguin, 1997.

———. *A War Imagined: The First World War and English Culture.* London: Bodley Head, 1990.

Ivanova, Iu. H. *Khrabreishchie iz prekrasnykh: Zhenshchiny Rossii v voinakh.* Moscow: Rossiiskaia Politicheskaia Entsiklopediia, 2002.

Jahn, Hubertus F. *Patriotic Culture in Russia during World War I.* Ithaca, N.Y.: Cornell University Press, 1995.

Jensen, Kimberly. "A Base Hospital Is Not a Coney Island Dance Hall: American Women Nurses, Hostile Work Environment, and Military Rank in the First World War." *Frontiers: A Journal of Women's Studies* 26, no. 2 (2005): 206–235.

———. *Mobilizing Minerva: American Women in the First World War.* Urbana: University of Illinois Press, 2008.

Johanson, Christine. "Autocratic Politics, Public Opinion, and Women's Medical Education during the Reign of Alexander II, 1855–1881." *Slavic Review* 38, no. 3 (September 1979): 426–443.

———. *Women's Struggle for Higher Education in Russia, 1855–1900.* Kingston, Ont.: McGill–Queens University Press, 1987.

Karpycheava, L. A. "Kto takie *sestry miloserdiia?* Ot istoricheskoi etimologii k sovremennomu kontekstu." *Pravoslavnyi Letopisets Sankt-Peterburga* 24 (2005): 11–28. http://www.omophor.ru/articles/kto-takie-sestry-miloserdiya-ot-istoricheskoy-etimologii-k-sovremennomu-kontekstu.

———. "Obshchiny sester miloserdiia i pravoslavnaia tserkov." http://www.omophor.ru/articles/obshchiny-sester-miloserdiya-i-pravoslavnaya-cerkov.

Khechikov, Iurii. *Angely-Khraniteli: Stranitsy istorii Otechestva.* Moscow: RIA DIUM, 1996.

Khristinin, Iu. N. "Ne radi nagrad, no radi tokmo rodnogo narodu." *Voenno-Istoricheskii Zhurnal* 1 (1994): 92–93.

Kohn, Stanislas. *The Cost of the War to Russia: The Vital Statistics of European Russia during the World War, 1914–1917.* New Haven, Conn.: Yale University Press, 1932.

Kolonitskii, Boris. *Tragicheskaia erotika: Obraz imperatorskoi sem'i v gody Pervoi mirovoi voiny.* Moscow: Novoe literaturnoe obozrenie, 2010.

Kozlovtseva, Elena N. "Moskovskie obshchiny sester miloserdiia vo vtoroi polovine XIX—nachale XX vekova." Dissertation, Moscow State University, 2006. http://www.temples.ru/kozlovtseva.php.

Krylova, Anna. *Soviet Women in Combat: A History of Violence on the Eastern Front.* Cambridge: Cambridge University Press, 2010.

Kuhlman, Erika. *Reconstructing Patriarchy after the Great War: Women, Gender, and Postwar Reconciliation between Nations.* New York: Palgrave Macmillan, 2008.

Kuznetskaia, L., and K. Mashtakova. *Mariia Ul'ianova.* Moscow: Molodaia gvardiia, 1979.

Lee, Janet. "A Nurse and a Soldier: Gender, Class, and National Identity in the First World War Adventures of Grace McDougall and Flora Sandes." *Women's History Review* 15 (March 2006): 83–100.

Leed, Eric J. *No Man's Land: Combat and Identity in World War I.* Cambridge: Cambridge University Press, 1979.

Lensen, George A., trans. and ed. *War and Revolution: Excerpts from the Letters and Diaries of the Countess Ol'ga Poutiatine*. Tallahassee, Fla.: Diplomatic Press, 1971.

Light, Sue. "British Military Nurses and the Great War: A Guide to Services." http://www.westernfrontassociation.com/great-war-on-land/casualties-medcal/1140-british-military-nurses-and-the-great-war-a-guide-to-the-services.html.

Lindenmeyr, Adele. "Public Life, Private Virtues: Women in Russian Charity, 1762–1914." *Signs: Journal of Women in Culture & Society* 18, no. 3 (Spring 1993): 562–592.

Lohr, Eric. "The Ideal Citizen and Real Subject in Late Imperial Russia." *Kritika: Explorations in Russian and Eurasian History* 7, no. 2 (Spring 2006): 173–194.

———. "The Russian Army and the Jews: Mass Deportation, Hostages, and Violence during World War I." *Russian Review* 60 (2001): 404–419.

Lopatkina, Nataliya L. *Kul'turologicheskie aspekty v razvitii sestrinskogo delo*. Kemerovo: Izdatelstvo Aksioma, 2009.

Marcus, Jane. "Corpus/Corps/Corpse: Writing the Body in/at War." In *Arms and the Woman: War, Gender and Literary Representation*, edited by H. M. Cooper, A. A. Munich, and S. M. Squier, 124–167. Chapel Hill: University of North Carolina Press, 1989.

Markwick, Roger D., and Euridice Charon Cardona. *Soviet Women on the Frontline in the Second World War*. London: Palgrave Macmillan, 2012.

Martin, Ian. "'When Needs Must': The Acceptance of Volunteer Aids in British and Australian Military Hospitals in World War I." *Health and History* 4, no. 1 (2002): 88–98.

Marwick, Arthur. *The Deluge: British Society and the First World War*. London: Bodley Head, 1965.

Melman, Billie, ed. *Borderlines: Genders and Identities in War and Peace, 1870–1930*. New York: Routledge, 1998.

Merridale, Catherine. "The Collective Mind: Trauma and Shell-Shock in Twentieth-Century Russia." *Journal of Contemporary History* 35, no. 1 (2000): 39–55.

Meyer, Alfred. "The Impact of World War I on Russian Women's Lives." In Clements et al., 208–224.

Molkina, O. I. *Nad nami Krasnyi krest*. Saint Petersburg: Ostrov, 2005.

Mosse, George. *Fallen Soldiers: Reshaping the Memory of the World Wars*. New York: Oxford University Press, 1990.

———. "Two World Wars and the Myth of the War Experience." *Journal of Contemporary History* 21, no. 4 (October 1986): 491–513.

Murray, Elizabeth. "Russian Nurses: From the Tsarist Sister of Mercy to the Soviet Comrade Nurse: A Case Study of Absence of Migration of Nursing Knowledge and Skills." *Nursing Inquiry* 11 (2004): 130–137.

Nawroz, Mohammad Yahya, and Lester W. Grau. "The Soviet War in Afghanistan: History and Harbinger of Future War?" *Military History*, September/October 1995. http://fmso.leavenworth.army.mil/documents/waraf.htm.

Norris, Stephen. *A War of Images: Russian Popular Prints, Wartime Culture, and National Identity, 1812–1945.* DeKalb: Northern Illinois University Press, 2006.

Orlovsky, Daniel. "Velikaia voina i rossiiskaia pamiat." In Smirnov et al., 49–57.

Pennington, Reina. *Wings, Women, and War: Soviet Airwomen in World War II Combat.* Lawrence: University Press of Kansas, 2001.

Petrone, Karen. "Family, Masculinity, and Heroism in Russian War Posters." In Melman, 95–119.

———. *The Great War in Russian Memory.* Bloomington: Indiana University Press, 2011.

Philips, Laura L. "Gendered Dis/ability: Perspectives from the Treatment of Psychiatric Casualties in Russia's Early Twentieth-Century Wars." *Social History of Medicine* 20, no. 2 (August 2007): 333–350.

Plamper, Jan. "Fear: Soldiers and Emotion in Russian Military Psychology." *Slavic Review* 68, no. 2 (Summer 2009): 259–283.

Polner, T. I. *Russian Local Government during the War.* New Haven, Conn.: Yale University Press, 1930.

Posternak, A. V. "Istorii obshchin sester miloserdiia." In O L. Leikinda, *Blagotvoritel'nost' v Rossii: Istoricheskie i sotsial'no-ekonomicheskie issledovaniia,* 311–318. Saint Petersburg: Liki Rossii, 2003.

———. *Ocherki po istorii obshchin sester miloserdiia.* Moscow: Izdatel'stvo Sviato—Dimitrievskii uchilishche sester miloserdiia, 2001.

Rachamimov, Alon. "'Female Generals' and 'Siberian Angels': Aristocratic Nurses and the Austro-Hungarian POW Relief." In *Gender and War in Twentieth-Century Eastern Europe*, edited by Nancy M. Wingfield and Maria Bucur, 23–46. Bloomington: Indiana University Press, 2006.

Ramer, Samuel C. "Feldshers and Rural Health Care in the Early Soviet Period." In Solomon and Hutchinson, 121–145.

Rogoza, Vladimir. "Pochemu Rimmu Ivanovu nazyvali Rossiskoi Zhannoi d'Ark?" *Shkola Zhizny, Posnavitel'nyi Zhurnal,* February 24, 2008. http://shkolazhizni.ru/archive/0/n-12952/.

Romaniuk, V. P., V. A. Lapotnikov, and Ia. A. Nakatis. *Istoriia sestrinskogo dela v Rossii.* Saint Petersburg: SPbGMA, 1998.

Rossiia v mirovoi voine, 1914–18 gg. (v tsifrakh). Moscow, 1925.

Rosslyn, Wendy, and Alessandra Tosi, eds. *Women in Nineteenth-Century Russia: Lives and Culture.* Cambridge, U.K.: Open Book Publishers, 2012.

Rothstein, Robert A. "Songs of Women Warriors and Women Who Waited." In *Embracing Arms: Cultural Representations of Slavic and Balkan Women in War*, edited by Helena Goscilo and Yana Hashamova, 179–204. Budapest: Central University Press, 2012.

Ruane, Christine. "Clothes Shopping in Imperial Russia: The Development of a Consumer Culture." *Journal of Society History* 28, no. 4 (Summer 1995): 765–782.

Ruthchild, Rochelle. *Equality and Revolution: Women's Rights in the Russian Empire, 1905–1917.* Pittsburgh, Penn.: University of Pittsburgh Press, 2010.

Rutherford, Ward. *The Russian Army in World War I.* London: Gordon Cremonesi, 1975.

Sanborn, Joshua. *Drafting the Russian Nation: Military Conscription, Total War, and Mass Politics, 1905–1925.* DeKalb: Northern Illinois University Press, 2003.

———. *Imperial Apocalypse: The Great War and the Destruction of the Russian Empire.* Oxford: Oxford University Press, 2014.

———. "Unsettling the Empire: Violent Migrations and Social Disaster in Russia during World War I." *Journal of Modern History* 77 (June 2005): 290–324.

Sarnecky, Mary T. *A History of the U.S. Army Nurse Corps.* Philadelphia: University of Pennsylvania Press, 1997.

Schönberger, Bianca. "Motherly Heroines and Adventurous Girls: Red Cross Nurses and Women Army Auxiliaries in the First World War." In Hagemann, 87–113.

Schultz, Christopher. "The Self Separated from Violence: Spectacle, Material Appropriation, and Voices of Resistance on the Western Front, 1914–18." *Canadian Journal of History* 46 (Winter 2011): 563–584.

Scott, Joan W. "The Evidence of Experience." *Critical Inquiry* 17, no. 4 (Summer 1991): 773–797.

Shevyrin, V. M. *Zemskii i gorodskoi soiuzy (1914–1917): analiticheskii obzor.* Moscow: INION RAN, 2000.

Showalter, Elaine. *The Female Malady: Women, Madness, and English Culture, 1830–1980.* London: Virago, 1987.

Siegelbaum, Lewis H. *The Politics of Industrial Mobilization in Russia, 1914–17.* London: Macmillan, 1983.

Sirotkina, Irina. "The Politics of Etiology: Shell Shock in the Russian Army, 1914–1918." In *Madness and the Mad in Russian Culture*, edited by Angela Brintlinger and Ilya Vinitsky, 117–129. Toronto: University of Toronto Press, 2007.

Smetankina-Gudkova, M. V. *Mat' Nonna: Sestra milioserdiia Rossiiskogo Krasnogo Kresta Lidiia Savel'evna Volkova (1896–1975).* Moscow: Biblioteka-fond "Russkoe Zarubezh'e," 2009.

Smirnov, N. N., et al., eds. *Rossiia i pervaia mirovaia voina: Materialy mezhdunarodnogo kollokviuma*. Saint Petersburg, 1999.

Soine, Aeleah. "The Relation of the Nurse to the Working World: Professionalization, Citizenship, and Class in Germany, Great Britain, and the United States before World War I." *Nursing History Review* 18 (2010): 51–80.

Solomon, Susan Gross, and John F. Hutchinson, eds. *Health and Society in Revolutionary Russia*. Bloomington: Indiana University Press, 1990.

Starks, Tricia. "*Papirosy*, Smoking, and the Anti-Cigarette Movement." In *Tobacco in Russian History and Culture: From the Seventeenth Century to the Present*, edited by Tricia Starks and Matthew Romaniello, 132–147. New York: Routledge, 2009.

Stites, Richard. "Days and Nights in Wartime Russia: Cultural Life, 1914–1917." In *European Culture in the Great War: The Arts, Entertainment, and Propaganda, 1914–1918*, edited by Aviel Roshwald and Richard Stites, 8–31. Cambridge: Cambridge University Press, 2008.

Stoff, Laurie. "The 'Myth of the War Experience' and Russian Wartime Nursing in World War I." *Aspasia: The International Yearbook of Central, Eastern, and Southeastern European Women's and Gender History* 6 (2012): 96–116.

———. *They Fought for the Motherland: Russia's Women Soldiers in World War I and the Revolution*. Lawrence: University Press of Kansas, 2006.

Stryker, Laurinda. "Mental Cases: British Shellshock—Politics of Interpretation." In Braybon, *Evidence*, 154–171.

Sudavtsov, N. D. "Geroina, protivopastavivshaia tevtonskoi zabronirovanmoi sile svoiu velikuiu liubiashchuiu dushu russkoi zhenshchiny." *Voenno-istoricheskii zhurnal*, no. 3 (2002): 47–52.

Summerfield, Penny. "Gender and War in the Twentieth Century." *International History Review* 19, no. 1 (February 1997): 4–15.

Tuve, Jeanette E. *The First Russian Women Physicians*. Newtonville, Mass.: Oriental Research Partners, 1984.

Ul'ianova, O. D. "Maria Il'inichna Ul'ianova." In M. I. Ul'ianova, *O V. I. Lenine i sem'e Ul'ianovkh*. Moscow: Izdat. Polit. Liter., 1989.

Vining, Margaret, and Barton C. Hacker. "From Camp Follower to Lady in Uniform: Women, Social Class and Military Institutions before 1920." *Contemporary European History* 10, no. 3 (November 2001): 353–373.

Vladimirsteva, N. I. "Iz vospominaniia sestry miloserdiia F. N. Slepchenko." *Otechestvennye arkhivi* 6 (1994): 58–72.

Wanke, Paul. *Russian-Soviet Military Psychiatry, 1904–1945*. New York: Routledge, 2005.

Watson, Janet. "Khaki Girls, VADs, and Tommy's Sisters: Gender and Class in First World War Britain." *International History Review* 19 (February 1997): 32–51.

Wood, Elizabeth A. *The Baba and the Comrade: Gender Politics in Revolutionary Russia.* Bloomington: Indiana University Press, 1997.

Youngblood, Denise. "Fade to Black: The Russian 'Bourgeois' Film Industry during War and Revolution." In *Russian Culture in War and Revolution, 1914–22. Book 1: Popular Culture, the Arts, and Institutions*, edited by Murray Frame, Boris Kolonitskii, Steven G. Marks, and Melissa K. Stockdale, 85–100. *Russia's Great War and Revolution* Series. Bloomington: Slavica Publishers of Indiana University, 2014.

INDEX